Innovating for Healthy Urbanization

Roy Ahn • Thomas F. Burke • Anita M. McGahan
Editors

Innovating for Healthy Urbanization

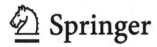 Springer

Editors
Roy Ahn
Division of Global Health and Human Rights
Department of Emergency Medicine
Massachusetts General Hospital
Boston, MA, USA

Thomas F. Burke
Division of Global Health and Human Rights
Department of Emergency Medicine
Massachusetts General Hospital
Boston, MA, USA

Anita M. McGahan
Rotman School of Management
University of Toronto
Toronto, ON, Canada

ISBN 978-1-4899-7812-7   ISBN 978-1-4899-7597-3   (eBook)
DOI 10.1007/978-1-4899-7597-3

Springer New York Heidelberg Dordrecht London

Springer Science+Business Media LLC New York is part of Springer Science+Business Media (www.springer.com)

Foreword

Urbanization is essentially the physical growth of urban areas as a result of rural migration. The United Nations projected that half of the world's population would live in urban areas at the end of 2008 (International Herald Tribune, Associated Press, February 26, 2008). By 2050, it is predicted that 64.1 % and 85.9 % of the developing and developed world, respectively, will be urbanized ("Open air computers," The Economist, October 27, 2012).

Urbanization has serious implications for health, and calls for innovations in global health professional education. Several health challenges needing urgent attention come to mind. The issue of human trafficking (and its implications for urban environments) is an emerging problem. With the decline in breastfeeding globally, a shift to fast foods, and the abandonment of traditional feeding practices, childhood malnutrition is bound to rise in urban areas. The need for innovations to address childhood malnutrition in urban environments, as well as newborn, childhood, and maternal health in urban resource-limited settings, cannot be overemphasized. Unscrupulous dealers and unfair trade practices have led to the proliferation of counterfeit drugs in low- and middle-income countries. This will have serious implications for the treatment of common conditions as well as drug resistance in urban environments. Therefore, there will be a need for more investments in diagnostic innovations in urban health settings. Due to poor planning and inadequate provision of basic services, an increasing number of urban populations in low- and middle-income countries are likely to be hard hit by climate change, noise pollution, and unintentional injury. The case for comprehensive, integrated, and standardized measures of health in cities cannot be overemphasized.

Overall, this book will go a long way in highlighting innovations to address these urbanization-related health issues.

School of Public Health   Dismas Ongore, M.B.Ch.B., M.P.H., Ph.D.
University of Nairobi
Nairobi, Kenya

Contents

Contributors

Emily Aaronson, M.D. Harvard Affiliated Emergency Medicine Residency at Brigham and Women's Hospital/Massachusetts General Hospital, Boston, MA, USA

Harvard Medical School, Boston, MA, USA

Roy Ahn, M.P.H., Sc.D. Division of Global Health and Human Rights, Department of Emergency Medicine, Massachusetts General Hospital, Boston, MA, USA

Harvard Medical School, Boston, MA, USA

Kendra Amico, M.D., M.Phil. Harvard Affiliated Emergency Medicine Residency at Brigham and Women's Hospital/Massachusetts General Hospital, Boston, MA, USA

Harvard Medical School, Boston, MA, USA

Patrick Beattie, B.S.E. Diagnostics for All, Cambridge, MA, USA

Paul Biddinger, M.D., F.A.C.E.P. Department of Emergency Medicine, Massachusetts General Hospital, Boston, MA, USA

Harvard Medical School, Boston, MA, USA

Susan M. Blaustein, Ph.D. The Earth Institute, Columbia University, New York, NY, USA

Thomas F. Burke, M.D., F.A.C.E.P., F.R.S.M. Division of Global Health and Human Rights, Department of Emergency Medicine, Massachusetts General Hospital, Boston, MA, USA

Harvard Medical School, Boston, MA, USA

Malcolm Clayton, B.A. Department of Diplomacy and World Affairs, Occidental College, Los Angeles, CA, USA

Lisa B. Collins, M.A. Division of Global Health and Human Rights, Department of Emergency Medicine, Massachusetts General Hospital, Boston, MA, USA

Kathryn Conn, B.A. Division of Global Health and Human Rights, Department of Emergency Medicine, Massachusetts General Hospital, Boston, MA, USA

Emily de Redon, B.A. Division of Global Health and Human Rights, Department of Emergency Medicine, Massachusetts General Hospital, Boston, MA, USA

David M. Dodson, M.B.A. Project Healthy Children, Cambridge, MA, USA

Melody Eckardt, M.D., M.P.H., F.A.C.O.G. Division of Global Health and Human Rights, Department of Emergency Medicine, Massachusetts General Hospital, Boston, MA, USA

Department of Obstetrics and Gynecology, Boston Medical Center, Boston, MA, USA

Boston University School of Medicine, Boston, MA, USA

David Elam, M.I.A. Johns Hopkins School for Advanced International Studies, Washington, DC, USA

Griffin Flannery, B.A. Division of Global Health and Human Rights, Department of Emergency Medicine, Massachusetts General Hospital, Boston, MA, USA

Hannah L. Harp, B.A. Division of Global Health and Human Rights, Department of Emergency Medicine, Massachusetts General Hospital, Boston, MA, USA

Boston University School of Medicine, Boston, MA, USA

Rosemary Hines, B.A. Division of Global Health and Human Rights, Department of Emergency Medicine, Massachusetts General Hospital, Boston, MA, USA

Laura Janneck, M.D., M.P.H. Cambridge Health Alliance, Cambridge, MA, USA

Harvard Medical School, Boston, MA, USA

Daniel Johnson, Ph.D. Indiana University Purdue University Indianapolis, Institute for Research on Social Issues, Indianapolis, IN, USA

Laurence Kornfield City and County of San Francisco, San Francisco, CA, USA

John D. Kraemer, J.D., M.P.H. Department of Health Systems Administration, Georgetown University School of Nursing & Health Studies and O'Neill Institute for National & Global Health Law, Georgetown University Law Center, Washington, DC, USA

George Luber, Ph.D. Centers for Disease Control and Prevention, Atlanta, GA, USA

Vijay Lulla, Ph.D. Indiana University Purdue University Indianapolis, Institute for Research on Social Issues, Indianapolis, IN, USA

Charles Mace, Ph.D. Diagnostics for All, Cambridge, MA, USA

Wendy Macias-Konstantopoulos, M.D., M.P.H. Division of Global Health and Human Rights, Department of Emergency Medicine, Massachusetts General Hospital, Boston, MA, USA

Harvard Medical School, Boston, MA, USA

Patricia L. McCarney, Ph.D. Department of Political Science, Global Cities Institute, John H. Daniels Faculty of Architecture, Landscaping, and Design, University of Toronto, Toronto, ON, Canada

Anita M. McGahan, Ph.D. Rotman School of Management, University of Toronto, Toronto, ON, Canada

Brett D. Nelson, M.D., M.P.H., D.T.M.&H. Division of Global Health and Human Rights, Department of Emergency Medicine, Massachusetts General Hospital, Boston, MA, USA

Harvard Medical School, Boston, MA, USA

Edward W.J. Pritchard, M.Phil. Division of Global Health and Human Rights, Department of Emergency Medicine, Massachusetts General Hospital, Boston, MA, USA

Natasha Prudent, M.P.H. Centers for Disease Control and Prevention, Atlanta, GA, USA

Genevieve Purcell, B.A. Division of Global Health and Human Rights, Department of Emergency Medicine, Massachusetts General Hospital, Boston, MA, USA

Laura A. Rowe, M.S., M.P.H. Project Healthy Children, Cambridge, MA, USA

Charles M. Salter, P.E. Charles M. Salter Associates, Inc., San Francisco, CA, USA

Ethan C. Salter, P.E. Charles M. Salter Associates, Inc., San Francisco, CA, USA

Gabe Shapiro, M.P.D. University of Southern California, Los Angeles, CA, USA

Elena Siegel, B.A. Department of Diplomacy and World Affairs, Occidental College, Los Angeles, CA, USA

Austin Stanforth, M.S. Indiana University Purdue University Indianapolis, Institute for Research on Social Issues, Indianapolis, IN, USA

Matthew Stewart, Ph.D. Diagnostics for All, Cambridge, MA, USA

Hanni Stoklosa, M.D. Division of Global Health and Human Rights, Department of Emergency Medicine, Massachusetts General Hospital, Boston, MA, USA

Harvard Medical School, Boston, MA, USA

Horacio R. Trujillo, M.Phil., M.B.A., Ph.D. Departments of Politics and of Diplomacy and World Affairs, Occidental College, Los Angeles, CA, USA

Leana S. Wen, M.D. M.Sc., F.A.A.E.M. Baltimore City Health Department, Baltimore, MD, USA

Faiza Yasin, M.P.H. Division of Global Health and Human Rights, Department of Emergency Medicine, Massachusetts General Hospital, Boston, MA, USA

Howard Zucker, M.D., J.D. Division of Global Health and Human Rights, Department of Emergency Medicine, Massachusetts General Hospital, Boston, MA, USA

Albert Einstein College of Medicine of Yeshiva University, Bronx, NY, USA

Introduction

Roy Ahn*, Thomas F. Burke*, and Anita M. McGahan

Innovating for Healthy Urbanization

The United Nations projects that the world's population will grow from 7 billion today to nearly 11 billion by the year 2100.[1] At the same time, cities will grow disproportionately, accounting for 80 % of humankind by 2100 (up from about 50 % today). The growth of cities presents unprecedented challenges, but also important opportunities. The concentration of human populations in increasingly dense urban areas raises the prospect of intensification of communicable diseases, while aging populations suggest a greater incidence of noncommunicable diseases in the future. On the other hand, cities can facilitate prevention, early diagnosis, and comprehensive treatment of health conditions through increased access to quality health services.

When we commissioned the chapters for this book, we envisioned that the contributing authors would advance understanding of the ways in which urbanization and health co-evolved. We had in mind that the book would point to the importance of early childhood education, sanitation systems, stable food supplies, personal security, and secure housing as important prerequisites and complements to classic health infrastructure. The chapters in this book certainly have delivered on this expectation.

---

*Roy Ahn and Thomas F. Burke serve as co-lead editors of this book.

[1] United Nations, Department of Economic and Social Affairs, Population Division (2013). *World Population Prospects*: *The 2012 Revision, Highlights and Advance Tables*. Working Paper No. ESA/P/WP.228.

R. Ahn, M.P.H., Sc.D. (✉) • T.F. Burke, M.D., F.A.C.E.P., F.R.S.M.
Division of Global Health and Human Rights, Department of Emergency Medicine,
Massachusetts General Hospital, Zero Emerson Place Suite 104, Boston, MA 02114, USA

Harvard Medical School, Boston, MA, USA
e-mail: RAHN@mgh.harvard.edu

A.M. McGahan, Ph.D.
Rotman School of Management, University of Toronto, Toronto, ON, Canada

What we did not fully anticipate were the ways in which the chapters would illuminate an entirely new way of thinking about the nature of health itself. Many chapters emphasize a conceptualization of health as resilience, and of cities as platforms for personal and community growth. This approach goes much further than evoking social determinants of health, by considering the complex interplay among environmental, economic, political, social, and health systems.

Numerous themes cut across the chapters:

1. Migrations indicate health challenges in both source and target communities.
   Several chapters in this book point to migrations as indicators of health challenges in source communities and as complicit in the emergence of new problems in targeted urban settings. For example, Rowe and Dodson report that migrants may escape chronic hunger but continue to face nutritional deficits in cities. Trujillo and colleagues allude to the frequent incidence of migration in escape from tribal conflict but focus primarily on the tragedy of urban violence, especially in cities where rapid population growth strains housing and other security systems. Ahn and colleagues describe the hazards of migration to the cities and the negative consequences of human trafficking. Beattie, Stewart, and Mace find that inadequate housing and sanitation systems mean that rapidly growing cities must contend with "persistent infectious disease" as well as a larger burden of non-communicable illness. Kraemer considers the significantly higher risk of unintentional injury as a major health challenge in urban settings as compared to rural communities.

   The implication? Urbanization does not guarantee improved health. Health systems must be constructed to address the specific problems that arise first from migration itself and subsequently with population density in cities. These problems arise in basic systems: food, water, housing, and security. And the chapters posit innovations to address many of these challenges in resourceful ways.

2. The chronic shortage of health professionals is worsening and compels a new vision for primary care in urban areas of developing countries.
   The shortage of health workers—including physicians, nurses, administrators, and specialists in almost every other domain of delivery—is well-described in the academic literature. The authors in this book focus on the consequences of the shortage for health in cities. Wen envisions "innovations in global health education" that involve not only extensive task shifting but also the training of a generation of providers specialized in the needs of the urban poor. Kraemer suggests the utility of a system adapted to the urban needs of low- and middle-income countries, where first responders are trained to provide sufficient care and reduce the risk of preventable death and disability, particularly from traffic accidents. Eckardt and colleagues, plus Nelson and colleagues, describe the need for training frontline health workers to bring about improvements in maternal, newborn, and child health in resource-limited settings.

   Some chapters address opportunities for improved governance in the delivery of care. Blaustein describes the necessity for coordination among nongovernmental agencies (NGOs) and for addressing gaps in the provision of primary care by these NGOs. McCarney and McGahan focus on the importance of the measurement of population health, and indicate that the measurement itself involves governance, simply through the act of data monitoring.

The general vision of primary care suggested by these analyses thus involves the construction of basic social systems in the interests of health. This act of construction depends primarily on effective governance through sound management and creative leadership in the deployment of human resources in low- and middle-income countries' urban settings.

3. Urbanization can simplify geographic access to care and can enable innovation that lowers the cost and improves the quality of diagnostic care.

Beattie, Stewart, and Mace argue that diagnostic innovations—and especially digitally-enabled diagnostics—create a basis for fundamental change in access to high-quality care. Their argument emphasizes the unique opportunities available in cities for implementing protocols that can be administered by trained health workers and monitored by specialists. Rowe and Dodson indicate that opportunities to improve nutrition in urban settings are legion, and Eckardt and colleagues pose a similar argument for maternal health in such settings. Kraemer and Trujillo and colleagues all suggest that innovative approaches that account for the density of the poor in urban settings—and that combat unsafe practices— can lead to better quality of urban life and lower costs in health delivery. Lulla and colleagues focus squarely and primarily on the opportunities associated with innovation in the delivery of care in urban settings. They identify the particular stressors on health tied to urban living, including pollution of all types. Salter and colleagues hone in on the innovations—present and future—that could mitigate a decidedly urban public health hazard: noise pollution.

Taken together, these chapters suggest that the opportunities for improving urban health arising from novel diagnostics include the implementation of effective protocols for administering familiar monitoring tests (such as on heart rate and glucose level), and the development of new devices and protocols that account specifically for health problems in urban slums. The latter may include, for example, diagnostics on asthma, toxic metals, and nutritional deficiencies, as well as on the psychological and social stresses that may accompany geographic dislocation.

4. Climate change has reshaped and will continue to reshape primary care, acute care, and disaster management.

Climate change influences urban health in myriad ways. Three are highlighted in the essays in this volume: food insecurity, air pollution, and weather disasters. Each has a direct impact on urban health and thus carries important consequences for health systems. Food insecurity is the primary subject of Rowe and Dobson's study on micronutrients. These authors show how the chronic absence of sufficient nutrition among the urban poor creates significant challenges for primary and acute care. Lulla and colleagues describe the relationship between climate change and air quality in urban locales. Janneck and Biddinger discuss the consequences of weather disasters for emergency and disaster management.

The requirements for innovation implied by these analyses are extensive. Building the capacity to deal with weather disasters requires unprecedented coordination at all levels of health systems. Addressing food insecurity requires integration between health and other essential systems in both the public and private sectors. Pollution is perhaps even more challenging, as its mitigation requires implementing controls as well as incentives in individual, private-sector, and public-sector institutions. Many of the chapters offer solutions to mitigate disasters of all types through the lens of innovation (e.g., Janneck and Biddinger's analysis of innovations in disaster management).

5. Increasing urban inequality, coupled with rising prices on basic goods such as food, raises the stakes on the design of inclusive systems.
   Many of the chapters specifically address the adverse consequences of inequity. Lulla and colleagues point to inequality, not only in the administration of health resources but also in vulnerability to health problems as a central facet of urban life. Trujillo and colleagues chronicle these vulnerabilities among the poor, particularly with regard to injury and personal violence. Wen describes inequality in the accountability of health providers—with systematically greater tolerance for poor health delivery when patients are vulnerable.

   What suggestions arise for addressing these challenges? McCarney and McGahan suggest that measurement of inequity itself is a step toward its mitigation because of the implicit importance attached to the conditions as a consequence of measurement. Kraemer highlights the need to address environmental hazards—such as substandard housing and workplace safety. Blaustein similarly points to the importance of inclusive systems.

6. Effective governance of health resources requires better data, accountability on health metrics, and innovation in health-system administration.
   Almost every chapter in this book asks for more accurate, timely, and relevant information on urban health challenges. Lulla and colleagues highlight the value of mapping and of comprehensive assessments as essential to the design of effective warning systems. Amico, Aaronson, and Zucker describe novel information technologies used to track pharmaceuticals through the supply chain in order to curb incidents of global drug counterfeiting. McCarney and McGahan focus on the promise of comparative measures that can allow city leaders to assess their performance relative to other jurisdictions with similar problems. Kraemer points to the importance of information on effective mechanisms for coordinating emergency response. Blaustein shows how better information would enable more effective and affordable solutions in the effective administration of resources in urban environments.

   Better information is only the first step in larger processes that each of these authors advocates. Overall, their vision is for more effective and creative governance of health systems. This vision requires persistence and determination in the allocation of decision rights, property rights, and financial claims on the provision of essential health services.

Summary

Human health in the twenty-first century begins and ends in cities. The purpose of this book is to explore the implications of massive urbanization for the health of human-kind—*and to unearth innovations to address the problems associated with urbanization and health*. As a whole, the chapters point to the potential for healthy cities that are rich in resources that matter for resilience: access to opportunity, better governance, equity, innovativeness, and actualization. In that vein, "innovations" are broadly construed as solutions that may include cutting-edge technology but often times may involve a lower-tech analog that is simple, elegant, and wholly impactful.

The implications for urban health systems are extensive: a new vision for the provision of primary care; urgency in addressing urban pollution and climate change; and improving accountability of health providers and especially of public- and private-sector leaders with the capacity to allocate resources to improve health systems.

On the whole, the chapter authors point to a future dominated by climate change, megacities, and resource scarcity. They call for creativity and innovation in the face of the challenges and simultaneously warn us against taking for granted that existing systems will work. Our current emphasis on access will give way to a broader agenda on equitability and fairness. Effective governance in the creation, stewardship, and allocation of scarce resources will be central to the resilience of cities and to the people who live within them.

Part I
Innovations to Address Specific Populations and Health

Chapter 1
Maternal Health Innovations and Urbanization

Melody Eckardt, Hannah L. Harp, Roy Ahn, Genevieve Purcell, Emily de Redon, Rosemary Hines, and Thomas F. Burke

Introduction

In 2014, nearly 300,000 women around the world will die from causes attributable to pregnancy and childbirth. An estimated 99 % of these maternal deaths occur in low- and middle-income countries. Most of these maternal deaths are caused by postpartum hemorrhage (PPH), infection, unsafe abortion, eclampsia, and obstructed labor. In stark contrast, in well-resourced settings, complications of pregnancy can usually be prevented or addressed successfully without death or disability to the

M. Eckardt, M.D., M.P.H., F.A.C.O.G. (✉)
Division of Global Health and Human Rights, Department of Emergency Medicine,
Massachusetts General Hospital, Zero Emerson Place Suite 104, Boston, MA 02114, USA

Department of Obstetrics and Gynecology, Boston Medical Center, Boston, MA, USA

Boston University School of Medicine, Boston, MA, USA
e-mail: MECKARDT@mgh.harvard.edu

H.L. Harp, B.A.
Division of Global Health and Human Rights, Department of Emergency Medicine,
Massachusetts General Hospital, Zero Emerson Place Suite 104, Boston, MA 02114, USA

Boston University School of Medicine, Boston, MA, USA

R. Ahn, M.P.H., Sc.D. • T.F. Burke, M.D., F.A.C.E.P., F.R.S.M.
Division of Global Health and Human Rights, Department of Emergency Medicine,
Massachusetts General Hospital, Zero Emerson Place Suite 104, Boston, MA 02114, USA

Harvard Medical School, Boston, MA, USA

G. Purcell, B.A. • E. de Redon, B.A. • R. Hines, B.A.
Division of Global Health and Human Rights, Department of Emergency Medicine,
Massachusetts General Hospital, Zero Emerson Place Suite 104, Boston, MA 02114, USA

© Springer New York 2015
R. Ahn et al. (eds.), *Innovating for Healthy Urbanization*,
DOI 10.1007/978-1-4899-7597-3_1

mother [1]. The major determinants of this enormous disparity in maternal survival are social, economic, and physical barriers to accessing quality health care.

The term "urban health advantage" refers to the general observation that health indices in urban settings are often better than in rural areas, due to physical proximity of healthcare facilities. However, with close examination, it is clear that the degree of poverty is more predictive of access to health care than actual geographic distance between patients and healthcare facilities [2]. Despite proximity, the urban poor often have limited access to health care and receive lower quality services because of their inability to pay [3, 4]. Additionally, the urban poor in high-density settings often suffer from low-quality public and private healthcare services, consequently disincentivizing desirable prevention and care-seeking behaviors of the population.

Novel, low-cost solutions are required in order to overcome the challenges unique to the growing phenomenon of global urbanization. This chapter will provide an overview of promising innovations in maternal health, via two themes: (1) increasing mothers' access to care, discussed in relation to the "Three Delays Model" [5], and (2) improving quality of maternal health care with a particular focus on addressing the major causes of global maternal mortality. In time, these innovations and others may become long-term solutions or may be replaced by new ideas. The innovations described in this chapter are examples of what is possible with fresh and creative approaches focused on saving the lives of our future mothers.

Background: Three Delays Model

The "Three Delays Model"—the product of multidisciplinary research by Thaddeus and Maine—is a framework for contextualizing the numerous determinants of maternal mortality. The model pinpoints three stages of the care delivery process at which delays are most likely to lead to maternal morbidity or mortality [5]. In the case of an obstetric complication, these delays include: (a) a delay in the decision to seek care at a health facility, (b) a delay in arrival at a health facility, and (c) a delay in the provision of adequate care once at the health facility [5].

Gabrysch and Campbell's "Still too far to walk" article is an updated review of the Three Delays Model that incorporates "socio-cultural factors, perceived benefit of a skilled birth attendant and economic and physical accessibility" to the maternal mortality framework (Fig. 1.1) [2]. Examining the frameworks presented in both pieces reveals that the causes of maternal mortality cannot be examined in isolation, but instead must be situated in social, cultural, structural, and economic contexts. The next section incorporates aspects of both frameworks, highlighting the interconnectedness of social determinants, structural barriers, and obstetric complications that contributes to maternal mortality.

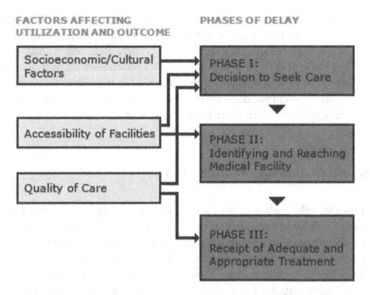

FACTORS AFFECTING
UTILIZATION AND OUTCOME

PHASES OF DELAY

Socioeconomic/Cultural Factors

PHASE I:
Decision to Seek Care

Accessibility of Facilities

PHASE II:
Identifying and Reaching Medical Facility

Quality of Care

PHASE III:
Receipt of Adequate and Appropriate Treatment

Fig. 1.1 Three Delays model (*Source*: http://www.unfpa.org/public/home/mothers/pid/4385)

Phase I: Decision to Seek Care

Delay in the decision to seek care begins with the time that it takes to first recognize an obstetric complication [6]. The speed of recognizing signs and symptoms of a complication, the use of traditional birth attendants (TBAs), and the woman's desire to deliver at home are all factors that affect the decision to seek care [6].

Women living in the lowest economic quintile have little education or autonomy and often are not able to access adequate skilled health care [7]. Instead, they utilize unskilled birth attendants who may not recognize complications and who lack a referral system. It has been established that a mother's education level directly correlates with her health-seeking behaviors before and during pregnancy [7–9]. A mother's basic understanding of pregnancy and childbirth increases the likelihood that she will identify abnormalities and potential complications during her pregnancy. Additionally, improving education for women has been shown to provide economic opportunities that increase the family financial resources available for maternal health care.

Delay in the decision to seek care is not only affected by a mother's education level, but also by the perceived benefit of skilled obstetrics services. The perceptions of whether delivering at a healthcare facility is beneficial are influenced by a number of factors, including a woman's understanding of the urgent nature of childbirth complications, awareness or trust of available interventions and treatments at health facilities, and prior experience with obstetric services [2]. Waiting times, positive or negative interactions with staff, facility infrastructure, and the availability of supplies within the facility, all contribute to whether women perceive seeking healthcare services as beneficial or necessary. The perceived benefit may be based solely on past individual as well as community experiences with healthcare facilities. This perceived benefit is then weighed against the individual financial, physical, and temporal costs in the decision to seek care. Often, these costs far outweigh the perceived benefit of seeking care until it is too late.

Innovations to Address the First Delay

Innovations that enhance a woman's ability to recognize pregnancy complications and strengthen the positive perception of obstetric services can reduce the first delay. A community midwife or birth attendant can assist a woman in recognizing the symptoms of an imminent emergency. However, TBAs and midwives do not always have the training or technical experience required to recognize these early signs. Thus, improving the level of training of birth attendants may improve the early recognition of potential complications, which increases the likelihood for a woman to seek a higher level of care more quickly [10].

Strengthening the communication and relationship between pregnant women, birth attendants, and skilled health providers can also increase the probability that a mother will seek care. Mobile health, or mHealth, is an innovation that greatly fosters communication and may provide point-of-care support. According to the World Bank, approximately three-quarters of the world's population now has access to a mobile phone [11]. The availability of mobile technology worldwide has allowed for mobile phones to serve as a platform for following up with patients, providing diagnostic testing, and fostering the exchange of information and education between community members and health specialists [12–15]. This communication and exchange of information promotes the involvement of women in their own care and enhances the knowledge of women about their health and pregnancy—all factors that can decrease delays in the decision to seek care.

Innovations have been developed that seek to address the financial constraints that are known to be barriers to accessing maternal health care. Several low-cost, financially-sustainable hospital systems have been developed worldwide to decrease the costs of maternity care with the hope of improving maternal mortality and morbidity rates. One of the most successful of these systems is the LifeSpring Hospital chain started in Hyderabad, India [16]. LifeSpring Hospitals are small (20–25 bed) facilities devoted to basic maternity and postpartum care [16]. Although subsidized originally by two corporations, LifeSpring Hospitals aims to create financially-sustainable facilities by providing a small repertoire of services with a tiered pricing plan. By outsourcing more critical cases to other facilities, relieving attending physicians of administrative duties, and running on a strict process-driven business model, LifeSpring Hospitals is able to offer high-quality maternity services at 30–50 % of the leading market price [16]. LifeSpring has provided health care to

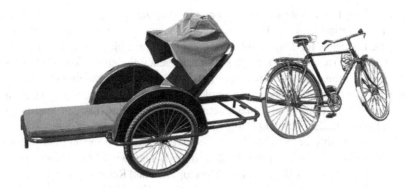

Fig. 1.2 The Zambulance, Zambikes, http://zambikes.org/what-we-do/

over 3.5 million low-income women in and around Hyderabad since its inception, and in 2010 it became the first healthcare chain to be adopted as a Business Call to Action partner [16].[1]

Phase II: Reaching the Health Facility

Once a decision is made to proceed to a health facility, barriers such as travel cost, distance, and transportation can delay an individual's ability to reach a healthcare facility. With many obstetric complications, distance to the facility and access to transportation can be a matter of life and death. Obstetric complications often present suddenly and must be addressed in a timely fashion in order to avoid dire consequences. Even though individuals living in urban areas may not be far from a health facility, poor roads, extreme traffic, and limited access to transportation can hinder a woman's arrival at a treatment facility [2].

Innovations to Address the Second Delay

Innovations that increase access to transportation are helping to avert morbidity caused by a delay in reaching the treatment facility. In Zambia, Zambikes is a company that has developed a two-wheeled ambulance trailer that can be attached to a bicycle or motorcycle (Fig. 1.2), providing safe and rapid transportation to healthcare

---

[1]Business Call to Action was created by the United Nations in 2008 and supported by multiple international donor agencies with "aims to accelerate progress towards the Millennium Development Goals (MDGs) by challenging companies to develop inclusive business models that offer the potential for both commercial success and development impact." (http://www.business-calltoaction.org)

facilities [17]. The Zambulance is integrated into the Ministry of Health's Safe Motherhood Initiative, with plans of being implemented countrywide. Similarly, in East Africa, Design for Development has constructed a bicycle-ambulance made out of bamboo. The Bambulance provides emergency transportation when motor-ized means of transportation are unavailable [18]. Since the Bambulance is made from locally-available bamboo and implemented locally, the innovation creates community-based training and manufacturing opportunities that can lead to jobs and local business development [18].

Similar to its role in the first delay, the advent of mobile technology provides novel applications to overcome the obstacles mothers face in reaching a health facility. For example, in Rwanda, the Adventist Development and Relief Agency has piloted an mHealth project to connect mothers to health facilities. This program uses SMS messaging as a way to deploy motorcycle ambulances when a pregnant woman requests assistance [19].

Phase III: Treatment

The third delay—the delay of proper treatment once at a facility—is perhaps the broadest and most complicated component of the Three Delays Model. Delayed treatment can be the result of supply inadequacies such as lack of medications and infrastructure for maintaining supplies (e.g., cold chain for preserving vaccinations and medications), inadequate treatment space, or an insufficient number of trained professionals [2]. The factors that drive the third delay are also directly connected to the first delay. Shortages of commodities, trained personnel, and user fees all contribute to disincentivizing healthcare-seeking behavior of mothers.

Inadequate supplies, equipment, and personnel are unfortunately common in resource-limited settings. The WHO considers skilled care attendance at delivery to be "the single most important factor in preventing maternal deaths" [2]. Although access to maternal care has increased in recent years, in 2014 only "46 % of women in low income countries benefit from skilled care during birth" [1]. Innovative solu-tions that increase quality training and retention of maternal healthcare providers are desperately needed.

Innovations to Address the Third Delay

The WHO recommends "task shifting" from doctors and midwives to properly-trained lower cadres as an effective way to extend health services to more women [20, 21]. Many countries and organizations around the world are designing and implementing innovative training programs focused on increasing the pool of avail-able skilled birth attendants. Some are training TBAs and including them in the formal health system as "professional midwives"; some are training TBAs to take on advocacy roles; and others are moving away from the use of TBAs in any capacity and instead focusing on increasing the numbers of fully-trained midwives [22].

A lack of equipment and supplies for safe and clean delivery contributes considerably to the third delay. "Maama Kits" (sometimes spelled "Maama" or "Mama") were developed in Uganda in order to make the basic requirements for childbirth available in a single low-cost kit. The kit, comprised of a plastic sheet, sterile gloves, razor blades, cord ligature, cotton, sanitary pads, tetracycline, and soap, is a simple and low-cost package for clean delivery [23]. In many countries, the components of the Maama Kit are items that a woman often is personally required to pay for, as individual pieces. The government of Uganda has integrated the kit into the essential drug distribution system as a free item to be distributed countrywide. Since implementation of the Maama Kit in Uganda, the rates of sepsis among women have been reduced (or even eliminated) in some regions [23]. The Maama Kit is an example of a simple low-cost package that equips providers and facilities with the ability to provide basic obstetric care, thereby decreasing the third delay.

In addition to the development of innovations such as the Maama Kit, it is critical to ensure that supply lines are functional and reliable. ColaLife is a creative delivery system innovation which uses packaging that fits into the empty space in Coca-Cola delivery crates (Fig. 1.3). Coca-Cola has opened their distribution channels to carry oral rehydration salts and zinc supplements to the most remote locations in the world [24]. One can imagine how ColaLife's shipping idea or something similar could be an innovative means for ensuring that clean birth kits are distributed widely.

Fig. 1.3 Kit Yamoyo Crate, ColaLife [24]

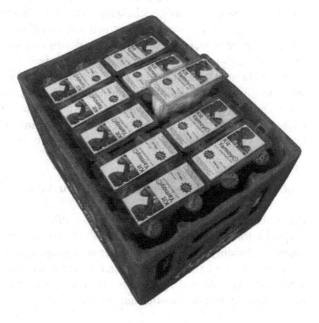

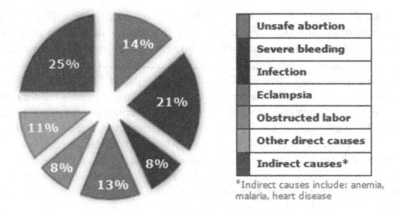

Fig. 1.4 (*Source*: UNFPA, http://web.lb.unfpa.org/mothers/obstetric.htm)

While severe shortages of skilled health workers, appropriate supplies, and affordable facility fees broadly cover the causes of the third delay, the bulk of innovations in this area center on creating low-cost means for bringing effective, specific medical treatments to women in low-resource settings. Many of these devices are "low-tech" adaptations of standard-of-care medical devices used in well-resourced tertiary care hospitals. In the following section, we discuss a few innovations that enable the prompt administration of medical treatment for the most common causes of maternal mortality, worldwide.

Globally, the most common medical causes of maternal death are hemorrhage, infection, obstructed labor, eclampsia, and complications of unsafe abortion (Fig. 1.4). While there are significant regional variations, these five conditions are consistently the primary causes of maternal deaths in low-and middle-income countries [25]. Additionally, considerable variations in causes of maternal death are often seen in rural versus urban settings. For example, women from rural Zimbabwe are more likely to die from abortion-related infection, while women from urban regions are more likely to die from infection subsequent to delivery [26]. In the next section, we identify the barriers to preventing each individual cause of death, and introduce a few innovations that are in early stages of development.

Innovations that Address Postpartum Hemorrhage

Effective interventions exist for addressing PPH emergencies in well-resourced hospital settings, but often are unavailable in poor countries. The standard clinical course for treating PPH begins with active management of the third stage of labor and then proceeds to massage of the uterus and the administration of treatment-dose uterotonic medications [27]. However, the uterotonic drugs that are standard of care in developed countries are often not available. Equipment required for the delivery

Fig. 1.5 Massachusetts General Hospital's Every Second Matters for Mothers and Babies-Uterine Balloon Tamponade™ (ESM-UBT™) Kit

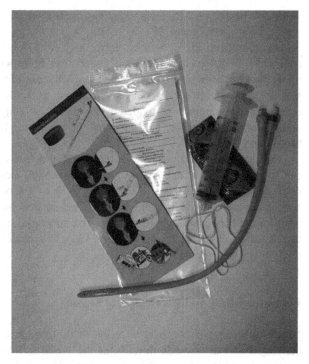

of uterotonics may also be difficult to access in informal settings. For example, oxytocin, the most commonly used and well-studied uterotonic, requires intramuscular injection or intravenous administration, and must be kept cold for long-term storage. Misoprostol, a uterotonic agent previously used principally for healing stomach ulcers which is available in a tablet form, is rapidly gaining widespread use but has unique challenges such as the common knowledge that it can be used to induce abortion. Below, three innovations to address PPH are described.

Massachusetts General Hospital's Division of Global Health and Human Rights[2] developed a PPH package called Every Second Matters for Mothers and Babies-Uterine Balloon Tamponade™ (ESM-UBT™) (Fig. 1.5). Unlike single-use UBT devices that are used in the United States and cost hundreds of dollars per device, the ESM-UBT kit costs $5, using components that are widely available. The uterine balloon kit consists of a condom tied to a Foley catheter and inflated with clean water through a syringe and one-way valve. When PPH cannot be controlled by medications, the ESM-UBT device is inserted through the cervix into the uterus and inflated with water to provide pressure against the walls of the bleeding uterus. This pressure provides a tamponade effect that halts the bleeding. MGH has successfully trained over 750 unskilled frontline healthcare workers in South Sudan on the

---

[2] Authors of this book chapter are all affiliated with the Massachusetts General Hospital.

PPH/UBT package [28] and has expanded the ESM-UBT to Kenya, Senegal, Sierra Leone, Ghana, and Nepal [28].

The non-pneumatic anti-shock garment (NASG) is a first-aid device made of neoprene and Velcro that compresses the lower body with nine segments closed tightly around the legs, pelvis, and abdomen. First used for PPH in 2002, the device may assist women to survive delays in transport to facilities for treatment. The circumferential compression provided by the NASG is thought to reduce vascular volume under the compressed areas, expand the circulating blood volume, and reduce blood loss [29].

An Australian group is developing an aerosol delivery system for oxytocin that can be inhaled by women from a simple, disposable device after childbirth. The delivery system avoids the need for refrigeration of oxytocin, which is a major concern in resource-limited health settings. The inhaled product would "negate the need for cold chain storage, remove the risk of needle stick injuries, and could be used by all levels of healthcare workers" [30]. The inhaled oxytocin product is currently under development.

Innovations that Address Puerperal Sepsis

Puerperal sepsis is a bacterial infection of the genital tract that occurs following delivery that then spreads throughout the blood stream. This type of infection accounts for 15 % of maternal deaths in developing countries [31]. If not adequately treated, puerperal infections can be fatal or have long-term health complications, such as chronic pelvic pain and infertility. Careful attention to "clean delivery," which includes clean (ideally sterile) instruments, clean hands, and proper disposal of soiled dressings, is crucial to prevent the spread of infection. However, many hospital facilities do not have access to sterile instruments or the equipment to sterilize them. The electricity required for traditional autoclaves is not available in many settings in the developing world. Often, health providers resort to boiling water or using alcohol swabs as crude sterilizing techniques.

Innovations that properly sanitize equipment without relying on electricity or other consumables, such as sterilizing gas, can potentially help decrease the burden of puerperal sepsis among mothers. For example, a solar-thermal-powered autoclave system, using energy from sunlight, can sterilize medical instruments in areas where electrical power is not available [32]. The solar-thermal-powered autoclave has been shown to produce enough steam to sustain the pressure and temperature levels that meet Centers for Disease Control and Prevention (CDC) sterilization requirements. Researchers from the University of Texas developed an autoclave that consists of a "Capteur Soleil" to produce steam from solar energy, a "hot plate" that harnesses the steam, and a commercially available thermal autoclave to sterilize equipment. This model does not require reliable electrical or gas sources, but it is still expensive at approximately US$2,100 [32]. A research team from MIT has developed the Solarclave as a low-cost alternative [33]. This solar-powered autoclave is comprised of pocket-sized mirrors, a bucket, and a pressure cooker—all parts that can be obtained in resource-limited settings at a low cost.

Innovations that Address Unsafe Abortion

Unsafe abortions occur worldwide, but are far more common in developing countries. In resource-limited settings, abortion laws are more restrictive, contraceptive use is less common, and women often are not allowed to make their own reproductive health decisions [34]. The World Health Organization (WHO) estimates that 22 million unsafe abortions take place annually, with 5 million women disabled each year as a consequence [35]. Abortion is often subject to a number of regulations, including those that restrict the time frame in which an abortion can be performed, require consent from family members, or mandate pre-abortion counseling. Since undergoing an abortion is not socially acceptable in most countries, women often seek abortions from providers willing to perform the procedures in confidence. These providers are often unskilled and perform procedures in unhygienic conditions with inadequate medical tools and supplies [34]. Unsafe abortions can lead to complications, such as uterine perforation, rectal fistula, bowel injuries, infection, hemorrhage, and death [36].

Unintended pregnancies can usually be prevented with the appropriate use of contraceptive technologies. However, in many countries, a lack of access to accurate information about available contraceptives and religious and cultural norms prevent women from accessing birth control [34]. Population Services International created an innovative toll-free hotline called "Ligne Verte," which provides confidential family planning and contraception information to individuals in 11 provinces of the Democratic Republic of the Congo. The hotline is staffed during normal business hours. Hotline staff members provide general information about birth spacing and contraceptives, dispel myths and rumors about family planning, and connect individuals with clinics where they can obtain contraceptives [37].

Since abortion is illegal or socially taboo in many developing countries, preventing unsafe abortion is a deeply complex issue. Scaling widespread contraceptive use and developing policies that protect vulnerable pregnant women are vital initial steps. In settings where abortion is legal, new surgical and medication-based abortion techniques—including manual vacuum aspiration (MVA) and misoprostol—are helping to reduce abortion-related morbidity and mortality for both elective terminations and incomplete, hemorrhaging miscarriages. (Miscarriage is called spontaneous abortion in the medical literature.) MVA replaces the more risky procedure of dilatation and curettage, while misoprostol is an effective, affordable, and easily available medication that will help induce uterine contractions that will then expel an early pregnancy. In Tanzania and Burkina Faso, MVA and misoprostol were compared for treatment of incomplete abortions [38, 39]. Both MVA and misoprostol effectively treated incomplete abortion [38]; however, in both studies, misoprostol had a higher rate of acceptability [39].

Innovations that Address Eclampsia

Eclampsia is one of the three leading causes of maternal mortality, accounting for more than 13 % of maternal deaths per year [40]. Eclampsia is the development of seizures in a woman whose pregnancy is complicated by preeclampsia—a condition specific to pregnancy involving body swelling, high blood pressure, and protein spilling from the kidney into the urine. Five to 10 % of pregnancies may be affected by preeclampsia. Effects of eclampsia or severe forms of preeclampsia include respiratory problems, heart failure, brain hemorrhage, and acute kidney failure. Effects on the infant include low oxygen and severe growth retardation. Other signs of preeclampsia include rapid weight gain, increased reflexes, visual changes, and upper abdominal pain [41]. The condition may develop rapidly in some women and can be missed between prenatal visits.

The only cure for preeclampsia or eclampsia is the delivery of the baby. However, to mitigate the impact of the disease process prior to delivery, magnesium sulfate ($MgSO4$) is administered as a treatment [40]. It is usually given intravenously or intramuscularly and is a low-cost, high-yield treatment that can prevent deaths. Unfortunately, magnesium is severely underused in developing countries for a variety of reasons due in part to the challenge of making the diagnosis.

A Congo Red Dot urine test is being developed by Dr. Irina Buhimschi of the Department of Obstetrics and Gynecology at Nationwide Children's Hospital (Cleveland, OH) for use as a simple, low-cost test to rapidly predict preeclampsia. The premise is that in preeclampsia, there are an increased number of misfolded proteins that are spilled into the mother's urine. These proteins have a strong affinity to the azo dye, Congo Red. Initial findings suggest high efficacy and portability of the test as an early diagnostic tool for preeclampsia [42].

Another diagnostic test in development is the Sensing Strip for preeclampsia developed by a chemical engineering team at Stanford University. The device is solar powered and comprised of carbon-based materials and flexible polymers. When biomarkers indicating the presence of eclampsia are detected, the strip creates an electrical current which triggers a signal [43].

Innovations that Address Obstructed Labor

When the presenting part of the fetus cannot move into the birth canal, a woman's labor is considered obstructed. Obstructed labor can cause severe and sometimes permanent injury to the uterus, bladder, rectum, and vaginal membranes and thereby increase a woman's risk for infection, hemorrhage, fistula, and death [44]. Malnutrition and diabetes are both risk factors for obstructed labor, both of which are recognized crises in the urban poor. Obstructed labor must be treated with either surgical delivery via cesarean section or by using specialized instruments such as vacuum extraction or forceps, neither of which may be possible in low-resource settings.

Most innovations to date that address the problem of obstructed labor, have focused on creating inexpensive and reusable vacuum delivery systems. Vacuum delivery devices attach to the fetal head using a suction cup, allowing the provider to pull the baby down the birth canal while the mother pushes. Standard vacuum delivery systems in well-resourced hospitals must be attached to engine-powered aspirators or expensive handheld pumps. In the past year, low-cost, self-contained vacuum delivery devices that require no external power source and are disposable have been developed. The most well-known model is the Kiwi® Complete Vacuum Delivery System with PalmPump or Kiwi® OmniCup, which uses a traction handle to create the suction needed to assist delivery, thereby eliminating the need for an electric pump [45]. The OmniCup is disposable and made of rigid plastic, reducing the risk of transmitting infection [45, 46].

The Odon device was invented by Jorge Odón, then a 52-year-old car mechanic living in Argentina. This device, now being further developed by WHO, is a low-cost technological innovation that facilitates vaginal delivery. Made of inexpensive film-like polyethylene material, the Odon device slides over the infant's head, redirecting descent and decreasing friction while allowing provider assistance to maternal pushing. The Odon device may be easier and safer to apply than forceps or the vacuum extractor [47]. It could play a significant role in low-resource settings that lack surgical capacity or personnel trained in the use of a vacuum extractor or forceps delivery [48]. Early simulation trials showed that the Odon device consistently facilitates immediate expulsion of the fetus [47]. Finally, an additional barrier to operative delivery for obstructed labor is the significant lack of available anesthesia services in resource-limited settings for emergency cesarean section. Massachusetts General Hospital has developed the Every Second Matters for Mothers and Babies-Ketamine™ package to address this gap for cesarean section and other painful reproductive health procedures. The package, which consists of a one-week training for non-anesthesia providers, an ESM-Ketamine kit of commodities, wall charts, and checklists is currently being piloted in Western Kenya. This disruptive innovation could dramatically increase the availability of safe ketamine anesthesia for emergency cesarean section and painful procedures when no anesthetist is available.

Conclusion

A number of disruptive innovations focused on reducing maternal mortality in resource-limited settings have been developed in the past few years. Adapting these innovations and developing new ones that are specific to the needs of urban settings is a growing challenge.

As seen in the LifeSpring Hospital system in India, innovations that target the first delay include sustainable business models that provide low-cost options for women seeking care. Innovations such as the Zambulance and the Bambulance enable rapid and safe transport of mothers to health facilities, thereby addressing the second delay. Innovations that target the third delay include training programs that promote "task shifting," simple and low-cost packages of supplies, such as the Maama Kit, and creative ways to enhance supply chain (e.g., ColaLife).

While most of the recent maternal health innovations are not specific to urban or rural settings—they are helpful in both settings—further improvements and new approaches will be needed to better understand the unique attributes of the urban setting. For example, cost barriers appear to be of greater importance in the urban setting; thus, future innovations supporting the urban poor will need to directly seek ways to decrease costs without harming quality of care.

Although many of the examples of maternal health innovations described in this chapter are remarkably exciting, no single innovation is likely to significantly reduce the rate of maternal mortality without proper integration into standard societal practices. A precondition for successful innovations in maternal health is sustained political commitment and business modeling that can facilitate the social, cultural, and economic changes necessary to make large inroads in reducing maternal mortality. For deaths from pregnancy-related conditions to be reduced or eliminated, governments will need to harness and integrate the most appropriate and impactful innovations.

References

1. Maternal Mortality [Internet]. WHO; 2012 May [cited 2014 January 01]. http://www.who.int/mediacentre/factsheets/fs348/en/
2. Gabrysch S, Campbell O. Still too far to walk: literature review of the determinants of delivery service use. BMC Pregnancy Childbirth. 2009;9:34.
3. Harpham T. Urban health in developing countries: what do we know and where do we go? Health Place. 2009;15:107–16.
4. Matthews Z, Channon A, Neal S, Osrin D, Madise N, et al. Examining the "urban advantage" in maternal health care in developing countries. PLoS Med. 2010;7(9):e1000327.
5. Thaddeus S, Maine D. Too far to walk: maternal mortality in context. Soc Sci Med. 1994;38:8.
6. Combs Thorsen V, Sundby J, Malata A. Piecing together the maternal death puzzle through narratives: the three delays model revisited. PLoS One. 2012;7(12):e52090.
7. McTavish S, Moore S, Harper S, Lynch J. National female literacy, individual socio-economic status, and maternal health care use in sub-Saharan Africa. Soc Sci Med. 2010;71(11):1958–63.
8. Alvarez JL, Gil R, Hernandez V, Gil A. Factors associated with maternal mortality in Sub-Saharan Africa: an ecological study. BMC Public Health. 2009;9:462.
9. Simkhada B, Teijlingen ER, Porter M, Simkhada P. Factors affecting the utilization of antenatal care in developing countries: systematic review of the literature. J Adv Nurs. 2008;61:244–60.
10. Campbell OMR, Graham WJ. Strategies for reducing maternal mortality: getting on with what works. Lancet. 2006;368:1284–99.
11. Mobile Phone Access Reaches Three Quarters of Planet's Population [Internet]. The World Bank Group; 2012 July 17 [cited 2014 Jan 14]. http://www.worldbank.org/en/news/press-release/2012/07/17/mobile-phone-access-reaches-three-quarters-planets-population
12. Mechael PH. The case for mHealth in developing countries. Innovations. 2009;4(1):103–18.
13. Tameat T, Kachnowski S. Special delivery: an analysis of mHealth in maternal and newborn health programs and their outcomes around the world. Maternal Child Health J. 2012;16:1092–101.
14. Speciale AM, Freytsis M. mHealth for midwives: a call to action. J Midwifery Womens Health. 2013;58:76–82.

15. Noordam AC, Kuepper BM, Stekelenburg J, Milen A. Improvement of maternal health services through the use of mobile phones. Trop Med Int Health. 2011;16(5):622–6.
16. LifeSpring Hospitals: Providing Affordable, High-quality Healthcare [Internet]. Business Call to Action; 2010 June [cited on 2014 January 14]. http://www.businesscalltoaction.org/members/2010/08/lifespring-hospitals/
17. Zambulance [Internet]. Zambikes; 2013 [cited 2014 January 14]. http://zambikes.org/why_zambulance/
18. The Project [Internet]. Bambulance; 2008 [cited 2014 January 14]. http://plippo.com/client/bambulance/project.html
19. GUHUZA—Connecting mothers to health care through group SMS [Internet]. Saving Lives at Birth Grand Challenge for Development; 2012 August 06 [cited 2014 January 14]. http://savinglivesatbirth.net/summaries/2012/169
20. World Health Organization, PEPFAR, and UNAIDS. Task shifting: rational redistribution of tasks among health workforce teams. 2008. http://www.who.int/healthsystems/TTR-TaskShifting.pdf
21. Pathmanathan I, et al. Investing in maternal health: learning from Malaysia and Sri Lanka. Human Development Network: Health, Nutrition, and Population Series (31 December 2003). The World Bank.
22. MacArthur C. Traditional birth attendant training for improving health behaviours and pregnancy outcomes: RHL commentary (last revised: 1 June 2009). The WHO Reproductive Health Library; Geneva: World Health Organization.
23. Maama Kit: Making childbirth clean and safer. WHO, Republic of Uganda Ministry of Health.
24. About ColaLife [Internet].Colalife; 2014 [cited on 2014 January 14]. http://www.colalife.org/about/colalife-about/
25. Leading and underlying causes of maternal mortality [internet]. Unicef; 2014 [cited on 2014 January 1]. http://www.unicef.org/wcaro/overview_2642.html
26. Mbizvo MT, Fawcus S, Lindmark G, Nystrom L. Maternal mortality in rural and urban Zimbabwe: social and reproductive factors in an incident case-referent study. Soc Sci Med. 1993;36(9):1197–205.
27. Anderson JM, Etches D. Prevention and management of postpartum hemorrhage. Am Fam Physician. 2007;75(6):875–82.
28. Nelson BD, Stoklosa H, Ahn R, Eckardt MJ, Walton EK, Burke TF. Use of uterine balloon tamponade for control of postpartum hemorrhage by community-based health providers in South Sudan. Int J Gynaecol Obstet. 2013;122(1):27–32.
29. Miller S, Bergel EF, El Ayadi AM, Gibbons L, Butrick EA, Magwali T, Mkumba G, Kaseba C, Huong NT, Geissler JD, Merialdi M. Non-pneumatic anti-shock garment (NASG), a first-aid device to decrease maternal mortality from obstetric hemorrhage: a cluster randomized trial. PLoS One. 2013;8(10):e76477.
30. Monash University. Inhaled oxytocin team wins prestigious Australian Innovation Challenge. 2 December 2013. http://www.monash.edu.au/pharm/about/news/archive/2013/australian-innovators.html. Accessed 31 Mar 2014.
31. Dellinger R, et al. Surviving sepsis campaign: international guideline for management of severe septic and septic shock. Intensive Care Med. 2008;34:1160–2.
32. Kaseman T, Bourbour J, Schuler DA. Validation of the efficacy of a solar-thermal powered autoclave system for off-grid medical instrument wet sterilization. Am J Trop Med Hyg. 2012;87(4):602–7.
33. Chandler DL. "Sterilizing with the Sun." MIT News. 26 February 2013. http://web.mit.edu/newsoffice/2013/sterilizing-with-the-sun-0226.html. Accessed 12 Jan 2014.
34. Faundes A. Unsafe abortion—the current global scenario. Best Practice Res Clin Obstetric Gynecol. 2010;24:467–77.
35. Safe Abortion: Technical and Policy Guidance for Health Systems. 2nd edition. Geneva: World Health Organization; 2012. 1, Safe abortion care: the public health and human rights rationale. http://www.ncbi.nlm.nih.gov/books/NBK138200/

36. Adler AJ, Filippi V, Thomas SL, Ronsmans C. Quantifying the global burden of morbidity due to unsafe abortion: magnitude in hospital-based studies and methodological issues. Int J Gynecol Obstetrics. 2012;118(2):65–77.
37. Population Services International. Ligne Verte Hotline: Using cell phones to increase access to family planning information in the Democratic Republic of Congo. January 19, 2010. http://www.psi.org/resources/research-metrics/publications/conference-presentation/ligne-verte-hotline-using-cell-phone
38. Dao B, et al. Is Misoprostol a safe, effective and acceptable alternative to manual vacuum aspiration for postabortion care? Results from a randomized trail in Burkina Faso, West Africa. BJOG, 2007.
39. Shwekerela B, et al. Misoprostol for treatment of incomplete abortion at the regional hospital level: results from Tanzania. BJOG. 2007.
40. Emergency Obstetric Care [Internet]. United Nations Population Fund; 2014 [cited 2014 January 14]. http://www.unfpa.org/public/cache/offonce/home/mothers/pid/4385;jsessionid=BB3BABE60A1A812D20C84071B99F3729.jahia02
41. Managing Eclampsia [Internet]. World Health Organization & International Confederation of Midwives; 2008. http://whqlibdoc.who.int/publications/2008/9789241546669_2_eng.pdf
42. Larson NF. Congo red dot urine test can predict, diagnose preeclampsia. Medscape Medical News, February 9, 2010. http://www.medscape.com/viewarticle/716741. Accessed 12 Jan 2014.
43. Pre-eclampsia sensing strip [Internet]. Maternal and neonatal directed assessment of technology; 2014. http://mnhtech.org/technology/technologies-in-development/ pre-eclampsia-sensing-strip/
44. Dolea C, AbouSahr C. Global burden of obstructed labour in the year 2000. In Global Burden of Disease 2000.World Health Organization, November 2001.
45. Groom KM, Jones BA, Miller N, Paterson-Brown S. A prospective randomised controlled trial of the Kiwi Omnicup versus conventional ventous cups for vacuum-assisted vaginal delivery. BJOG. 2006;113:183–9.
46. Attilakos G, Sibanda T, Winter C, Johnson N, Draycott T. A randomised controlled trial of a new handheld vacuum extraction device. BJOG. 2005;112:1510–5.
47. The World Health Organization Odon Device Research Group. Feasibility and safety study of a new device (Odon device) for assisted vaginal deliveries: study protocol. Reprod Health. 2013;10:33.
48. Requejo JH, Belizan JM. Odon device: a promising tool to facilitate vaginal delivery and increase access to emergency care. Reprod Health. 2013;10:42.

Chapter 2
Innovations in Low- and Middle-Income Countries for Newborn and Child Health

Brett D. Nelson, Lisa B. Collins, and Edward W.J. Pritchard

Overview of Newborn and Child Health

A leading health priority worldwide is the improvement of newborn and child health. Children represent a particularly vulnerable group and carry a disproportionate share of the global burden of disease. UN Millennium Development Goal (MDG) 4 focuses specifically on improving newborn and child health through the reduction of under-five mortality rates by two-thirds between the years 1990 and 2015 [1]. Unfortunately, MDG 4 is the most off track of any of the eight MDGs; only 31 countries will likely meet this goal, and many countries have worse child mortality rates today than they did in 1990.

Currently, approximately 6.6 million children under the age of five die each year worldwide. The vast majority of these deaths occur in resource-limited countries [2]. In fact, 94 % of the world's childhood deaths occur in just 60 low- and middle-income countries, with approximately 50 % of child mortality occurring in sub-Saharan Africa [3]. Furthermore, recent evidence suggests that the growing subset of children in these countries who live in the urban setting are becoming increasingly at risk relative to those in the rural setting [4]. The historical "urban advantage" of children living in urban environments is rapidly diminishing in the face of rapid urban growth, overcrowding, poor sanitation, environmental pollution, and limited access to affordable healthcare in urban settings.

B.D. Nelson, M.D., M.P.H., D.T.M.&H. (✉)
Division of Global Health and Human Rights, Department of Emergency Medicine,
Massachusetts General Hospital, Zero Emerson Place Suite 104, Boston, MA 02114, USA

Harvard Medical School, Boston, MA, USA
e-mail: brett.d.nelson@gmail.com

L.B. Collins, M.A. • E.W.J. Pritchard, M.Phil.
Division of Global Health and Human Rights, Department of Emergency Medicine,
Massachusetts General Hospital, Zero Emerson Place Suite 104, Boston, MA 02114, USA

© Springer New York 2015
R. Ahn et al. (eds.), *Innovating for Healthy Urbanization*,
DOI 10.1007/978-1-4899-7597-3_2

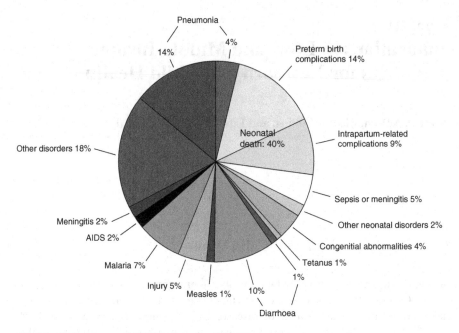

Fig. 2.1 Global causes of childhood deaths, 2010 [5]

Most childhood deaths in urban settings, as well as globally, result from treatable and preventable causes. The most common causes of childhood mortality are newborn causes (40 %), acute respiratory infections (14 %), diarrheal illness (10 %), malaria (7 %), injury (5 %), and AIDS (2 %) (Fig. 2.1). Meanwhile, child malnutrition, while typically not categorized as a direct cause of mortality, is believed to contribute to up to half of all childhood deaths.

Although there is still much to accomplish in improving newborn and child health worldwide and increasingly in urban environments, notable progress has been made over the last several decades. Innovations and technologies have played a significant role in those improvements. Cost-effective interventions have been developed that can save many newborn and child lives, and additional innovations are being developed each year.

The aim of this chapter is to introduce the reader to leading innovations that are saving thousands and even millions of lives annually. We have selected for discussion five general categories of newborn and child health innovations, including innovations related to newborns, childhood rehydration, nutrition, vitamins, vaccinations, and HIV/AIDS. Particular focus is given to innovations that are ideal for an urban environment, in that they are simple, easy to use, low cost, and require little infrastructure or training.

Newborn Health

Of all childhood deaths under the age of 5 years, 40 % occur within the newborn period, or the first 28 days of life. Worldwide, 3.1 million newborns die each year, and, as with other causes of childhood mortality, the overwhelming majority of these newborn deaths occur in resource-limited settings. Not included among these deaths is an approximately equal number of "stillbirths" [6]. Recent research shows that a large proportion of deaths considered stillbirths in low- and middle-income countries can actually be saved and are, therefore, apparently miscategorized as nonviable [7].

The three leading causes of newborn deaths worldwide are perinatal asphyxia (or failure of the newborn to take the first breath of life), complications associated with prematurity, and infections [8]. Fortunately, simple, cost-effective interventions are available to prevent most perinatal deaths. Well-accepted interventions include antenatal care, skin-to-skin care, facility-based deliveries, management of maternal complications, access to operative deliveries, and neonatal resuscitation [9, 10]. However, while solutions for reducing perinatal mortality exist, there have been significant limitations in establishing them in resource-limited settings [11, 12].

In this section, we discuss newborn health innovations that strive to decrease newborn mortality while overcoming some of the historic barriers to implementation in resource-limited settings.

Newborn Resuscitation Algorithms and Equipment

Arguably one of the most impactful and effective interventions in medicine is the use of newborn resuscitation for the management of perinatal asphyxia. In developed countries, simple resuscitation procedures are sufficient for managing up to 99 % of newborns [13, 14]. Nevertheless, these approaches that are effective in developed countries were historically not easily transferrable to settings with significantly fewer resources and fewer trained staff.

Thanks to a renewed commitment to improving newborn health worldwide, significant progress is being made in the management of perinatal asphyxia in low- and middle-income countries. This progress includes advances in resuscitative algorithms, devices, and training equipment that address the unique needs of this setting, including limited financial resources, fewer trained personnel, and poor supply chains. Furthermore, some clinical approaches to newborn resuscitation may need to be adapted, particularly for care outside of tertiary referral centers. For example, resuscitation recommendations in resource-limited settings frequently stop short of chest compressions, intubation, and other advanced resuscitative efforts, given lack of resources and the poor access to supportive critical care.

In June 2010, an initiative known as "Helping Babies Breathe" (HBB) introduced an evidence-based approach to newborn resuscitation in resource-limited settings [15, 16]. HBB was developed by the American Academy of Pediatrics, in collaboration with the World Health Organization (WHO), US Agency for International Development, Save the Children, the US National Institute of Child Health and Development, and many other partners. This new approach uses interactive training and simplified algorithms to train providers in effectively managing asphyxia during the first minutes of each newborn's life. HBB has quickly received wide endorsement and has become a central, global strategy for reducing newborn mortality and achieving MDG 4 [17].

HBB and other birth asphyxia programs have largely focused on building capacity among facility-based urban and rural providers, which is consistent with the general priority to improve the proportion of deliveries attended by skilled birth attendants in health facilities. However, in many areas of the developing world, a large number of deliveries still occur within the communities among unskilled birth attendants, like traditional birth attendants. In such areas, where the cadre of skilled birth attendants is nearly nonexistent and will likely take decades to be effectively established, interim training of unskilled birth attendants may be necessary [18, 19]. In South Sudan, for example, the overwhelming majority of deliveries still occur at home among unskilled birth attendants [20]. As this newly independent country works to build essential, facility-based skilled birth capacity, targeted training of community-based providers is occurring. The Massachusetts General Hospital's Division of Global Health and Human Rights, in partnership with the Ministry of Health of South Sudan, developed an innovative training program for community-based health workers called Maternal, Newborn, and Child Survival (MNCS) [21]. MNCS aims to improve the identification, initial management, and referral for the leading causes of maternal, newborn, and childhood mortality. The program utilizes setting-appropriate training, evidence-based checklists (Fig. 2.2), and reusable equipment and commodities. In contrast to HBB, MNCS is specifically intended for community-based, largely nonliterate, healthcare cadres [22]. Critical evaluation has shown that the program has improved frontline provider knowledge, practices, and referral to healthcare facilities.

Complementing these new setting-appropriate algorithms are innovations in resuscitative devices and training equipment. Historically, implementation and dissemination of newborn resuscitation management were significantly limited by inaccessible and prohibitively expensive equipment. Bag-mask resuscitation devices (for ventilating asphyxia newborns) and bulb suction devices (for clearing newborn airways) that are used in developed countries are frequently single-use items, and a bag-mask device can cost upward of $100 USD or more [23]. Traditional newborn training mannequins were also exorbitantly expensive, costing hundreds or thousands of dollars, and were, therefore, impractical in resource-limited settings.

Coinciding with the development of HBB—and critical to its success—was the production by Laerdal Medical of innovative and affordable resuscitative equipment that was designed specifically for resource-limited countries and that includes a reusable bag-mask device, bulb suction, and newborn training resuscitator [24]. The bag-mask device and bulb suction are boilable after each use and together cost less than $20 USD, making the equipment much more accessible to healthcare facilities and providers in resource-limited countries [25]. Laerdal's training resuscitator,

Fig. 2.2 Example of an MGH MNCS newborn resuscitation algorithm for nonliterate, community-based providers [22]

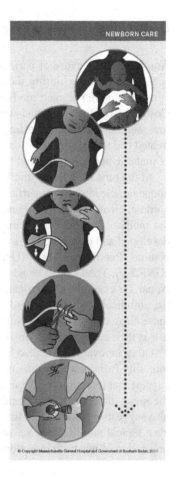

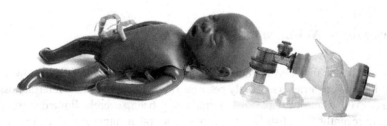

Fig. 2.3 Laerdal's affordable training mannequin and resuscitative equipment for low- and middle-income countries [22]

named NeoNatalie (Fig. 2.3), can be inflated with air or filled with water and includes functioning lungs and umbilical cord pulse, depending on the model. NeoNatalie ($50 USD) greatly decreases the barriers to training providers and to building much-needed healthcare capacity in the settings where the vast majority of birth asphyxia-related deaths are occurring.

Controlling Newborn Infections

Another leading cause of perinatal mortality is infection. These infections may be acquired prenatally, during the course of delivery, or postnatally. Antenatal interventions among pregnant mothers can reduce the likelihood of perinatal infections. Cost-effective interventions, which are recommended for all pregnant women in low- and middle-income settings, include tetanus toxoid vaccinations, insecticide-treated bed nets (for prevention of malaria), intermittent preventive treatment (IPT) of malaria, and screening and treatment for syphilis.

At the time of delivery, the WHO advocates for "six cleans": clean hands of the attendant, clean delivery surface, clean blade for cutting the umbilical cord, clean cord tie, clean towels to dry and then wrap the newborn, and a clean cloth to wrap the mother [26]. Several of these come as part of clean delivery kits, which are developed and distributed by a large number of organizations, including the United Nations Population Fund (UNFPA) and the United Nations Children's Fund (UNICEF). The kits can be adapted to meet unique local conditions and culture. In Nepal, for example, kit advocates discovered the traditional local practice of cutting the umbilical cord upon a hard surface, such as a coin [27]. Therefore, included in these clean delivery kits in Nepal was a clean plastic coin that practitioners could use as their cutting surface instead.

Other innovations are also being tested and introduced to reduce morbidity and mortality from newborn infections. Recent large trials in Bangladesh and Pakistan suggest that infections of the umbilical stump may be reduced by 20–40 % through the application of 4 % chlorhexidine solution to the stump [28, 29]. Another research also suggests a possible role for community-based administration of antibiotics and even topical emollients (e.g., sunflower oil) to the newborn for the treatment and prevention of newborn infections [30, 31].

Innovations in Newborn and Child Critical Care

Due to insufficient financial and human resources, critical care medicine in low- and middle-income countries has largely been restricted to large tertiary referral hospitals, and, even when available, it has frequently been severely limited in scope. However, recently established innovations, and other innovations currently in development, promise to expand the reach of critical care medicine and improve newborn and child health care in resource-limited countries beyond tertiary referral hospitals. Included among pediatric critical care advances are setting-appropriate innovations in ventilation, monitoring, thermoregulation, phototherapy, and infection control. It should also be noted that many of these innovations are also used among other patient populations beyond the newborn period.

Newborns who are significantly ill or premature may need ongoing respiratory support. This support can come in the form of supplemental oxygen, continuous positive airway pressure (CPAP), and mechanical ventilation. Oxygen concentrators can provide safe and affordable oxygen to patients by removing nitrogen from ambient air and supplying concentrated oxygen up to 10 L per minute. These machines do, however, require a continuous electrical supply, which may not always be feasible in many resource-poor settings. More significant respiratory support can be provided with CPAP machines and newborn ventilators. Some of these machines may even include features such as variable selection of oxygen concentrations, optional power by car batteries, ability to monitor and regulate newborn temperature, simplified settings for staff without high levels of newborn training, and simple design and parts to facilitate local repair.

Technology around newborn care is quickly evolving with new innovations being developed each year. Other examples of recent newborn innovations include vital sign monitoring/screening equipment (e.g., pulse oximetry, temperature monitoring, hemoglobin screening, jaundice screening, etc.), inexpensive newborn scales, incubators, warming cocoons, and jaundice phototherapy.

Rehydration

Discussion of childhood rehydration must begin with mention of one of the most notable child health innovations worldwide: oral rehydration therapy (ORT) for the prevention and management of dehydration. Identified by the *Lancet* as "potentially the most important medical advance" of the twentieth century, this example illustrates well the great potential for simple innovations to save millions of childhood lives each year [32].

Dehydrating diarrheal illness is among the leading causes of childhood mortality in low- and middle-income countries and is responsible for up to a million childhood deaths each year [5]. Diarrhea can be particularly concerning within urban settings where there is frequently overcrowding, contaminated water, and inadequate sewage systems. MDG 4 specifically addresses the need to revitalize efforts against diarrhea. The primary tool in managing diarrheal illness and its resulting dehydration is ORT, which consists of a simple solution of water, salts, and sugars [32]. First investigated in the 1940s, developed further over subsequent decades by cholera researchers in Bangladesh and India, ORT was ultimately endorsed in 1978 by the WHO as the cornerstone for fighting diarrheal illness.

The physiologic effectiveness of the ORT relies on a simple salt-sugar solution creating an osmotic gradient across the intestinal wall. As a result of the gradient, water is absorbed much more effectively into the body than would otherwise occur without the solutes. The patient is, therefore, more readily rehydrated. In fact, ORT has been shown to be as effective as intravenous (IV) rehydration in mild and moderate dehydration and is more readily available and affordable [33]. Largely as a result of ORT, the number of annual deaths in children aged 0–4 decreased by 3.1 million between 1979 and 1995 [34].

Although oral rehydration is the preferred route for rehydrating children (when clinically appropriate and tolerated), there are a number of alternative rehydration strategies that have advantages in specific circumstances. These alternative rehydration routes include IV, nasogastric, intraosseous, intraperitoneal, subcutaneous (or hypodermoclysis), and proctoclysis rehydration [35].

Nutrition

Children typically have less nutritional reserve than adults and are, therefore, particularly susceptible to malnutrition. Both a cause and a manifestation of poverty, malnourishment contributes to up to half of under-five deaths globally. Approximately 826 million people in the world are malnourished, 792 million of which are in the developing world, and malnutrition is on the rise in urban settings [36]. Poor nutrition depletes children of essential nutrients, rendering them underweight, weakened, and vulnerable to infections. It is estimated that feeding children an adequate diet would prevent one million deaths per year caused by pneumonia, 800,000 caused by diarrhea, 500,000 caused by malaria, and 250,000 caused by measles [37].

Various ready-to-use therapeutic foods (RUTF) have been developed to assist with acute malnourishment. Plumpy'Nut, the first RUTF developed by Nutriset in 1996, is intended specifically for the treatment of severe acute malnutrition. Described by Save the Children as a "miracle cure," Plumpy'Nut is a peanut-based paste with sugar, vegetable fat, and skimmed milk powder, enriched with vitamins and minerals, providing 500 kcal per sachet. As a ready-to-use food, Plumpy'Nut requires no preparation, no dilution in water prior to use, no cooking, and can be consumed directly from the sachet. Another RUTF, BP-100, acts similarly as a high-nutrient supplement and can be served either as a biscuit or as porridge when mixed with water. Neither BP-100 nor Plumpy'Nut requires the addition of water, eliminating the need for dilution instructions or the need for clean water, which is frequently unavailable in urban settings. Cooking and other preparations can also be avoided [38]. A joint declaration in May 2007 by the WHO, UNICEF, World Food Programme (WFP), and the UN Committee on Nutrition recommended RUTF as an essential community-based management of severe acute malnutrition [39].

An additional innovation for addressing childhood malnutrition is the mid-upper arm circumference (MUAC) tape (Fig. 2.4), which is an inexpensive and effective way of screening for malnourishment (specifically, marasmic malnutrition) in children ages 6–59 months. This simple tape is wrapped around the child's upper arm, midway between the tip of the shoulder and the tip of the elbow, and uses color-coding to indicate whether the child is likely suffering from malnourishment: red suggests severe malnourishment, orange suggests moderate malnourishment, yellow suggests a risk for malnourishment, and green suggests adequate nourishment. Many children in a community can be quickly screened using the MUAC tape and referred as indicated to a health facility for additional diagnosis and management. The WHO and UNICEF define non-edematous severe acute malnutrition either by a MUAC measurement of less than 115 mm or by a weight-for-height z-score less than −3 [40].

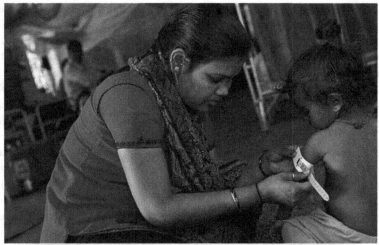

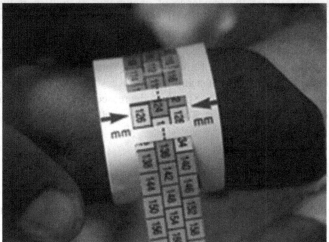

Fig. 2.4 Mid-upper arm circumference (MUAC) tape for the screening of childhood marasmic malnutrition (*Source*: Nick Cunard/CHI-Photo/Rex Features. Available at: http://www.telegraph. co.uk/health/expathealth/9017878/Expat-guide-to-India-health-care.html)

Micronutrient Fortification

Micronutrient and vitamin deficiencies have been identified as the "hidden hunger" of the developing world [41]. Inadequate levels of vitamin A, iron, zinc, and insufficient intake of fruits and vegetables can deprive children of essential nutrients, rendering them more vulnerable to a plethora of morbidities including blindness, scurvy, stunting, lower IQ, and death. The Copenhagen Consensus project on hunger and malnutrition reported that efforts to provide vitamin A, iodine, iron, and zinc rendered greater advantage than malaria, water, or sanitation programs [42]. Vitamin A supplementation is recognized as one of the most cost-effective interventions for improving child survival [37]. The WHO estimates that worldwide 100–140 million children are vitamin A deficient, causing 1–3 million deaths per year [43]. These children suffer a dramatically increased risk of death, ear infection, respiratory disease, and illness, especially from measles and diarrhea. As part of the global call to action, the UN Special Session on Children in 2002 set as one of its goals the elimination of vitamin A deficiency and its consequences by the year 2010. Studies have found that a single oral dose of vitamin A given to children shortly after birth can reduce their risk of death by 15 % [44]. A combination of vitamin A with vaccines has proven particularly successful. In 1987 the WHO advocated for the combined administration of vitamin A with the measles vaccine in countries where vitamin A deficiency is problematic.

Zinc supplementation used in conjunction with ORT has significantly reduced diarrhea and pneumonia among children. It has been observed that a weekly dose of 70 mg not only reduces the incidence of pneumonia, overall mortality is also reduced by 85 % [45]. The Sprinkles Global Health Initiative developed a home fortification solution in an attempt to treat micronutrient deficiencies among young children and other vulnerable groups at risk. Sprinkles are sachets containing a blend of micronutrients in powder form that can be sprinkled onto semi-solid foods in the home. Clinical trials in Ghana and Western Kenya have shown that even with low and infrequent use, Supplefer Sprinkles decreased rates of anemia, iron, and vitamin A deficiency in children in a resource-poor setting [46].

Nutrition and mHealth

Several studies indicate a growing adoption rate of information and communication technologies in the developing world. A common proxy for this is the use of mobile phones. In a world almost entirely covered in mobile phone networks, it is not surprising that international development efforts are increasingly focused on leveraging this technology to improve program reach [47]. RapidSMS, a collaboration among Columbia University and UNICEF, explored the use of mobile phones as a tool to collect and transmit child nutrition information via text messages (SMS). Utilizing an open-source software platform, the mobile phone was presented as an electronic input device for health workers, permitting the transmission of data directly to a central server at the national government level (Fig. 2.5). The pilot study of RapidSMS demonstrated that government and development workers benefited from real-time data access and analysis. Health workers received instant feedback messages confirming the information sent and provided additional directions if malnutrition was indicated by the data received.

UNICEF has also used the RapidSMS platform for field data collection purposes in Ethiopia to monitor the supply and distribution of the ready-to-use food Plumpy'Nut.

Child #	Sex	Age	Weight	Height	% Weight for Height	MUAC	Oedema	Diarrhoea
70	M	24	7.5	66.5		13.5	N	N
28	F	13	6.7	55.4		12.1	N	N
42	F	42	8.6	65.8		13.8	Y	N

Example of original paper-based form

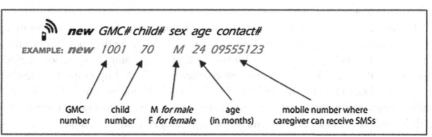

Example of RapidSMS text message for registering a child

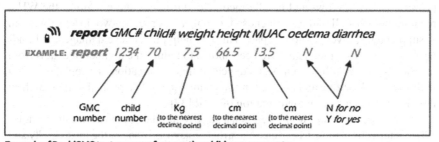

Example of RapidSMS text message for reporting child measurements

Fig. 2.5 RapidSMS is a mobile phone-based platform that can be used for data collection (*Source*: UNICEF Malawi and UNICEF Innovations. Using mobile phones to improve child nutrition surveillance in Malawi. June 2009. Available at: http://www.sipa.columbia.edu/academics/concentrations/epd/documents/UNICEFFinalReport_2009.pdf)

Vaccinations

Approximately 2.5 million under-five deaths are averted each year by immunization against diphtheria, pertussis, tetanus (DPT), and measles [48]. Global vaccination coverage is improving: 130 countries have been able to administer all three primary doses of the DPT vaccine to 90 % of children aged one and younger. Nevertheless, it has been reported that in 2010, over 19 million children still did not get all three primary doses of DPT vaccination. Childhood vaccination rates in urban settings have waned, while overcrowding has increased the risks for communicable, vaccine-preventable diseases. In this section, we examine innovative methods that have been adopted to deliver vaccination across resource-poor countries.

Measles is one of the primary preventable childhood diseases continuing to claim the lives of thousands of children worldwide. The WHO estimates that more than 95 % of measles deaths occur in low-income countries with weak health infrastructures [49]. Measles is a highly-contagious, serious disease caused by a virus in the paramyxovirus family and is spread person-to-person through coughing, sneezing, or close or direct contact with infected nasal or throat secretions. It is particularly worrisome in population-dense environments, such as urban slums or refugee camps. Before 1980, before widespread vaccination, measles caused an estimated 2.6 million deaths each year.

Fortunately, accelerated immunization activities have had a major positive impact on reducing measles deaths. From 2001 to 2011, more than one billion children aged 9 months to 14 years who live in high-risk countries were vaccinated against the disease. Measles vaccination resulted in a 74 % drop in measles deaths between 2000 and 2010, worldwide [49, 50]. The vaccine is safe, effective, and inexpensive, costing less than one US dollar to immunize a child against measles. In April 2012, a Global Measles and Rubella Strategic Plan was launched, which aimed to entirely eliminate measles and rubella in at least five WHO regions. In addition, implementation of vitamin distribution alongside measles vaccination has proven effective in low- and middle-income countries. In these regions, the WHO recommends that all children diagnosed with measles receive two doses of vitamin A supplements, given 24 hours apart. This can help prevent eye damage and blindness. Vitamin A supplements have been shown to reduce the number of deaths from measles by 50 %. It has even been advocated that fortification or supplementation with vitamin A or zinc and measles immunization should be pushed to their highest possible levels before supplementation of food [37].

The prevalence of diarrheal illness can also be reduced through vaccine innovations. While numerous pathogens can cause diarrhea, rotavirus is one of the most deadly and has been identified as the most common cause of diarrhea in children in the developing world [51]. Traditional hygiene measures have proven ineffective in fully combating the devastating effects of the virus, which also causes vomiting, rendering attempts of hydration provided by oral rehydration therapies ineffective. It has been estimated that nearly 85 % of rotavirus-related deaths occur in the developing world [52].

The rotavirus vaccine was initially accepted for use in 14 countries in the Americas and Europe only. In 2005, the WHO's Strategic Advisory Group of Experts (SAGE) stated that they were not yet in a position to make a global recommendation about the use of rotavirus vaccines. However, a clinical trial, funded in part by the Global Alliance for Vaccines and Immunization (GAVI), alongside PATH, WHO, GlaxoSmithKline (GSK), and research institutions in low-socioeconomic settings of South Africa and Malawi, found that the vaccine significantly reduced severe diarrhea episodes due to rotavirus. Results revealed that vaccines with even moderate efficacy have the potential to prevent a substantial number of childhood deaths in regions where rotavirus has deadly consequences, predominantly Africa and Asia [53]. In 2009, the WHO recommended that rotavirus vaccination—Rotarix (GSK) and RotaTeq (Merck)—be included in all national immunization programs worldwide [54]. SAGE also emphasized the importance of providing rotavirus vaccination in the context of improvement of water quality, hygiene, and sanitation, and provision of oral rehydration solution and zinc supplements.

Another vaccine-preventable childhood illness is polio. In 2003, Dr. Gro Harlem Brundtland, Director-General of WHO, reported that there was no moral or economic justification for any child anywhere in the world to be crippled by polio [55]. Four countries—India, Afghanistan, Pakistan, and Nigeria—are still endemic for polio. Cases of polio remain highest in India, where, by 2003, 85 % of new polio cases were identified. The polio vaccine, which contains the three strains of poliovirus, can protect a child for life. Vaccination against polio commenced in 1978 in India with the Expanded Program on Immunization (EPI). A collaboration between the WHO and the Indian Government introduced the National Polio Surveillance Project, and strategies involved immunizing children less than 3 years with a single dose of oral polio vaccine at polio booths all over the country on two national immunization days. Children that were not immunized were targeted through house-to-house search.

Pneumococcal vaccines prevent certain forms of pneumonia, the leading vaccine-preventable killer of children under the age of five. It is estimated that 700,000–1 million children under the age of five die of severe pneumococcal infections [56]. However, the effectiveness of the vaccine in children under 2 years of age remains unclear—unfortunately excluding the use of the vaccine in the most important target group for pneumococcal vaccines: the youngest children in low- and middle-income countries [57].

A number of diseases continue to evade vaccination. *Plasmodium falciparum* malaria, a major cause of infectious mortality, presents a great challenge to vaccine developers [58]. Vaccine prototypes have entered clinical trials. The RTS,S/AS01 *Plasmodium falciparum* malaria vaccine has been celebrated as the first malaria vaccine. The vaccine, developed by a public-private partnership between GlaxoSmithKline and PATH Malaria Vaccine Initiative and supported by the Bill & Melinda Gates Foundation, is primarily for use in infants and young children in sub-Saharan Africa. It has been predicted to become available in 3 years, but there is no vaccination presently being utilized to combat this deadly disease. Challenges are not merely scientific; delivery methods, partnerships between governments and educational departments, and funding and political commitment remain imperative difficulties pertaining to the availability of any vaccinations.

HIV/AIDS

HIV has devastating consequences for children in low- and middle-income countries and is one of the primary contributing factors that keep the poorest on our planet poor. At the end of 2009, it was estimated by the WHO that 2.5 million children were HIV positive, the majority of whom live in sub-Saharan Africa [59]. Prevention of HIV infection is paramount in combating the virus, and preventing new HIV infections in children is the only long-term sustainable way to conquer the HIV epidemic. With by far the most common cause of infection in children being vertical transmission from mother to infant during and after pregnancy, much research has been tailored toward the prevention of mother-to-child transmission (PMTCT) of HIV. Using existing interventions, PMTCT can be reduced to 2 % or lower. However, these interventions are rarely fully accessible in low- and middle-income countries. Meanwhile, for the children already infected with the virus, only 500,000 are estimated to be receiving antiretroviral therapy, leaving a further two million children untreated. Innovations in the diagnosis, treatment, and management of children infected with HIV are continually sought.

In this next section, we look at the innovations in PMTCT of HIV, diagnosis of HIV in children in low-income countries, pediatric treatment and management of the virus, and what is being done to overcome the many barriers faced by children affected by the HIV epidemic.

PMTCT, ARV Prophylaxis, and Breastfeeding

The most common cause worldwide for children acquiring the HIV infection is through mother-to-child transmission (MTCT). Prevention of MTCT of HIV has enabled efficacious and effective prophylactic treatment of HIV-positive mothers and represents the best hope to reduce HIV in children. Prophylactic prevention strategies include prevention of in utero and intrapartum transmission of HIV infection with antiretroviral therapy as well as prevention of postnatal transmission in breastfeeding.

A number of evidence-based approaches and innovations for preventing transmission by breastfeeding have been developed and deserve discussion. In the developed world (e.g., North America, Europe, etc.), mothers with HIV are strongly discouraged from breastfeeding their children. However, in low- and middle-income countries, the WHO recommends that all mothers—including those with HIV—exclusively breastfeed their newborns during the first 6 months of life. Although at first glance the ethics of these contrasting guidelines may seem puzzling, research now clearly shows that the health risks to the newborn are less from being breastfed by an HIV-positive mother than from using milk substitutes. Substitutes to breastfeeding, such as newborn formulas, are frequently prohibitively expensive in resource-limited settings and, more importantly, greatly expose the newborn to formula mixed with unclean water. Diarrheal illness represents a greater health threat to these newborns than HIV transmission. Furthermore, milk substitutes lack the very useful maternal antibodies and ideal nutrition found in breast milk.

Several innovations have, therefore, been introduced to reduce the transmission of HIV to children while exclusively breastfeeding. Efforts have included breast milk pasteurization, breast milk banking, extended postnatal antiretroviral therapy, and other approaches for reducing HIV transmission via breast milk [60]. Breastfeeding nipple shields have also been utilized in reducing MTCT of HIV. The

JustMilk project, for example, is presently aiming to provide a modified nipple shield that could deliver antiretroviral drugs to the infant for prophylaxis against infection or release an edible microbicide into breast milk that directly reduces HIV infectivity in the milk [61].

There is also ongoing research into the effectiveness of extended postnatal anti-retroviral prophylaxis during breastfeeding. A Cochrane review in 2009 concluded that although complete avoidance of breastfeeding is efficient in preventing MTCT of HIV, it has significant associated morbidity, including diarrheal disease when formula is prepared without clean water. Therefore, they recommend two interventions to prevent transmission if breastfeeding is initiated: (1) exclusive breastfeeding during the first few months of life; and (2) chronic antiretroviral prophylaxis to the infant (nevirapine alone or nevirapine with zidovudine) [62]. It is hoped that additional research efforts in this field can further maximize the number of healthy, thriving, HIV-free children around the world [60].

Diagnosis of HIV in Children

In resource-limited countries, diagnosing children and newborns with HIV remains challenging. In these settings, other infections and malnutrition may mimic the signs and symptoms of AIDS, and diagnosis is complicated by the fact that infants retain maternal antibodies for up to 12–18 months after birth [63]. The enzyme-linked immunosorbent assay (ELISA) HIV tests used for adult diagnosis in resource-limited settings do not distinguish between maternal and infant antibodies. RNA polymerase chain reaction (PCR) and other assays to detect the virus remain too expensive for use in resource-poor settings. Consequently, in some parts of sub-Saharan Africa, practical clinical diagnosis is based on the integrated management of childhood illness (IMCI) algorithm developed by the WHO and UNICEF [64]. IMCI permits trained providers to recognize symptoms consistent with HIV infection.

One of the greatest innovations in the diagnosis of HIV in children and infants has come in the use of dried blood spot testing (Fig. 2.6). Unlike traditional blood collection, a dried blood spot sample is easy to prepare in resource-limited settings and can be stored and shipped to central testing facilities without refrigeration. A study performed in South Africa found that the Roche Amplicor assay for diagnosing HIV from dried spot testing had a sensitivity of 100 % and a specificity of 99.6 %, making it incredibly precise in diagnosing and ruling out HIV infection [65]. For this reason, HIV DNA PCR tests on dried blood spots have a massive potential to improve healthcare delivery to HIV-affected children in low-resource settings.

Universal screening of infants for HIV infection in an immunization clinic has had some positive results. Among 646 mothers bringing infants for immunizations, 584 (90.4 %) agreed to HIV testing of their infant and 332 (56.8 %) subsequently returned for results. Furthermore, most mothers interviewed said they were comfortable with testing of their infant at immunization clinics and would recommend it to others [66].

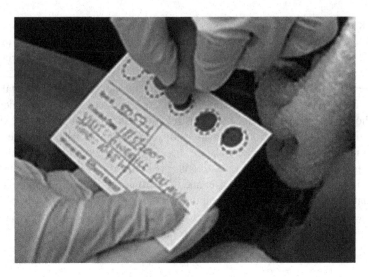

Fig. 2.6 Nurse takes a sample from a child using dried blood spot testing (©UNICEF/ NYHQ2009-0733/ Nesbitt. http://www.unicef.org/aids/index_51950.html)

As many people in low- and middle-income countries do not have access to laboratory services, point-of-care (POC) tests for the diagnosis of HIV and other infections are becoming increasingly available. POC tests, requiring no laboratory equipment and minimal training, are now available for HIV infection, syphilis, and malaria. Nevertheless, these tests should be used in conjunction with clinical status, history, and risk factors of the person being tested.

Treatment of Children with HIV

Several barriers exist to the proper diagnosis and management of pediatric HIV. UNICEF reports that distance from a health facility, poor transportation, lack of supplies and medications, limited trained staff, cost of services, and stigma are a few of the obstacles keeping people from being tested or receiving treatment [67]. These barriers are present in many urban settings.

As a result, HIV-positive children are often not diagnosed nor treated. Despite growing research on the efficacy of HIV treatment in children and the need for antiretroviral therapy (ART) to be commenced early in infants, pediatric HIV treatment has remained overshadowed by adult HIV treatment in resource-poor settings [68]. According to UNAIDS data, only 37 % of adults receive HIV receive treatment, whereas only 28 % of eligible children are on this life-saving therapy [69]. In some low- and middle-income countries, the disparities are even more marked.

To overcome these disparities, some focus has been directed toward a greater emphasis on family-directed services in order to improve treatment of children in resource-limited settings [70]. A recent systematic review found the use of a home-based nursing scheme improved ART adherence. However, in other studies, peer-support groups for adolescents have not demonstrated effectiveness in improving adherence. Much more research is needed to improving pediatric adherence to ART [71].

HIV infection remains heavily stigmatized throughout the world, and people living with HIV infection continue to face discrimination. Stigma and discrimination are considered major barriers to HIV prevention, diagnosis, and care-seeking behavior [72]. A study in Zambia reported HIV/AIDS-related stigma in schools came in forms of rejection, gossip, and taunts [73]. HIV/AIDS-related stigma forces the epidemic underground and is one of the main reasons that people do not wish to know their HIV status, contributing to vertical transmission to children. Stigma-reduction interventions exist, although they are frequently demoted to the bottom of HIV/AIDS program priorities [74]. These interventions include counseling, cognitive-behavioral therapy, support groups, empowerment, home-care teams, community education, and policy development [75].

Mobile phone technology has also been utilized to improve HIV awareness and enhance behavior change. Text to Change, a nonprofit in Uganda, utilized mobile messaging to increase awareness around HIV/AIDS [76]. The intervention included a multiple-choice quiz related to HIV awareness that was sent by text message to more than 15,000 people in southwest Uganda. During the weeks after the awareness quiz text, there was a 40 % increase in HIV testing in the region. Nevertheless, the impact that this intervention had on children specifically is not known, and UNICEF cautions that relying significantly on technology to raise awareness may not reach the poorest, most vulnerable subgroups, for whom technology is not an option.

Other mHealth innovations for addressing the HIV epidemic include patient tracking, relay of centralized laboratory results, patient ART adherence reminders, provider support and guidelines, continuing medical education, and data collection.

Conclusion

Newborns and children in resource-limited settings are among society's most vulnerable groups. Children in dense urban environments are at particular risk. Fortunately, effective innovations to improve newborn and child health exist and are currently saving millions of lives each year. Table 2.1 summarizes examples of innovations discussed in this chapter. These innovations include interventions for newborns, childhood rehydration, nutrition, vitamins, vaccinations, and HIV/AIDS. Improving availability and access to these solutions is an important priority worldwide.

Table 2.1 Examples of child health innovations discussed in this chapter

Summary table of example innovations
Newborn health
Setting-appropriate resuscitation algorithms
Reusable bag-mask device
Reusable bulb suction
Newborn training mannequin
Oxygen concentrators
Vital sign monitoring/screening equipment
Skin-to-skin care
Facility-based deliveries
Infection
Insecticide-treated bed nets
Intermittent preventive treatment for malaria
Screening and treatment for syphilis
Clean delivery kits
4 % chlorhexidine solution to the umbilical stump
Tetanus toxoid vaccination
Measles vaccination
Rotavirus vaccination
Oral polio vaccination
Pneumococcal vaccination
Dehydration
Oral rehydration therapy
Alternative rehydration methods, including intravenous, nasogastric, intraosseous, intraperitoneal, subcutaneous (or hypodermoclysis), and proctoclysis
Malnutrition
Ready-to-use therapeutic foods (RUTF) (e.g., Plumpy'Nut)
Mid-upper arm circumference (MUAC) tape
Vitamin A supplementation
Zinc supplementation
RapidSMS
HIV/AIDS
Breast milk pasteurization
Breast milk banking
Postnatal antiretroviral therapy
ELISA HIV tests
IMCI algorithm
Dried blood spot testing
Point-of-care testing
"Text to Change"

References

1. Lozano R, Wang H, Foreman KJ, Rajaratnam JK, Naghavi M, Marcus JR, Dwyer-Lindgren L, Lofgren KT, Phillips D, Atkinson C, Lopez AD, Murray CJ. Progress towards Millennium Development Goals 4 and 5 on maternal and child mortality: an updated systematic analysis. Lancet. 2011;378(9797):1139–65.
2. Inter-agency Group for Child Mortality Estimation. Levels and trends in child mortality: Report 2012. UNICEF: New York. 2012. Presentation: United Nations expert group meeting on population distribution, urbanization, internal migration and development. 21–23 January 2008. http://www.un.org/esa/population/meetings/EGM_PopDist/Madise.pdf
3. Black RE, Morris SS, Bryce J. Where and why are 10 million children dying every year? Lancet. 2003;361:2226–34.
4. Fotso JC, Ezeh AC, Madise NJ, Ciera J. Progress towards the child mortality MDG in urban sub-Saharan Africa: the dynamics of population growth, immunization, and access to clean water. BMC Public Health. 2007;7:218.
5. Liu L, Johnson HL, Cousens S, Perin J, Scott S, Lawn JE, Rudan I, Campbell H, Cibulskis R, Li M, Mathers C, Black RE, for the Child Health Epidemiology Reference Group of WHO and UNICEF. Global, regional, and national causes of child mortality: an updated systematic analysis for 2010 with time trends since 2000. Lancet. 2012;379:2151–61.
6. Lawn JE, Blencowe H, Pattinson R, Cousens S, Kumar R, Ibiebele I, Gardosi J, Day LT, Stanton C. Lancet's Stillbirths Series steering committee. Stillbirths: Where? When? Why? How to make the data count? Lancet. 2011;377(9775):1448–63.
7. Msemo G, Massawe A, Mmbando D, Rusibamayila N, Manji K, Kidanto HL, Mwizamuholya D, Ringia P, Ersdal HL, Perlman J. Newborn mortality and fresh stillbirth rates in Tanzania after helping babies breathe training. Pediatrics. 2013;131(2):e353–60.
8. Lawn JE, Kerber K, Enweronu-Laryea C, Cousens S. 3.6 million neonatal deaths–what is progressing and what is not? Semin Perinatol. 2010;34(6):371–86.
9. Lee AC, Lawn JE, Cousens S, Kumar V, Osrin D, Bhutta ZA, Wall SN, Nandakumar AK, Syed U, Darmstadt GL. Linking families and facilities for care at birth: what works to avert intrapartum-related deaths? Int J Gynaecol Obstet. 2009;107(Suppl 1):S65–85, S86–8.
10. Newton O, English M. Newborn resuscitation: defining best practice for low-income settings. Trans R Soc Trop Med Hyg. 2006;100(10):899–908.
11. Lawn JE, Yakoob MY, Haws RA, Soomro T, Darmstadt GL, Bhutta ZA. 3.2 million stillbirths: epidemiology and overview of the evidence review. BMC Pregnancy Childbirth. 2009;9 Suppl 1:S2.
12. Lawn JE, Lee AC, Kinney M, Sibley L, Carlo WA, Paul VK, Pattinson R, Darmstadt GL. Two million intrapartum-related stillbirths and neonatal deaths: where, why, and what can be done? Int J Gynaecol Obstet. 2009;107 Suppl 1:S5–19.
13. Kattwinkel J, editor. Textbook of neonatal resuscitation. Elk Grove Village: American Academy of Pediatrics and American Heart Association; 2006.
14. American Heart Association and American Academy of Pediatrics. 2005 American Heart Association (AHA) Guidelines for Cardiopulmonary Resuscitation (CPR) and Emergency Cardiovascular Care (ECC) of pediatric and neonatal patients: neonatal resuscitation guidelines. Pediatrics. 2006;117:e1029–38.
15. American Academy of Pediatrics. Helping babies breathe. http://www.helpingbabiesbreathe.org/
16. International Liaison Committee on Resuscitation. The International Liaison Committee on Resuscitation (ILCOR) consensus on science with treatment recommendations for pediatric and neonatal patients: pediatric basic and advanced life support. Pediatrics. 2006;117(5):e955–77.
17. UNICEF. MDG 4: Reduce child mortality. http://www.unicef.org/progressforchildren/2007n6/index_41806.htm
18. Sibley LM, Sipe TA. Transition to skilled birth attendance: is there a future role for trained traditional birth attendants? J Health Popul Nutr. 2006;24(4):472–8.

19. Sibley LM, Sipe TA, Brown CM, Diallo MM, McNatt K, Habarta N. Traditional birth atten-
    dant training for improving health behaviours and pregnancy outcomes. Cochrane Database
    Syst Rev. 2007;(3):CD005460.
20. Ministry of Health, Republic of South Sudan. Health sector development plan, 2011–2015:
    transforming the health system for improved services and better coverage. 1 March 2011.
21. Nelson BD, Fehling M, Eckardt MJ, Ahn R, Tiernan M, Purcell G, Bell S, El-Bashir A, Walton
    EK, Ghirmai E, Burke TF. Maternal, Newborn, and Child Survival (MNCS): An innovative
    training package for building frontline health worker capacity in South Sudan. South Sudan
    Med J. 2011;4(4):80–2.
22. Nelson BD, Ahn R, Fehling M, Eckardt MJ, Conn KL, El-Bashir A, Tiernan M, Purcell G,
    Burke TF. Evaluation of a novel training package among frontline maternal, newborn, and
    child health workers in South Sudan. Int J Gynecol Obstet. 2012;119:130–5.
23. PATH, USAID. Practical selection of neonatal resuscitators, Version 3: a field guide. May
    2010. http://www.path.org/publications/detail.php?i=1565
24. Laerdal. NeoNatalie: Realistic and affordable training and therapy. http://www.laerdal.com/
    binaries/AEVJNCXO/NeoNatalie-Brochure-310510.pdf
25. Laerdal. NeoNatalie. http://www.laerdalglobalhealth.com/neonatalie.html
26. Lawn J, Kerber K (Eds.). Opportunities for Africa's newborns: practical data, policy and pro-
    grammatic support for newborn care in Africa. WHO. 2006. http://www.who.int/pmnch/
    media/publications/africanewborns/en/index.html
27. PATH. A brief overview of the purpose, development, and evaluation of clean delivery kits.
    Nairobi: PATH; 1999.
28. Arifeen SE, Mullany LC, Shah R, Mannan I, Rahman SM, Talukder MR, Begum N, Al-Kabir
    A, Darmstadt GL, Santosham M, Black RE, Baqui AH. The effect of cord cleansing with
    chlorhexidine on neonatal mortality in rural Bangladesh: a community-based, cluster-
    randomised trial. Lancet. 2012;379(9820):1022–8.
29. Soofi S, Cousens S, Imdad A, Bhutto N, Ali N, Bhutta ZA. Topical application of chlorhexi-
    dine to neonatal umbilical cords for prevention of omphalitis and neonatal mortality in a rural
    district of Pakistan: a community-based, cluster-randomised trial. Lancet. 2012;379(9820):
    1029–36.
30. Zaidi AK, Ganatra HA, Syed S, Cousens S, Lee AC, Black R, Bhutta ZA, Lawn JE. Effect of
    case management on neonatal mortality due to sepsis and pneumonia. BMC Public Health.
    2011;11 Suppl 3:S13.
31. Darmstadt GL, Saha SK, Ahmed AS, Ahmed S, Chowdhury MA, Law PA, Rosenberg RE,
    Black RE, Santosham M. Effect of skin barrier therapy on neonatal mortality rates in preterm
    infants in Bangladesh: a randomized, controlled, clinical trial. Pediatrics. 2008;121(3):522–9.
32. Water with sugar and salt. Lancet. 1978;2:300–01.
33. Spandorfer P, Akessandrini EA, Joffe MD, Localio R, Shaw KN. Oral versus Intravenous
    rehydration of moderately dehydrated children: a randomized, controlled trial. Pediatrics.
    2005;115(2):295–301.
34. Pierce NF. How much has ORT reduced child mortality? J Health Popul Nutr. 2001;
    19(1):1–3.
35. Rouhani S, Meloney L, Ahn R, Nelson BD, Burke TF. Alternative rehydration methods: a
    systematic review and lessons for resource-limited care. Pediatrics. 2011;127(3):e748–57.
36. Mason JB, Musgrove P, Habicht JP. At least one third of poor countries' burden is due to mal-
    nutrition: working paper no. 1. Disease Control Priorities Project. Fogarty International Center,
    National Institute of Health. 2003.
37. Edjer TT, Moses A, Black R, Wolfson L, Hutubessy R, Evans DB. Cost effectiveness analysis
    of strategies for child health in developing countries. BMJ. 2005;331(7526):1177.
38. Médecins Sans Frontières. BP-100™ vs Plumpy-Nut. http://www.compactforlife.com/upload/
    BP-100vsPlumpyNut.pdf
39. World Health Organization, World Food Programme, United Nations System Standing
    Committee on Nutrition, The United Nations Children's Fund. Community-based manage-

ment of severe acute malnutrition: a joint statement by the World Health Organization, the World Food Programme, the United Nations System Standing Committee on Nutrition and the United Nations Children's Fund. May 2007. http://www.unicef.org/publications/files/ Community_Based_Management_of_Sever_Acute_Malnutirtion.pdf

40. World Health Organization, UNICEF. WHO child growth standards and the identification of severe acute malnutrition in infants and children. 2009. http://www.who.int/nutrition/publica-tions/severemalnutrition/9789241598163_eng.pdf

41. Jamil KM, Rahman AS, Bardhan PK, Khan AI, Chowdhury F, Sarker SA, Khan AM, Ahmed T. Micronutrients and anaemia. J Health Popul Nutr. 2008;26(3):340–55.

42. Hoddinott J, Rosegrant M, Torero M. Hunger and malnutrition: investments to reduce hunger and undernutrition. International Food Policy Research Institute: Washington, DC. April 9, 2012.   http://copenhagenconsensus.com/Files/Filer/CC12%20papers/Hunger%20and%20 Malnutrition.pdf

43. Neidecker-Gonzales O, Nestel P, Bouis H. Estimating the global cost of vitamin A supplemen-tation: a review of the literature. Food Nutr Bull. 2007;29:307–16.

44. Klemm RD, Labrique AB, Christian P, Rashid M, Shamim AA, Katz J, Sommer A, West Jr KP. Newborn vitamin A supplementation reduced infant mortality in rural Bangladesh. Pediatrics. 2008;122(1):e242–50.

45. Temple VJ, Masta A. Zinc in human health. PNG Med J. 2004;47(3–4):146–58.

46. Suchdev PS, Ruth LJ, Woodruff BA, Mbakaya C, Mandava U, Flores-Ayala R, Jefferds ME, Quick R. Selling sprinkles micronutrient powder reduces anemia, iron deficiency, and vitamin A deficiency in young children in Western Kenya: a cluster-randomized controlled trial. Am J Clin Nutr. 2012;95(5):1223–30.

47. Horvath T, Azman H, Kennedy GE, Rutherford GW. Mobile phone text messaging for promot-ing adherence to antiretroviral therapy in patients with HIV infection. Cochrane Database Syst Rev. 2012 Mar 14;3:CD009756.

48. UNICEF. State of the World's Children, 2012. UNICEF:New York. February 2012. http:// www.unicef.org/sowc2012/pdfs/SOWC%202012-Main%20Report_EN_13Mar2012.pdf

49. WHO. Measles. http://www.who.int/mediacentre/factsheets/fs286/en/

50. Jones G, Steketee RW, Black RE, Bhutta ZA, Morris SS, Bellagio Child Survival Study Group. How many child deaths can we prevent this year? Lancet. 2003;362(9377):65–71.

51. UNICEF. Tracking progress in maternal, newborn, and child survival: the 2008 Report. UNICEF:New York. 2008. http://www.who.int/pmnch/Countdownto2015FINALREPORT-apr7.pdf

52. PATH. New rotravirus vaccines, more hope: development of new vaccines is critical to protect-ing children everywhere. 2010. http://path.org/projects/rotavirus_vaccine.php

53. WHO. Rotavirus vaccines in the developing world: update on clinical trials in Africa and Asia. http://www.who.int/vaccine_research/about/gvrf/Neuzil%20presentation.pdf

54. WHO. Global use of rotavirus vaccines recommended. http://www.who.int/mediacentre/news/ releases/2009/rotavirus_vaccines_20090605/en/index.html

55. WHO. WHO Director-General calls India 'number 1' polio eradication priority. http://www. who.int/mediacentre/news/releases/2003/pr30/en/index.html

56. Sergio AC, Soares de Moura AT, Berkelhamer JE. Overview of the global health issues facing children. Pediatrics. 2012;129(1):1–3.

57. Mathew JL. Pneumococcal vaccination in developing countries: where does science end and commerce begin? Vaccine. 2009;27(32):4247–51.

58. Hill AV. Vaccines against malaria. Philos Trans R Soc Lond B Biol Sci. 2011;366(1579):2806–14.

59. World Health Organization. Paediatric HIV and treatment of children living with HIV. World Health Organization. 2011. http://www.who.int/hiv/topics/paediatric/en/index.html

60. Young SL, Mbuya MN, Chantry CJ, Geubbels EP, Israel-Ballard K, Cohan D, Vosti SA, Latham MC. Current knowledge and future research on infant feeding in the context of HIV: basic, clinical, behavioral, and programmatic perspectives. Adv Nutr. 2011;2(3):225–43.

61. Just Milk. Combating mother-to-child HIV transmission. http://justmilk.org/
62. Horvath T, Madi BC, Iuppa IM, Kennedy GE, Rutherford G, Read JS. Interventions for preventing late postnatal mother-to-child transmission of HIV. Cochrane Database Syst Rev. 2009 Jan 21;(1):CD006734.
63. Louisirirotchanakul S, Kanoksinsombat C, Likanonsakul S, Sunthornkachit R, Supanit I, Wasi C. Patterns of anti-HIV IgG3, IgA and p24Ag in perinatally HIV-1 infected infants. Asian Pac J Allergy Immunol. 2002;20 (2):99.
64. Horwood C, Liebeschuetz S, Blaauw D, Cassol S, Qazi S. Diagnosis of paediatric HIV infection in a primary health care setting with a clinical algorithm. Bull World Health Organ. 2003;81(12):858–66.
65. Sherman GG, Stevens G, Jones SA, Horsfield P, Stevens WS. Dried blood spots improve access to HIV diagnosis and care for infants in low-resource settings. J Acquir Immune Defic Syndr. 2005;38(5):615–7.
66. Rollins N, Mzolo S, Moodley T, Esterhuizen T, Van Rooyen H. Universal HIV testing of infants at immunization clinics: an acceptable and feasible approach for early infant diagnosis in high HIV prevalence settings. AIDS. 2009;23(14):1851–7.
67. UNICEF. Children and AIDS: innovations in HIV treatment, prevention and care. http://www.unicef.org/aids/index_51950.html
68. Violari A, Cotton MF, Gibb DM, Babiker AG, Steyn J, Madhi SA, Jean-Philippe P, McIntyre JA, CHER Study Team. Early antiretroviral therapy and mortality among HIV-infected infants. N Engl J Med. 2008;359:2233–44.
69. UNAIDS. Chapter 4: HIV treatment. 2010 Global Report. http://www.unaids.org/documents/20101123_GlobalReport_Chap4_em.pdf
70. Rochat TJ, Bland R, Coovadia H, Stein A, Newell ML. Towards a family-centered approach to HIV treatment and care for HIV-exposed children, their mothers and their families in poorly resourced settings. Future Virol. 2011;6(6):687–96.
71. Bain-Brickley D, Butler LM, Kennedy GE, Rutherford GW. Interventions to improve adherence to antiretroviral therapy in children with HIV infection. Cochrane Database Syst Rev. 2011;(12):CD009513.
72. Brown L, Macintyre K, Trujillo L. Interventions to reduce HIV/AIDS stigma: what have we learned? AIDS Educ Prev. 2003;15(1):49–69.
73. Bond V, Chase E, Aggelton P. Stigma, HIV/AIDS prevention, and mother-to-child transmission in Zambia. Eval Prog Plann. 2002;25:347–56.
74. Mahajan AP, Sayles JN, Patel VA, Remien RH, Sawires SR, Ortiz DJ, Szekeres G, Coates TJ. Stigma in the HIV/AIDS epidemic: a review of the literature and recommendations for the way forward. AIDS. 2008;22 Suppl 2:S67–79.
75. Heijnders M, Van Der Meij S. The fight against stigma: an overview of stigma reduction strategies and interventions. Psychol Health Med. 2006;11:353–63.
76. Ingraham N. Children and AIDS: Innovations in HIV treatment, prevention and care. UNICEF. November 30, 2009. http://www.unicef.org/aids/index_51950.html

Chapter 3
Addressing Micronutrient Malnutrition in Urban Settings

Laura A. Rowe and David M. Dodson

Introduction

There is increasing dialogue around the dichotomy that a world dominated by urban settings and urban populations can offer. On the one hand, cities provide increased opportunity to benefit from education and job opportunities, health and social services, and other consolidated and efficient delivery systems (i.e., if one can access them). For those who cannot access these benefits, the threats can be daunting: suboptimal environments, poor dietary options, and increased exposure and risk to infectious and chronic disease.

A 2010 global report published jointly by the World Health Organization (WHO) and the United Nations Human Settlements Programme (UN-HABITAT) offers four broad, overarching factors that can influence the health of the urban poor, including "food security and food quality" [1]. Access to nutritious foods for those living in poor urban settings is often more of a problem than the availability of these foods; there may be plenty of healthy options available, but they may be difficult to find or unaffordable.

This chapter describes a proven and effective strategy to impact food quality in urban settings through the implementation of national, mandatory food fortification programs. By leveraging what large sectors of the urban population already have access to and are already consuming on a regular basis, no new delivery mechanisms are needed, limited behavior change is required, and no additional responsibilities are placed on the healthcare system. A country can consistently reach large portions of its population, including many of the most vulnerable, with enough

L.A. Rowe, M.S., M.P.H. (✉) • D.M. Dodson, M.B.A.
Project Healthy Children, 125 Cambridge Park Drive, Suite 301,
Cambridge, MA 02140, USA
e-mail: lrowe@projecthealthychildren.org

© Springer New York 2015   41
R. Ahn et al. (eds.), *Innovating for Healthy Urbanization*,
DOI 10.1007/978-1-4899-7597-3_3

essential vitamins and minerals to positively and significantly impact nutritional status. This is exactly what food fortification aims to do.

Now more than ever, under the context of expanding urbanization in the developing world [2], we face the challenge of tackling growing rates of urban malnutrition and chronic disease. Both burdens have roots in a lack of essential vitamins and minerals. Food fortification has proven to be one of the most cost-effective interventions to address micronutrient malnutrition in the developing world—it is particularly relevant for the urban poor because of this population's high consumption of centrally processed foods [3], limited access to micronutrient-rich foods [4], disproportionately high burden of disease [1], and strong reliance on a consolidated food delivery system.

Based on Project Healthy Children's experience assisting governments to design and implement national food fortification programs, this chapter describes: (1) micronutrient malnutrition, particularly in the context of urban settings, (2) multiple interventions that exist to address this form of malnutrition, (3) why food fortification is a well-suited strategy for urban populations, (4) broad steps necessary to design a program, and (5) critical components needed to successfully implement a national food fortification program in urban settings, including lessons learned from past programs.

Background: Global Micronutrient Malnutrition

Micronutrient malnutrition, also referred to as "hidden hunger" due to the fact that it can exist without any clinical manifestations, occurs most commonly among populations that consume a low *quality* or unvaried diet, regardless of the amount of calories consumed. Such diets are often lacking in nutrient-rich foods (meat, eggs, fish, fruit, vegetable, legumes) and occur in settings where populations rely heavily on one or two low-cost but bulky staple foods, such as cereals, roots, and tubers containing few micronutrients [5]. It can also occur among those who rely heavily on poor-quality, highly processed foods [1], which is often the case in poor urban settings. Inadequate dietary intake can be compounded by the presence of dietary inhibitors (compounds such as phytic and oxalic acid and tannins found in certain foods) and health conditions such as intestinal parasites, malaria, diarrhea, acute respiratory tract infection, HIV, and obesity, inhibiting nutrient absorption. Evidence suggests that *over two billion* people worldwide suffer from this "hidden hunger" [6].

What is the impact? The WHO has identified iodine, iron, vitamin A, and zinc deficiencies as serious health risk factors [7] responsible for a significant portion of the global burden of disease and an enormous drain on national economies. Annually 1.1 million children under the age of five die due to vitamin A and zinc deficiencies, with vitamin A deficiency representing 6.5 % of the global child mortality burden [8]. Iron deficiency causes over 600,000 stillbirths and neonatal deaths every year and more than 100,000 maternal deaths during pregnancy [9]. Each year, 300,000 children are born with one of the most common and severe kinds of birth defects, known as neural tube defects (NTDs). NTDs result in an open spine (spina bifida), an open skull (encephalocele), or a lack of a brain (anencephaly), due to maternal folate deficiency [10]. Seventy five percent of these cases could be prevented with sufficient folate intake [10] at a cost of less than five cents per person per year [11].

Poor urban populations living in crowded and unsanitary living conditions where infections thrive are at a greater disadvantage than their rural counterparts. Dismal living conditions wreak havoc on the immune system, weakening its ability to ward off infection and increasing the risk of diarrhea, pneumonia, measles, and malnutrition [1]. Concentrated living conditions increase the chance of spreading airborne diseases to family members and the community, while the lack of latrines in confined urban settings increases the chance of spreading disease through human waste. This makes having an inadequate supply of micronutrients that much riskier—and an adequate supply that much more powerful in these settings.

If one survives the effects of micronutrient malnutrition, there are often lasting adverse impacts on education, productivity, and health [12]. The micronutrient health of a child has an enormous impact on that child's long-term cognitive ability. During the early stages of life in utero and up to 5 years of age, irreversible developmental delays can occur if proper micronutrients are not available. For example, although pregnant women require hardly a pinch of iodine a day (220 µg or 0.00022 g) [13], 18 million babies are born each year mentally impaired due to maternal iodine deficiency, which leads to a loss of up to 15 IQ points and an earning potential at least 20 % less than their healthy counterparts [12]. This outcome cannot be reversed in later years, since the small window of growth and development for the brain is missed and/or compromised. This undermines the impact of schooling and explains why children can attend classes year after year without progressing [14]. In light of this, it is worrisome that the development community (i.e., bilateral and multilateral aid commitments) spends roughly US$5.6 billion a year in aid-related education programs [15] when students may lack the ability to retain information or concentrate as a result of vitamin and mineral deficiencies.

The same needs hold true for vitamin A. Less than 1 mg of vitamin A per day is needed to maintain proper health [16], yet each year, 350,000 cases of childhood blindness occur, and countless diseases persist (as a result of vitamin A's impact on the immune system) due to insufficient intake [6]. It has been estimated that undernutrition (including micronutrient malnutrition) contributes to at least 53 % of deaths associated with infectious disease among children in the developing world [2]—a remarkable statistic, given the resources spent to battle and treat infectious diseases, when prevention could cut these deaths in half.

Early in life, undernutrition permanently changes or reprograms the body's structure, physiology, and metabolism [17]. This reprogramming alters biological mechanisms such as the distribution of blood flow; the production of insulin, growth hormones, and glucose tolerance; cholesterol metabolism and blood coagulation; fat tissue distribution; renal functioning; and vascular structure [18]. All of this increases the risk of developing noncommunicable diseases (NCDs) later in life, such as diabetes, cancer, and cardiovascular disease [18–20]. This is of particular concern in urban settings where obesity and NCD rates are increasing due to changes in diet and physical activity [21, 22]. In fact, overweight and obesity are no longer only problems of the developed world. As of 2005, the prevalence of overweight and obesity exceeded that of undernutrition in the majority of 37 different developing countries [17].

A vicious cycle emerges: the presence of disease increases the risk of micronutrient malnutrition by hindering absorption of key nutrients, just as undernutrition and vitamin and mineral deficiency increase the risk of infectious and chronic disease by preventing the proper functioning of the immune system and other critical metabolic processes. Individuals who lack essential nutrients in utero but are exposed to excess calories in childhood and adolescence (an increasingly common scenario given the demographic shift from rural to urban settings) risk an even greater threat of chronic disease [17, 23].

Finally, annual GDP losses attributable to micronutrient deficiencies are estimated to be 2–3 % for developing nations [24], equivalent to direct costs of US$20–30 billion [12]. However, this number excludes losses attributable to chronic disease [25].

Interventions to Address Micronutrient Malnutrition

Four main strategies to address micronutrient malnutrition have been endorsed by the WHO and the United Nations Food and Agriculture Organization (FAO) [5]: dietary diversity and nutrition education, supplementation, food fortification, and disease control measures. Most recently, biofortification has been introduced, but no global recommendations have yet been established.

Dietary Diversity/Nutrition Education

Dietary diversity and nutrition education initiatives encourage increasing the quantity and range of micronutrient-rich foods consumed through, for example, the creation of kitchen gardens, provision of seeds and/or fertilizer to households, and encouraging nutritious food selection and preparation [5, 16]. Improving dietary diversity allows many nutrients found naturally in foods to complement one another and assist in efficient absorption. Proper infant feeding is a critical component to nutrition education. Exclusive breastfeeding for the first 6 months of life and adequate complementary feeding after 6 months of age are vital during the formative years of a child's life. Proper infant and young child feeding will determine, to a large extent, the future health of that child and should be given concerted attention regardless of other micronutrient strategies developed.

However, the bioavailability of nutrients within particular diets should be considered. Populations consuming large amounts of tea, coffee, beans, and wheat products are at risk of not absorbing enough nutrients, due to naturally occurring substances found in these products that inhibit absorption of minerals, which increases the risk of deficiency. Similarly, iodine is obtained naturally from the soil or water from which food is grown. If a region's soil is deficient in iodine, so will any food that is grown in it, and there is little that can be done through the alteration of farming practices or consumption patterns to compensate for the poor iodine status of soils.

Dietary diversity and nutrition education are considered long-term approaches. The time it takes to change behavior, to increase accessibility and consumption of nutrient-rich foods, and to defend against potential outside factors that could derail its success (e.g., environmental conditions, such as drought, and economic situations, such as changes in individual household income because of illness and/or market price fluctuations, all of which can prevent the growing, purchase, and consumption of nutrient-rich foods) makes this a strategy that should be given focused attention *while* implementing other initiatives.

Supplementation

Supplementation is the periodic provision of relatively high amounts of a specific vitamin or mineral in the form of a capsule or pill. While in theory supplementation could be provided for an entire population, it has only been proven to be cost effective as an intervention targeting vulnerable populations, such as pregnant and postpartum women and young children. Supplements are often distributed during national child health days or national immunization days.

Although the health benefits of supplementation programs are usually rapid, success is contingent upon a number of factors: financial resources to procure the relatively expensive capsules; a means of distributing the tablets to the vulnerable population, usually through already established healthcare delivery systems (however, this excludes those who cannot or do not access to healthcare services); and individual compliance with supplement regimes, which is often a barrier, due to such side effects as gastrointestinal issues or perceived consequences of supplementation [5, 26] (e.g., intentions other than improving health status such as sterilization). Furthermore, since many pregnancies are unplanned, supplementation with iron and folic acid will not reach many adolescent girls and women at the time they need it most—preconception.

Supplementation is considered a short-term approach to addressing micronutrient deficiencies because of this intervention's quick impact but high expense—as much as ten times that of fortification in some settings (because of the labor-intensive nature of the program) [27, 28]. However, in many cases, there will always be groups, such as pregnant women, who need to consume more of a particular nutrient than can be provided by diet alone.

Food Fortification

Food fortification is the addition of one or more essential nutrients to food. These nutrients are added (whether or not the nutrients are normally contained in the food) during the production process in order to prevent or correct a demonstrated nutritional deficiency in the population or target group [29]. The goal is to choose centrally processed staple foods that are consumed in relatively consistent amounts throughout the year by the vast majority of the population, particularly the most vulnerable (e.g., women of childbearing age and children under 5 years of age).

Fortificants (vitamins and minerals) must be selected such that, when added to the food, they produce little to no organoleptic changes (i.e., in taste, smell, look, texture). Although this has been an obstacle in the past, technological advances have produced compounds that have successfully addressed these concerns. Since much of the implementation relies on the food industry's established delivery system, fortification has the potential to efficiently reach very large portions of the population.

Fortified foods, consumed on a regular and frequent basis, maintain body stores of nutrients more efficiently and effectively than occasional, high-dose supplementation [30]. Fortification also lowers the risk of multiple deficiencies due to the interconnectedness of multiple micronutrients added or already within the food. For example, a deficiency in vitamin A could cause a deficiency in iron because of the biological mechanisms that connect these nutrients[1] [13, 31, 32]. Additionally, fortified products are likely to contain levels of micronutrients that come close to levels that should be obtained from a regular, healthy diet [30].

Success of a fortification program, considered a longer-term approach, is contingent upon a number of factors: most notably which vehicle and type of fortificants are chosen, the ability of implementing partners to effectively coordinate the private and public sector, and the presence of a strong monitoring system. Although it takes longer to see immediate impacts, the sustainability of this strategy is often unrivaled. It will not, however, reach those living in remote rural areas or for other reasons that prevent the consumption of industrially processed food unless implemented at a small-scale level. Recent work by Project Healthy Children in the development of fortification at small-scale mills is currently being implemented and tested at scale in Tanzania.

---

[1] Vitamin A deficiency can cause iron deficiency due to vitamin A's role in mobilizing iron stores, increasing absorption, and turning stem cells into red blood cells, while iron deficiency may inhibit the effectiveness of iodine, since iron is needed in the first few steps of thyroid hormone synthesis.

Disease Control Measures

Many common diseases found in the developing world, such as diarrhea, measles, pneumonia, and malaria, decrease the body's ability to absorb and metabolize consumed micronutrients [33]. As a result, disease can indirectly cause micronutrient malnutrition. This leads to a downward spiral in an individual's health status as disease suppresses the immune system and reduces the ability to retain important stocks of micronutrients required by the body to fight off existing and future infection. Finally, disease suppresses appetite, further reducing micronutrient levels. Although disease control measures do not directly increase the intake of micronutrients, they do mitigate the effects of micronutrient malnutrition by improving absorption and usage rates by the body.

Disease control measures usually include deworming, immunizations, water and sanitation control, and control of diarrhea and acute respiratory infections. For example, the treatment of hookworm infection reduces iron loss, thereby complementing strategies to improve iron status [16]. Similarly, measles adversely affects vitamin A metabolism, interfering with how efficiently vitamin A is used and stored within the body [34, 35]. The presence of HIV can also have a significant impact on micronutrient status because of the body's decreased absorptive abilities when infected with this virus. Protein-energy malnutrition can impact vitamin A [36–38] status through several different mechanisms, one being the prevention of transport protein synthesis, which inhibits the use of the body's stored vitamin A. These are a few examples of how disease states and exposures can influence our body's ability to maintain optimal levels of micronutrients.

Biofortification

Biofortification is a strategy that breeds crops to increase their nutritional value. This can be done through conventional selective breeding (transgenic splicing) or genetic engineering [39]. Biofortification improves plant characteristics by altering the makeup of the plant's seed. This approach is advantageous, because it has the potential to reach those who cannot access the healthcare system or centrally processed foods. It has the potential to be extremely sustainable if the seed stock is saved and reused. However, the unknown consequences of changing environmental factors and genetic engineering, the question of farmer acceptance, and the fact that this strategy is still in initial stages of development leave biofortification as a potential solution for the future.

Pros and Cons of These Strategies

Successfully addressing micronutrient malnutrition depends largely on the right mix of tools chosen for a particular country setting and the right people and organizations identified to lead implementation [14, 16]. Each strategy targets a different subgroup of the population, some larger than others, and each will supply a different percentage of the needed nutrient gap that exists. In general, fortification and supplementation hold the most promise for urban settings, while biofortification and dietary diversity may prove to be the best strategies for rural populations. Implementers in each country should understand how different strategies complement and affect one another. For example, the successful implementation of a fortification program may eliminate the need for portions of the population to receive supplementation. In Nicaragua [40] and Guatemala [41], where the supply of vitamin A-fortified sugar complemented vitamin A supplementation for children under 36 months of age every 6 months, xerophthalmia was eliminated in Guatemala, and vitamin A deficiency in Nicaragua was drastically reduced. The fortification program in these two countries removed the need to provide vitamin A supplementation to older children and postpartum women [42] since their needs were met through the fortification program alone. Similarly, if direct micronutrient improvement strategies are implemented without attention to reducing disease, the impact on micronutrient status will be less than expected (Table 3.1).

Monitoring the impact of each strategy is important from a public health perspective to avoid supplying the population with unneeded nutrients, and from a monetary perspective, to avoid expenditures on overlapping programs that may no longer be needed.

Why Food Fortification Is Particularly Well Suited for Urban Settings

Food fortification programs come in many different forms [5]: targeted, market-driven, mass, and small-scale. Targeted programs involve the fortification of specific foods to benefit very specific portions of the population. Market-driven or voluntary programs involve manufacturers voluntarily deciding to fortify their product based on anticipated market demand. Mass fortification refers to the fortification of widely consumed foods by the general population and usually comes in the form of a mandatory program, as declared by the government. It is especially suited for urban populations. Small-scale fortification involves implementation at village level mills, allowing for those who do not consume centrally processed food to benefit. The bulk of this discussion will focus on mass fortification programs because of their proven impact and reach.

Food fortification programs implemented in urban settings stand out among other micronutrient-specific interventions for the following reasons: unparalleled reach [43] and need [1]; a reliance on a consolidated delivery system [30] that ensures access and eases monitoring; and proven impact.

Unparalleled reach and need. The goal of a fortification program is to reach the vast majority (≥80 %) of the population in any geographic area with that population's daily needs of essential vitamins and minerals [44]. This is done most effectively among populations that regularly consume similar centrally-processed foods

Table 3.1 Key micronutrients—sources, functions, and consequences of deficiency

Micronutrient	Food sources	Functions	Consequences of deficiency
Iodine	Seafood, dairy, navy beans, eggs, breast milk (affected by maternal status)	• The thyroid gland uses iodine to make thyroid hormones, which in turn directs brain development • Particularly essential in the developing fetus for proper brain development	• Annually, 18 million babies are born mentally impaired due to maternal iodine deficiency • Leading cause of preventable mental retardation • Decreases IQ by as much as 15 points
Iron	Red meats, poultry, seafood, eggs, legumes, tomato, dark green leafy vegetables (kale, collard greens, spinach, pumpkin leaves), nuts, breast milk (not affected by maternal status)	• Essential for hemoglobin and red blood cell production, oxygen transport, and immune function • Critical during childbirth and infancy	• 136,000 women and infants deaths / year • Leading cause of death in childbirth • 1.6 billion people suffer reduced productive capacity due to anemia • Impairs the mental development of 40–60 % of children in the developing world
Vitamin A	Cassava leaves, kale, collard greens, plantains, spinach, cabbage, liver, carrots, tomato, mango, squash, sweet potato, dairy, eggs, breast milk (affected by maternal status)	• Regulates immune system • Essential for vision, growth, and reproduction	• 1 million premature child deaths a year • Leading cause of preventable blindness among children • Compromises immune systems of 40–60 % of children under 5 in the developing world • Absence during critical periods of fetal development can lead to central nervous system defects
Zinc	Goat, beef, liver, shellfish, poultry, dairy, eggs, whole grains, peanuts, legumes, cabbage, spinach, breast milk (not affected by maternal status)	• Essential for immune function • Important in growth and repair of tissue	• 450,000 deaths of children under five a year • Addressing even mild cases in children can reduce incidence of diarrhea, which kills 9 million children a year, by 27 %, acute respiratory infection by 15 %, and child mortality by 6 % • Has been linked to rates of stunting and to anemia

(continued)

Table 3.1 (continued)

Micronutrient	Food sources	Functions	Consequences of deficiency
Folic acid (vitamin B9)	Liver, seafood, dairy, green leafy vegetables (spinach, okra), eggplant, cabbage, legumes, beans, lentils, nuts, breast milk (not affected by maternal status)	• Critical to the development of fetus and fetal DNA • Helps form red and white blood cells	• Due to maternal folate deficiency, 300,000 babies are born a year with severe birth defects • Associated with 1 in every 10 adults deaths from heart disease • Absence during critical periods of fetal development can lead to central nervous system defects

delivered through established delivery channels (a situation that mirrors urban settings). These populations' high consumption of centrally-processed food (due to low cost and accessibility) and limited consumption of micronutrient-rich foods (due to high cost and inaccessibility) make it possible to effectively deliver a needed public heath good to the majority of the urban population.

As populations move from rural to urban environments, there is a corresponding shift from traditional foods, such as native whole grains and cereals, to more refined, high-fat, and high-sugar foods low in essential nutrients. This is most often found in poor urban settings but can also be prevalent among the well-off (despite higher income levels). Inherent to urban lifestyles is a dependence on highly-refined foods because of limited access to natural sources of micronutrients [4]. As a result, the importance and reliance on industrially processed foods increase with urbanization [3]. This becomes all the more relevant in the wake of rising food prices. When financial crises hit, these low-nutrient, refined staple foods, for the most part, remain stable in the diet of the urban poor at the expense of dietary diversity and nonfood expenditures, such as health care and education [45]. In other words, when finances get tight, poor urban populations tend to maintain a consistent purchase and consumption of refined staple foods while reducing their intake of varied food, such as vegetables and meats. When compared to their rural counterparts, the urban poor often have lower health status [1] that is attributable to compromised immune systems (due to poor sanitation and contaminated water, crowded living, poor diet, and limited access to healthcare). Malnourished children in particular have poorly developed immune systems, making them more susceptible to diseases, such as diarrhea, pneumonia, malaria, and measles. This situation is exacerbated in poor urban settings, because children are presented with the challenge of starting life with a faltering immune system (being malnourished) in a setting that requires an exceptionally strong immune system for survival. When comparing rural and urban regions, the inequity in chronic malnutrition among poor urban children less than five years of age is particularly extreme throughout Africa [1]. Finally, it has been found that slum dwellers throughout the developing world have less access to health resources, more illness, and shorter life spans than those in any other segment of the population [1].

For urban-dwelling individuals who do not have access to centrally processed foods (estimated to be less than 20 % of the total) because of production preferences, cost, and/or location, small-scale fortification is becoming an increasingly viable option. Although the technology involved and the implementation required for small-scale fortification are in initial pilot phases, preliminary data [46, 47] suggest promising coverage and impact for rural, remote populations and, potentially (although there is no research on this to date), high-density urban slums. Urban slums fall geographically within urban areas, but, in some settings, these individuals may not access the same market channels as the rest of the urban population, presenting an unusual pairing of population concentration and consumption patterns more closely resembling those of their rural counterparts.

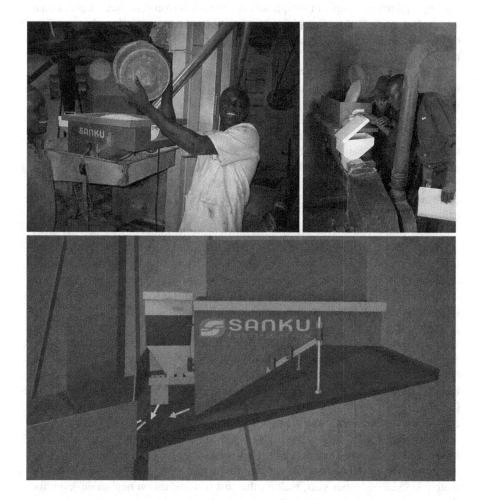

Small-scale fortification pilot project. Project Healthy Children. Tanzania 2013

Consolidated delivery system. Although urban settings tend to consolidate risk for disease, they also consolidate services and means of delivering those services. Fortification takes advantage of this consolidation; it is a public health intervention that, instead of working through traditional health sector channels, is adopted by and delivered through the private sector (i.e., food producers) using its delivery expertise [14]. By taking advantage of commodities urban inhabitants already access and improving the nutritional content of these commodities, the issue of access to affordable, nutritious foods is addressed. At the same time, this method allows the often overburdened healthcare system to be free from the responsibility of implementation. Few other interventions operate in this manner.

A consolidated delivery system also allows for efficient monitoring of fortified foods. Although most urban settings contain a number of markets where fortified foods may be sold, these markets are contained within a specific geographic area, making it relatively simple to sample and test the foods to ensure they meet national standards. Likewise, these samples can in most cases be traced back to the manufacturing source, since facilities are often located in urban settings where issues of noncompliance can be addressed in a timely manner.

Cost-effectiveness and proven impact. Food fortification programs have proven to be one of the most cost-effective [5, 48], and sustainable stand-alone interventions to impact global welfare [49] (not just health). In 2008, a group of economic experts came together—five of whom were Nobel laureates—to identify priorities that would address the ten greatest global challenges. The economists were asked the best ways of advancing global welfare, particularly that of developing countries, assuming an additional $75 billion of resources were available over a 4-year period [49]. At the end of their deliberations, guided heavily by consideration of economic costs and benefits, food fortification (salt iodization and flour fortification, specifically) ranked in the top three.

Taking into account lives saved, disabilities prevented, loss of productivity costs averted, and cost to implement and sustain the program over many years, fortification offers an extremely cost-effective strategy. Evidence indicates that the benefits of investing in fortification far outweigh the costs [48]. Horton and Ross [48] found the cost-to-benefit ratio of iron fortification to be 6:1 for effects on physical productivity (e.g., the benefits that adequate iron has on labor-intensive activities). This jumps to 36:1 when cognitive benefits are included, one of the greatest returns for any intervention. In other words, every dollar spent on fortification results in $6 or $36 in benefits to the economy. Salt iodization has a 30:1 [6] to 70:1 [48] cost-to-benefit ratio. This compares with vitamin A supplementation, which has a cost-to-benefit ratio of 8:1–17:1, and zinc supplementation, which has a ratio of 6:1–14:1 [6], and the annual cost per person ranges from US$1.00 to 2.60. The average annual cost per person for fortification can range from US$0.002 to 0.97, depending on the added nutrients and the chosen vehicle [11]. Fortification costs are either absorbed by the manufacturer or passed through to the consumer. To put this into perspective, the population at the bottom of the world's economic pyramid lives on approximately US$250–350 per year, making the cost of fortification negligible, even for the poorest populations.

Although annual cost-per-person estimates have not yet been generated for bio-fortification, quantifications have been estimated using Disability-Adjusted Life Years (DALYs). Cost-per-DALY-saved for biofortification ranges from US$10–120 [50], which is comparable to supplementation (US$9–250) [6, 48] and fortification (US$22–60) [48].

The Chilean flour fortification program provides a powerful example of fortification's cost-effectiveness. Implemented in 2000, it was found that Chile's mandatory wheat flour fortification with folic acid only needs to prevent two neural tube defects (estimated to cost $120,000 per child for care from birth to age eighteen) to recoup more than the annual cost of the nationwide flour fortification program (costing $0.15 per metric ton, or $175,000 per year, to fortify the entire country's ration of flour) [51].

Fortification programs have proven to have a remarkable impact on reducing micronutrient deficiencies in numerous locations across the world. Success can be defined in terms of the impact a program has on specific biomarkers, as outlined in the "impact" column in the table below. However, supplying an adequate amount of bioavailable nutrients to the identified target population (i.e., closing the nutrient gap to allow for sufficient additional intake of the needed micronutrients) is the true definition of a successful program and is what allows for "impact" to occur [3].

Country	National program	Impact
Guatemala [52]	• Sugar fortification with vitamin A began in 1975. The program became mandatory in 1998	• Vitamin A deficiency, measured by serum retinol levels, decreased from 22 to 5 % in 1 year
Chile [53, 54]	• In 2000, mandatory fortification of wheat flour with folic acid was introduced	• Within 1 year of the program, blood folate levels in women of reproductive age increased three to fourfold
		• The neural tube defects (NTDs) decreased by 40 %
Costa Rica [55]	• Mandatory fortification of wheat flour was introduced in 1997 and corn flour in 1999 with folic acid and other micronutrients	• After 2 years, an 87 and 63 % decrease was seen in folic acid deficiency in urban and rural areas, respectively, as measured by serum folate levels
		• Neural tube defects decreased by 74 %
South Africa [56]	• In 2003, mandatory fortification of maize and wheat flour with folic acid was introduced	• Overall neural tube defects decreased by 30 %; spina bifida, specifically, dropped 41.6 %
Tanzania [57]	• One of numerous successful salt iodization programs: In the early 1990s, Universal Salt Iodization (USI) was adopted in Tanzania	• By 2004, total goiter prevalence fell from 25 to 6.9 %
Canada [58, 59]	• In 1998, mandatory fortification of grain products with folic acid was introduced	• Four years later, the rate of neural tube defects decreased by 46 %

(continued)

Country	National program	Impact
China [55]	• An iron efficacy study: In 2007, iron was added to soy sauce. An efficacy trial was conducted among 14,000 men, women, and children	• All age and sex groups receiving iron as NaFeEDTA in soy sauce had significantly higher hemoglobin levels, lower prevalence of anemia, and higher ferritin levels than controls
United States [60]	• In 1998, the FDA introduced mandatory folic acid fortification of grain products	• Studies indicate at 19 % decrease in the number of births with neural tube defects since the introduction of mandatory folic acid fortification
		• The incidence of elevated total plasma homocysteine has also declined, a biomarker of folate deficiency and a risk factor for cardiovascular disease

What Is Needed to Design and Implement a National Fortification Program? Lessons Learned from PHC

The trajectory of a food fortification program is largely determined by how the program's design is approached. As a result, the process should be given considerable attention and analysis. The methodology offered in the next sections, based on extensive experience throughout much of Africa and parts of Central America, accomplishes two goals: it systematically identifies overarching areas that have proven inherent to fortification programs, and it presents an organizational structure for tackling these areas [14]. Overlooking components of this methodology may derail or delay the initiative, at the very least. In the worst case scenario, program sustainability and impact may be lost altogether.

First and foremost, to ensure sustainability, it is critical to secure political support and government buy-in. Once this has been attained (often through the signing of a memorandum of understanding between the implementing agency and the home ministry), design and implementation can begin.

With government buy-in in place, the process of designing and implementing a nationwide mandatory food fortification program involves three phases: *research*, *design*, and *implementation*. The research or data collection phase captures a clear and concise picture of what the health, nutrition, consumption, and political environments look like in addition to the domestic food production vs. imported food scenario. This step creates a blueprint to guide the program and includes foundational data on nutrition policy and legislation, food fortification standards, industry implementation, and government monitoring and social marketing [14]. The design phase utilizes the information gathered in the research phase to answer the question: what needs to be done based on what we know exists or does not exist within the specific focus areas? For example, which foods are most appropriate for fortification with what micronutrients and at what levels? Where should fortification as a strategy be included in existing national policies? What government bodies are responsible for monitoring and inspecting foods? The implementation phase ensures safe, effective fortified foods reach the target population through active industry engagement in a way that can be appropriately monitored, measured, and adjusted for as population needs change [14]. Broadly speaking, there are ten steps that need to be taken into consideration throughout the process:

Research and analysis
Step 1. Determine the population's micronutrient status and consumption patterns
Step 2. Map the flow of imports and domestic staple food production
Design and development
Step 3. Convene a national fortification alliance
Step 4. Draft fortification policy
Step 5. Draft and pass fortification regulation
Step 6. Draft and disseminate national fortification standards
Implementation
Step 7. Engage industry
Step 8. Create a monitoring system and train inspectors
Step 9. Promote consumer advocacy
Step 10. Design impact evaluations

Note: There is inherent crossover of many steps within the three different phases, and each step does not necessarily need to follow the order indicated above. This table is meant simply to serve as a guide to critical elements needing focused attention

Research and Analysis

Step 1: Determine the population's micronutrient status and consumption patterns. Obtaining up-to-date nationwide data on the prevalence of nutrient deficiencies and food consumption patterns is the first step in gaining an understanding of the population's nutritional needs and eating habits. This data will be used to draft country-specific fortification standards.

By isolating which vitamins and minerals the target population is deficient in, the appropriate nutrients to add to foods can be considered. Although populations in the same geographic region often present with similar micronutrient deficiencies (i.e., deficiencies in iron, vitamin A, or zinc), a one-size-fits-all approach is not recommended [4]. While harmonizing standards with neighboring countries is important, at this stage each country should be considered as a unique cohort in order to identify the nutrients the specific population needs. For example, due to the consumption of beans, chickpeas, and lentils in many sub-Saharan African countries, folate deficiencies may not be as persistent as they are perceived to be in this region. However, since folate deficiency is rarely measured, it is often added to fortified products without understanding whether there is a true need [42]. At the same time, it is important to understand the implicit interconnectedness that multiple micronutrients have with one another, as mentioned earlier (i.e., a deficiency in vitamin A can cause iron deficiency, while iron deficiency may inhibit the effectiveness of iodine) [13, 31, 32].

The status of micronutrient malnutrition in a country can often be obtained from already established nationwide studies that contain nutrition-specific information such as national Demographic and Health Surveys (DHS) or Multiple Indicator Cluster Surveys (MICS). Obtaining micronutrient deficiency data from these national studies is generally straightforward and simply involves obtaining the study results from the government and identifying the required data. When this information is unavailable or out of date, national micronutrient surveys should be conducted.

Although foods targeted for fortification depend on the specific setting, appropriate food vehicles generally include common staples such as maize and wheat flour, cooking oil, sugar, salt, bouillon cubes, soy sauce, and rice. However, taking a country-specific approach to determining consumption patterns is equally important. Consumption studies answer important questions that pertain to who consumes how much of what, and when. For example, do mothers eat more grams of flour per day than children? Is the coverage of sugar consumption higher among men than women? Is rice consumed throughout the year or only during a particular season? This data provides critical insights into which foods are best suited for fortification. It also allows for the drafting of fortification standards that consider those who consume the least and those who consume the most, guaranteeing safety while simultaneously ensuring impact.

Consumption and coverage data should be collected in a quick and cost-effective manner using, for example, a Food Fortification Rapid Assessment Tool (FRAT) or data derived from Household Income and Expenditure Surveys (HIES). The FRAT is designed specifically to obtain consumption information for fortification programs. It combines simplified 24-hour recall and food frequency questionnaires to delineate the consumption and usage patterns of potential fortification food vehicles [61]. It is designed to provide the minimum amount of information needed to set fortification standards.

Consumption information obtained from Household Income and Expenditure Surveys (HIES) is considered to be "implied consumption" data, since the amount consumed per person is calculated based on the amount of food purchased. Alternately, it is sometimes possible to piggyback on other national food security or market surveys to infer or directly obtain consumption information. This was the case in Liberia for PHC, where fortification-specific consumption questions were included in WFP's Comprehensive Food Security and Nutrition Survey to obtain up-to-date information in an extremely cost-effective manner, since it took advantage of a tool that was already being deployed.

There are five factors taken into consideration when identifying the best staple foods for fortification to ensure food reaches the greatest number of people in the target population:

Coverage: The food should be consumed by a large proportion of the population and be eaten in most or all geographic regions of the country.

Consumption: The amount consumed should be relatively constant, regardless of location or season, making it possible to supply roughly the same amount of micronutrients to all consumers.

Cost: The selected food should be inexpensive, to ensure even the least well-off have proper access to fortified foods.

Central Processing: Ideally, the food should be processed in a relatively small number of large facilities to facilitate monitoring and ensure consistent implementation.

Compatibility: The addition of micronutrients should cause no discernible change in taste, appearance, or coloring of the food, and there should be minimal loss of micronutrients during typical processing or cooking of the food.

Consumption surveys also provide vital information on regional differences, storage conditions, and procurement patterns of staple products. They answer questions such as: Do individuals in rural areas purchase their maize flour, or is it grown and/or processed at home or in the village? Are consumption and coverage patterns different in rural vs. urban areas? How are staple products stored within households? This information is vital to shaping the design and implementation of a program that will have a measurable impact. For example, in Malawi, after working with the government to conduct a FRAT survey, PHC found that although *nsima* (maize porridge) is a mainstay of the Malawian diet (regardless of urban or rural setting or individual economic status), only a fraction of the population consumes *centrally processed* maize flour (instead, maize is grown and processed at home or at small rural mills). As a result, although consumption and coverage were found to be high, it proved to be an inappropriate vehicle for mass fortification.

Storage patterns of staple products within a household are important to consider because of the instability of many micronutrients when exposed to heat, light, and/or moisture. If cooking oil, for example, is routinely sold or stored in clear containers, the amount of added vitamin A will need to be considered when formulating standards because of the potential degradation of that vitamin A once it is exposed to light. In other cases, altering the packaging used by manufacturers and/or distributors may be necessary to protect the vitamin A from these exposures.

Finally, it is important to consider any consumption variation that may exist between rural and urban regions. For example, in Uganda, the consumption of wheat flour was found to be significantly higher in urban areas than in rural areas. This urban subset was also found to be mildly deficient in B vitamins because of a lack of natural B vitamin sources and a high consumption of micronutrient-poor products (despite higher levels of wealth) [4]. This data provided important insights into which vehicles and which micronutrients should be targeted to address the needs of this urban population.

These examples highlight the foundational nature of this initial data collection for the design and efficacy of the program. If there are significant errors in this information, an impractical vehicle may be chosen for fortification—or an inappropriate amount of fortificant may be added to the food.

Step 2. Map the flow of imports and domestic staple food production. Imported foods subject to fortification will be held to the same national fortification standards as domestic producers. Initially the food flows should be mapped to identify where domestic production is taking place, what staple products are imported, from where, and to what level. One must understand the extent to which imported products may already be fortified and then determine whether the standards aspired to are close enough to the existing level of imports. In general, to the extent fortification standards can be harmonized with existing neighboring standards, the better (even if it requires some adjustment to the ideal, national standard).

Setting the stage to engage with these players is vital to ensure clear communication channels are established around regulatory expectations; required testing, monitoring, and labeling; technical and/or financial assistance needed to scale up production (predominately for domestic producers); and timing of implementation.

Design and Development

Step 3. Convene a national fortification alliance. Getting the right people around the same table and communicating on a consistent basis represent some of the biggest programmatic challenges for fortification initiatives. Due to the multi-sector nature of this strategy, a guiding body that meets on a regular basis and involves all partners and players is essential to ensure communication channels are established, activities are harmonized, and roadblocks addressed. This is a particularly important step, since the individuals and agencies involved in fortification have likely never had to coordinate or communicate with each other before; a national alliance (often referred to as a National Fortification Alliance, or NFA) provides this common platform. The leadership or chairmanship that is elected to guide this alliance is equally important. Without an individual to motivate and mobilize the multiple parties involved, and without the ability to maintain focus and ensure action from a group where consensus is often difficult to attain, the success of the program will be in jeopardy. Such national alliances are oftentimes the single factor that allows programs to overcome otherwise intractable issues. More attention will be given to this important component in the following sections.

Step 4. Draft fortification policy. Food fortification as a strategy should be written into national health and nutrition policies and harmonized with other ongoing nutrition interventions. As already discussed, fortification is only one means of addressing micronutrient malnutrition. Most countries use multiple approaches to fight this battle. As a result, fortification should be incorporated as a complementary approach to existing measures, such as supplementation, dietary diversification, disease control, and biofortification.

A fortification strategy is often included in national micronutrient strategies or imbedded in more comprehensive national nutrition action plans. This inclusion in national policy is important to ensure the program sustains itself through political or economic changes [62] while enabling future program alterations, as population needs change over time. For example, it may be deemed unnecessary to continue supplementation to specific demographic groups receiving both fortification and supplementation interventions because of potential overlap in less vulnerable groups. In light of available impact results, both programs should be reviewed and altered as necessary to avoid redundant programming. Regardless of where fortification is included in national policy, it is critical to ensure it is drafted in a way that describes specifically what must be done to implement, to monitor, and to adjust the program over time. In other words, the strategy must be "actionable."

Step 5. Draft and pass fortification regulation. Mandatory programs ensure a fair market for producers and guarantee the maximum coverage of fortified foods. Each country is likely to require its own unique legal or regulatory path, given the powers vested with various branches of the government (e.g., Ministry of Health vs. Ministry of Trade), existing laws or standards that may already be in place governing food safety standards (e.g., Bureau of Standards regulations, laws currently enforced, executive decrees), and the structure of the government. For example, in Rwanda, PHC initially believed legislation needed to be passed for mandatory fortification, and considerable time and effort were expended lobbying for such legislation within the two elected chambers. However, PHC eventually came to realize that a "ministerial decree," signed by the President, was a more streamlined approach to passing food safety and security laws. In the case of Honduras, PHC found existing laws in effect that had to be changed or repealed before a more efficient regulatory structure could be put in place. Since food fortification is often a new concept within a country, the right answer may not be obvious to the governmental constituents or, in other cases, may first need to be "invented."

Equally important, incorporating a framework that allows food standards to be amended in a relatively straightforward manner will prove useful if and when future needs require changes to the law (such as was the case in Honduras). The identification of an in-country champion to advocate for fortification has assisted numerous past and current programs through what can often be a long, bureaucratic process to get legislation/regulation written, approved, and passed. This champion will also prove to be useful for moving other stalled works streams forward.

Understanding what is required to put in place the best legal framework will vary from country to country and may not be readily apparent. This step is often the most time-consuming and therefore requires patience and effort to carefully navigate the country's legal system; doing so allows for identification of the most enduring (and efficient) method of promulgating and enforcing mandatory food fortification.

Step 6. Draft and disseminate national fortification standards. Key stakeholders will be needed in order to draft national standards for the staple foods to be fortified. These standards will determine which micronutrients should be included and at what levels, by using the up-to-date deficiency and consumption data collected. By matching country-specific needs and intake, the levels should ensure the fortified food is safe for all (taking into account those who consume the most) and effective in improving health (taking into account those who consume the least).

The most appropriate forms of fortificants (i.e., nutrients) should also be decided on in the standards creation process. Chosen fortificants should be of the highest quality, taking into consideration cost and bioavailability of both the fortificant form and the population's diet [3]. In some cases, the most bioavailable fortificant may also be the most expensive. In these cases, it will be necessary to weigh the pros and cons of best price vs. most bioavailable. For example, sodium iron ethylenediamine-tetraacetic acid (NaFeEDTA) is the most bioavailable form of iron to use in fortification, since it is unaffected by dietary inhibitors present in the diet; it also tends to be the most expensive. However, other factors will need to be considered. Since NaFeEDTA is so bioavailable, lower amounts of it are required to meet established standards when compared to less bioavailable forms, such as ferrous sulfate or fumarate. This is particularly true for diets high in dietary inhibitors that render iron unavailable to the body. As a result, the type of diet the target population consumes should be considered in light of the fortificant forms chosen.

Drafted standards should then be harmonized with regional standards in order to preclude any barriers to trade. In some cases, standards will need to be approved or ratified by regional bodies before they are endorsed nationally, as was the case in Rwanda, where country-specific standards had to be presented and approved by the East Africa Community (EAC) before they were officially endorsed by the country. Mapping the process for standards approval will be useful for facilitating movement. Once appropriate authorities have approved the standards, the country's identified authority on food inspections should disseminate copies of the standards to each domestic producer and importer, where appropriate. The standards should include a grace period, whereby industry will be given a specified window of time to scale up their facilities before they are held to consequences of noncompliance. In many cases, this will include communicating to industry the necessary steps required to apply for a national fortification logo (indicating that their product is fortified to the national standard and approved by food-inspecting authorities, and communicating to the public that the product contains healthy micronutrients).

Implementation

Step 7. Engage industry. While fortifying staple foods may be well understood by some facilities, the process may be new to certain sectors of the food industry. As a result, the private sector should be guided through the process of procuring, financing, and incorporating the necessary equipment and vitamin and mineral premix into their production lines (and through the process of establishing a strong quality assurance and quality control system). Industry should be given technical assistance on how to ensure equipment is dispensing the appropriate amount of premix during the fortification process, how to test the final product for compliance to standards, when to send samples out for quantitative testing, and what to expect from national regulatory bodies required to take samples for external validation.

In the case of Rwanda, PHC was able to introduce food processors to the Global Alliance for Improved Nutrition's (GAIN) Global Premix Facility, where they were given expert advice on the best places to source affordable, quality premix and equipment. Smaller industries concerned about the initial capital needed to purchase equipment and premix were connected with organizations that assisted them in securing loans for up-front costs.

Step 8. Create a monitoring system and train inspectors. The appropriate government agencies should establish a national monitoring system that ensures samples are collected and analyzed from domestic production sites, importation sites, markets, and households on a regular basis. Food inspectors should be trained on how and when to collect samples, how to test fortified products, and how to deal with issues of noncompliance. They should ensure fortification labeling is clear and accurate. It is important that the fortification level, which food inspectors should be testing, and which differs, depending on the location (i.e., domestic facilities, border sites, markets, and households), is clearly defined.

Data should be consolidated so that reports can be generated and performance can be reviewed on a periodic basis. In Malawi, PHC created a comprehensive national monitoring tool that consistently pools monitoring data (by brand) from domestic facilities, border sites, and markets. This tool allows reports to be quickly generated in order to observe where levels may be failing and to ensure action is taken in a timely manner. Pooling collected data on fortified products also elucidates any discrepancies that may exist among agencies that are collecting the same information. For example, in one particular country setting, data collected on the percentage of imported iodized salt at the border was found to differ significantly, depending on whether the data came from the Revenue Authority or the Bureau of Standards.

Step 9. Promote consumer advocacy. Consumer advocacy helps consumers understand the benefits of the fortified foods they are buying and assists industry in increasing consumer demand for its new product. It is generally the government's responsibility under mandatory fortification programs to communicate the health benefits of fortified foods to the public. This social marketing is usually included in Ministry of Health and/or Consumer Association public health messaging and can include radio spots, TV advertisements, billboards, and the engagement of community leaders. A fortification logo, along with guidelines on its use and application, is often designed or adopted from the region to designate the new products as "fortified."

Without a communication strategy in place, products risk customers not understanding the benefits of the new ingredients and/or consumer speculation and fear of fortified products on the market. It is equally important that health campaigns do not advocate or encourage increasing the consumption of fortification vehicles, because consumption levels of these foods (i.e., salt, oil, sugar, and refined flours) are often already too high, particularly in urban areas [3], and can contribute to the development of chronic diseases, such as obesity and cardiovascular disease. However, to date, this has not been an issue with fortified foods.

Step 10. Design impact evaluations. Finally, after monitoring has ensured fortified products have reached ≥80 % coverage, impact evaluations should be conducted to measure change in micronutrient status. Consumption of the fortified food, however, should not be a proxy measure for program success. The identification of appropriate measurement indicators is vital, as is making sure that the initial pre-fortification data was collected in a way that allows for comparison. Appropriate measurement indicators should be based on the proportion of the nutrient gap that is being filled by the fortified products and the percent of each age and demographic group's daily needs (Estimated Average Requirement (EAR) or Recommended Nutrient Intake or (RNI)) that the fortified foods aim to meet [42].

Overarching Components Necessary for Success

Due to fortification's extraordinary low cost and sustainability, the "bang for your buck" that national, mandatory programs offer is unrivaled. Moreover, the inherent structure of the program makes for a natural fit within poor urban settings. Yet despite decades of widespread success in many parts of the world and unparalleled cost-effectiveness and sustainability, fortification programs are often missing from national agendas for the same reasons that they are so successful—namely, the need for:

1. Interagency coordination within the government
2. Strong in-country leadership
3. Government and private sector coordination and commitment
4. A robust monitoring and surveillance system [14]

Although these components were introduced in the ten-step fortification process described above, they warrant greater attention, because they are so often overlooked throughout the design and implementation. The key to success lies in knowing how to orchestrate and balance the multiple players and initial demands required to solidify these elements as effective program components.

Strong interagency coordination and the identification of in-country leadership. The very nature of a fortification program requires that individuals and agencies that do not normally communicate and collaborate work together to chart and agree upon a course for fortification. This is often a challenge, in and of itself. In the beginning, a "home" agency is typically identified within which the program is housed, usually the Ministry of Health. This home ministry must work to collaborate with numerous other ministries, including (but not limited to) the Ministry of Trade and Commerce, the Bureau of Standards, the Ministry of Justice, the Ministry of Agriculture, the Ministry of Finance, the Revenue Authority, and the Legislative Branch. In addition to these governmental agencies, consumer associations and importers of staple foods must be involved throughout the process. Constituents outside of government must be active contributors. This often includes UN agencies and international nongovernmental organizations (INGOs), such as the United Nations Children's Fund (UNICEF), World Food Programme (WFP), WHO, FAO, and the World Bank. Finally, there is the private sector, which requires an untraditional collaboration between businesses that likely never before had to deal with the realm of public health interventions, government ministries, or INGOs and UN agencies. Ensuring these multiple players are willing to communicate across disciplinary boundaries while speaking a common language is essential.

One means of accomplishing this coordination is through the creation of a NFA. This mechanism brings together all parties involved in fortification—from the very initial design stages to the final evaluation stages—on a regular basis to ensure coordination and harmonization of fortification-related activities. This is arguably one of the most valuable components of a fortification program, since such a convening body provides, in many cases, the only common touch point these actors will have with one another.

The leadership and funding of this convening body is a critical matter not to be overlooked. Guiding the national alliance should be an individual from a ministry or local agency or institution that possesses an unwavering ability to convene, lead, and ensure action. The individual that is identified is often more important than the agency to which the individual belongs. The importance of this leadership cannot be underestimated; programs have thrived and faltered based on the presence (or lack) of this leadership.

Inevitably there will be monetary resources needed to hold regular meetings. Although the level of funding will vary depending on the country setting (some countries will require substantial funding for customary meeting per diems, while other programs will simply require funding for logistics, such as food, tea, or meeting space), the source or multiple revolving sources should be identified and agreed upon immediately after an alliance is created. A lack of an identified funding mechanism has derailed projects and caused implementation to be delayed for years.

Government commitment to a mandatory program. The importance of government commitment to fortification through its inclusion in national strategies and through the creation of consumer advocacy campaigns has already been covered in this chapter. Less attention, however, has been given to fortification as a mandatory program.

Since it is the industry's responsibility to make the necessary production line changes to incorporate fortification and purchase the vitamin and mineral premix, all of which have an impact on the product's cost structure, a mandatory program is important for industry compliance and to ensure a level playing field for all producers. A level playing field prevents potential price differences across different brands that could disincentivize facilities from producing—or consumers from purchasing—the fortified product. In fact, it is often industry that pushes for mandatory programs to preclude any barriers within the market. Such a program ensures imported- and domestically-produced commodities comply with established fortification standards, enables consistent monitoring, and sends clear signals to trade partners [14].

As new staple food production facilities come online, a mandatory program ensures expectations to fortify are established, standards and guidelines for monitoring are in place, and the mechanisms for ordering vitamin and mineral premix are well defined. With multiple facilities requiring premix, the purchase price for industry may be more economical than if only a few facilities were ordering, because of options available for bulk purchasing. Finally, in some cases, opportunities exist to procure low-interest rate loans for equipment in conjunction with premix purchasing.

Although there are some food manufacturers willing to voluntarily fortify, due to a perceived market advantage or a desire to influence the health of the community, such an approach is generally not sustainable (as it depends upon the goodwill of a given food processor) and creates inconsistent coverage, with some producers fortifying and others not fortifying. As a result, the impact on micronutrient status can be compromised.

Although mandatory programs have proven to be the most sustainable form of fortification programming, what happens when the implementation of a mandatory program is met with resistance? The limitations of voluntary programs have already been outlined; inconsistent coverage and limited industry participation reduce the impact of these programs. In light of this, and despite the fact that such an idea has not been attempted to date, it is worth considering the implications of a program based on market incentives. By providing an incentive, such as a tax break, producers may be encouraged (and enticed) to begin fortification. The goal would be to make sure that the incentive is enough to guarantee that fortified products maintain the same price as their unfortified counterparts (in effect, making it undesirable *not* to fortify), in conjunction with strong consumer advocacy. Despite the fact that this approach necessitates a very different cost structure (i.e., the need to fund the incentive), which by nature may limit the sustainability of the program, it may offer a viable alternative to voluntary programs. Required costs could be shared between government and private donors, industry, and/or UN agencies, depending on the specific situation.

Regardless of the type of program—whether mandatory, voluntary, or some new form of a market incentive approach—government should consistently lead the process, all fortifying facilities should be held to established national regulatory standards, and a strong governmental monitoring system should be put in place to make sure the program is safe and effective.

Reliance on a committed private sector. Cooperation from the private sector, as fortification's sole mode of delivery, is an essential programmatic linchpin. It is imperative that industry is involved in the initial planning stages, for the following reasons: so they understand the program's importance, why it is a government priority, the vital role they will play, and what expectations they will be held to. Since industry, in most cases, will be expected to pick up fortification costs on their own, it is important that industry understands all implications of the program. Hearing industry-specific concerns and receiving feedback is vital to preventing later obstacles. The role of government in the social marketing of fortified products and the subsequent increase in demand that will presumably result should be clearly communicated to industry players.

A committed private sector is particularly relevant when there are delays in passing fortification regulation. Industries are often willing to retrofit their facilities and begin production before legislation is passed if they know it will be mandatory in the near future (and if they know consumer education is taking place). This is desirable and should be encouraged, because the legislative process is often slow and bureaucratic; this also assumes that standards have been drafted and monitoring systems have been established. Delays in approving regulation have, in the past, delayed programs by years.

Obtaining a market advantage is another benefit to early industry initiation, assuming government has begun advocacy campaigns to educate consumers about the benefits of fortification. In an ideal situation, once one industry succeeds in getting a fortified product on the market, others will want to follow to ensure they don't lose their customer base. Without appropriate advocacy, however, there is a chance that just the opposite will happen—customers see a product different from their normal purchase, or one with a slight price difference, and they will not fully grasp the health benefits of it (they might even have fears that the added fortificant will do harm). As a result, they turn to other, nonfortified products to purchase. This scenario presents a good case for why mandatory programs with social marketing components, both from the public and private sector, are beneficial. Ministries of Trade and/or Commerce should conduct industry-specific advocacy to encourage the value-added aspect of the initiative, particularly when the regional market is saturated with fortified products.

Robust monitoring and evaluation system. A robust monitoring and evaluation system is the true test of a successful program. All initial structures may be in place, policy may be adopted, regulation may be established, and premix may be bought and used, but if the final product does not meet the established fortification standards, if the nutrients are not available to the target population, or if there is no way to monitor compliance, the program will not have the anticipated nutritional impact.

Internal monitoring. Robust monitoring must first take place at the industry level, within staple food production facilities. Industry must establish quality assurance and quality control measures for the premix being added and the final fortified product. Staff should routinely sample and test to ensure compliance. In short, this process generally includes ensuring the following: premix is appropriately stored and always available within the facility (i.e., away from light, moisture, and heat); premix is properly added to the flour and discharged in accordance with the flow of the food being fortified; the ratio of product produced to premix used is close to the theoretical ratio calculated; frequent qualitative testing (every 2–4 hours for large mills) occurs; composite samples are created every hour for daily qualitative testing; and external quantitative testing of these composite samples takes place on a monthly or quarterly basis, depending on the size of mill [63–65].

External monitoring. At the same time, the government's regulatory agencies must monitor and enforce compliance. This is often the weakest component of a program and should be given focused attention. National monitoring bodies should outline a clear plan with specific training for appropriate inspectors on how to sample and test fortified products. Government food inspectors should make routine visits to facilities to review industry's internal test results, conduct their own on-site qualitative analyses, and obtain samples to be tested quantitatively at an external facility. For facilities just beginning fortification, external inspections should occur each month. For more established facilities, external inspections should occur at least three times a year [64]. Results should be communicated back to industry management in a timely manner (and appropriate enforcement steps taken) if samples or procedures indicate noncompliance.

Government inspectors are also responsible for collecting samples of fortified products at importation sites, in market places, and in households. Establishing the appropriate range of levels that should be detected in fortified products at each location must be communicated to inspectors. The level of addition required in the factory will be different from that required within households because of overage included at the production level to account for natural and expected nutrient degradation that occurs by the time the product reaches the household [42]. If this communication of required testing levels does not take place, the monitoring exercise will be of little use to the program and a waste of time and money for the government.

This interim monitoring is critical to any program. Results ensure inspectors are inspecting and provide further insight into whether the correct amounts of nutrients are being added, whether a better chemical form of the nutrient should be used, or if particular brands are consistently noncompliant. Monitoring allows managers to correct program shortcomings *before* long-term surveillance or impact studies occur. It saves time, money, valuable resources, and lives. Imagine, if in 3–5 years, an impact study is conducted, and results indicate fortified products had no impact on rates of iron or vitamin A deficiency because of a miscalculation in the nutrient lost during transport. This simple error could have been caught if products had been consistently tested and monitored prior to the impact study.

Only after industry and government monitoring have established consistent coverage and compliance should an evaluation or surveillance system be put in place to evaluate the change in micronutrient status or other identified outcomes or indicators in the target population. Coverage should be a sustained ≥80 % for at least 1 year in order to detect an initial effect; however, the program should be continued indefinitely in order to maximize impact [44].

Identifying the appropriate impact indicator is critical to defining success. The choice of indicator should be dictated by: (a) the percent of the Estimated Average Requirement (EAR) that the program provides to different gender, age, and physiological groups; and (b) other confounding factors that may be present, such as infection, inflammation, or seasonality [42]. For example, according to Dary, the additional intake of 60 % EAR of iron is necessary to detect changes in secondary indicators (such as serum ferritin, which depends on metabolic conditions), whereas an intake of 90 % EAR of iron is necessary to detect changes in tertiary indicators (such as anemia) [66]. If these factors are not considered together, inappropriate indicators may be chosen that deem the program a failure, when in fact the wrong indicator was used to measure impact.

Learning from Past Programs

Finally, success requires a thorough understanding of why current and past programs have thrived or faltered. Despite the fact that fortification has been a powerful force in addressing vitamin and mineral deficiencies around the world since the

1920s, there have been programs that have been less than successful and that have faltered due to missteps and oversights. Understanding why is critical.

Malawi's National Fortification Alliance. In the early 2000s, Malawi's government implemented a national food fortification program. This program soon began to falter, due largely to a lack of strong leadership required to guide the country's NFA, in addition to a lack of a sustainable funding strategy for the alliance. Project Healthy Children's engagement in Malawi began as a result of the government's desire to reinvigorate the NFA to enable it to move the program forward. Restructuring the NFA, which included enhanced coordination and communication among players and the identification of strong leadership to guide activities and address identified roadblocks, largely changed the direction of the program. Shortly after reinvigorating the alliance, Malawi's sole sugar manufacturer began producing fortified sugar, and the country's cooking oil, wheat, and maize flour facilities were only months away from achieving the same. Although Malawi's fortification progress cannot be attributed solely to the revitalization of the national alliance, it was a powerful contributor to overcoming obstacles and engaging other players that worked to facilitate progress, all of which allowed the program to achieve new heights.

The role of government in Zambia's sugar fortification program. In 1998, with encouragement from the government, Zambia's largest domestic sugar producer began fortifying sugar with vitamin A. With an influx of less expensive sugar already on the market, Zambia's sugar producer was encouraged by the fact that the government was willing to enact legislation that would ensure only fortified sugar was sold. However, fortification legislation in Zambia was delayed for months, and once enacted, there was inadequate regulation to monitor fortification, because of weak customs enforcement and little support for advertising and education from the government. As a result, significant amounts of lower-cost, smuggled sugar eroded the market, jeopardizing the profitability of Zambia's sugar producer. Although Zambia's Fortification Task Force (its equivalent of a national alliance) aided in resolving many of these issues [67], the influx of cheap, unfortified sugar came close to derailing the country's fortification program. This serves as an excellent example of the importance of government involvement in the creation of a mandatory program and the establishment of strong, consistent enforcement and monitoring. Without a level playing field and common ground rules, it becomes exceedingly difficult for industry to comply with established standards without adversely affecting the bottom line.

Rwanda's early industry engagement. In 2007, Rwanda's government adopted a national food fortification program. However, passing fortification regulation (which, in the case of Rwanda, is in the form of a Ministerial Decree) is, as of February 2013, still pending final approval. This has prevented most industries from taking up fortification, even though all other systems are in place. Without a mandatory program, a level playing field cannot be guaranteed.

Despite this situation, Rwanda's largest maize flour producer began to voluntarily fortify a portion of their product, based on market demand from schools and the WFP. Although it is too early to tell, this early industry engagement, if coupled with strong consumer advocacy from the Ministry of Health or the Consumer's Association, could be enough to usher other industries into fortifying their products before regulation is passed (in order to compete with a more desirable product on the market).

Measuring impact in Zambia. When it came time to measure the impact of Zambia's sugar fortification program, serum retinol was used as the biomarker of choice. However, results indicated no change in serum retinol measurements before and after sugar fortification. The program was, therefore, deemed unsuccessful. What was not considered, however, were the high rates of infection present in the target population, which impacts the release of serum retinol binding protein from the liver and the absorption of vitamin A [42, 68]. As a result, serum retinol should not have been the indicator of choice to measure the impact of the program. Instead, retinol in breast milk or a proxy indicator (such as reduced mortality) should have been used to measure change in nutrient status [42]. Because of a poor choice in outcome indicators, the program risked losing government support.

Choice of fortificant as a recurring problem. After evaluating wheat flour iron fortification programs in 78 different countries, Hurrell et al. concluded that only nine of the 78 programs reviewed were likely to have a significant positive impact on iron status because of the low bioavailability or nonrecommended form of iron that was used throughout the programs [69]. This is a critical point to understand, because numerous programs have repeated this mistake over and over again. If the bioavailability of the diet and/or the fortificant form used are not carefully considered, changes in nutritional status will be limited. This can lead to "failed" programs, when in fact the misstep was simply in the choice of the fortificant.

The two situations above are two examples that point to the growing importance of reviewing all components of the program when outcomes are not as expected: was bioavailability of the nutrient taken into consideration, was increased intake of the nutrient measured, was the right vehicle chosen in regard to reach and coverage, was the correct biomarker to measure impact chosen, and was the correct level used to measure the nutrient concentration of food at the industry vs. household level? Of course, it is better to address these issues before outcomes are actually measured, but these components are often overlooked and frequently lead to disappointing results in the final phases of the program.

Nevertheless, as is the case in any post-implementation study, it is important to recognize that the survey, at best, can only be indicative of what might be occurring as a result of fortification. Absent a control group, placebos, and other standard testing tools, there is no way to positively attribute an improvement in micronutrient status, or lack thereof, to the food fortification program. For example, improvements or deteriorations in diet caused by economic fluctuations or location (urban vs. rural), and the reduction or increase in disease as a result of improvements in sanitation or outbreaks of disease, may all play a role in influencing study outcomes. As a result, these factors should be carefully observed (and controlled for) to the extent possible in order to obtain a clear understanding of what programmatic components may be working—and what needs improvement.

Conclusion

Over the next 25 years, it is estimated that most of the world's growth will be in urban populations of low- and middle-income countries throughout Africa and Asia [21]. It is within these poor urban settings that macronutrient and micronutrient malnutrition is on the rise, and where infection rates are disproportionately high [1]; where industrially processed foods have an increasing role; and where native whole grains and other micronutrient-rich foods are being replaced with refined flours, sugar, and oil [4]. By 2030, NCDs will cause over three quarters of all deaths worldwide [17], of which micronutrient deficiencies will be an inextricable component.

This situation provides a set of conditions that could arguably create a perfect storm for increasing rates of disease and malnutrition, and points to the importance of maintaining a strong focus on identifying flexible, creative, and cost-effective strategies targeted at the urban sector to prevent what may be an ever-growing number of vitamin and mineral-deficient global citizens. The inherent need among the urban poor cannot be argued.

At the same time, there exists an opportunity to reach these individuals through existing delivery channels and through commodities they are already consuming. By taking advantage of what already exists, micronutrient-rich foods can be delivered to over 80 % of the population, which has powerful implications for individual lives: immune systems could be bolstered enough to ensure the body can successfully face challenges posed by urban settings; infections, such as pneumonia, measles, and diarrhea, could be prevented; and the billions of dollars spent on education may translate into knowledge that is retained and usable. Individual country economies could save, on average, over $30 billion a year.

Food fortification programs (which are some of the most uniquely designed interventions that exist today to address micronutrient deficiencies) have proven to fit the bill for improving the quality of food and, consequently, the health of the urban poor, in places where the need is high and the delivery system is already in place. One might believe that fortification programs are actually designed with the urban poor specifically in mind. However, this can only happen if countries are willing to put the time and effort into their careful design and implementation, managing and leading them, and sustaining them over time.

With multiple actors involved, and with competing demands and incentives at play, maintaining focus and patience throughout the process is vital. This becomes even more important with the inevitably sensitive issues that arise from dealing with the private sector's bottom line, a persistent and critical public health issue, and a nation's food supply. As a result, upholding a broad perspective of the program's goals and how to measure them, while maintaining a clear understanding of individual agendas and how the project must bridge multidisciplinary commitments, becomes the real art of implementation.

Why spend billions of dollars on curative interventions when the world health community and local governments could spend an order of magnitude less on preventative measures? We have a responsibility to leverage what we already know works to influence a situation that could otherwise result in the further deterioration of the lives of the urban poor and the health of national economies.

Appendix: Macronutrients vs. Micronutrients

It was not until the 1980s that efforts to address malnutrition shifted from a focus solely on a lack of protein and calories (known as protein-energy or "macronutrient" malnutrition) to one focused on a lack of vitamins and minerals (known as "micronutrient" malnutrition) [5]. Macronutrients are carbohydrates, proteins, and fats. Micronutrients are essential vitamins and minerals, such as iron, folic acid, zinc, vitamin A, and iodine, required in only small amounts yet remain critical to the human body for proper health and development. The body cannot produce most micronutrients, so they must be obtained directly from the diet.

How Is Food Actually Fortified?

Although the process of adopting fortification differs for production facilities depending on the food being fortified and the current state of the facility, the major premise remains the same: 1) the food processor identifies required changes that must take place, which generally includes source and cost of needed equipment, source and cost of premix (i.e., blend of vitamins and minerals based on established national standards), and required process line alterations; and 2) the food processor establishes internal quality assurance and quality control measures that continually test the safety and efficacy of the premix and fortified product.

Step 1: Identification of equipment needs, premix, and process line changes. The introduction of fortification into a facility's production line can happen, even if a plant is already operating. Fortunately, most modern facilities already have the equipment needed for fortification [70]. Dosifiers, used to accurately dispense the correct amount of premix, are often already used to add ascorbic acid and vitamin E for food preservation purposes. The same holds true in many cases for mixers, which are important in fortification to ensure the premix is mixed equally into the final product. Where this is not the case, it is a relatively straightforward process to add a dosifier and appropriate mixing devices. The establishment of quality assurance and quality control measures specific to fortification will be outlined in Step 2. For facilities that do need to purchase new equipment, dosifier costs can range from $1,000–20,000, depending on the kind of dosifier chosen (i.e., volumetric, gravimetric, or loss-of-weight, in order of expense). Mixing units can range from $2,000–10,000. The cost of premix, where the bulk of fortification costs fall, will depend on the type and number of nutrients added and the amount of product that is produced. Rice fortification is the only process where the number of micronutrients added does not affect cost because of the comparatively high price of purchasing rice kernels for extraction methods.

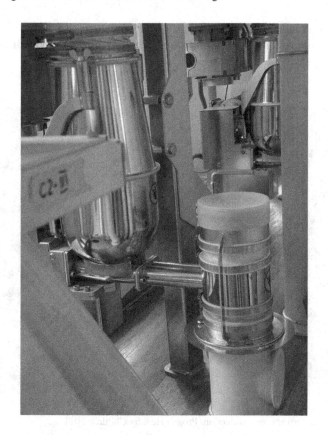

Large-scale mill dosifier. Project Healthy Children 2011

Taking wheat flour as an example, using 2008 prices, it costs $268 to produce one metric ton (MT) of wheat flour and $312 to buy one MT of wheat flour. The cost of premix to fortify this wheat flour falls between $1.50 and $3.00 per MT when fortifying with iron, folic acid, and other B vitamins [51], which is an infinitesimal portion of the production costs. This rises to $8 per MT when vitamin A is added [63]. Fortificant cost can, however, range up to $15–20 per MT, depending on the vehicle being fortified, production capacity of the facility, and other addition factors. To put metric tons into perspective, a large-scale flour production facility may produce in the range of 48 MT per day or greater. In most cases, however, production within these large facilities is more on the magnitude of 250 MT per day.

Premix should be sourced from companies that have already received quality approvals from global nutrition bodies. For example, the Global Alliance for Improved Nutrition (GAIN)'s Global Premix Facility has already approved a number of companies around the world as quality premix supplies and is available to provide procurement assistance to facilities as needed.

The timing of premix addition into the production line is important to consider (due to premix's sensitivity to heat) and needs to be thoroughly mixed in with the final product. Premix should be added before any processing steps that require high temperatures to avoid nutrient degradation but before the final product is mixed (to ensure homogeneity).

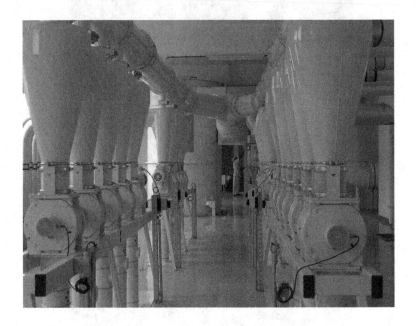

Large-scale flour fortification production. Project Healthy Children 2011

Step 2: *Establish internal quality assurance and quality control measures.* Fortification quality assurance and quality control measures are needed to ensure the product meets the established national standard for safety and efficacy. These measures should be incorporated into the production facility's already established protocols for hygiene and safety. The East, Central, and Southern African (ECSA) Community has established quality assurance and quality control guidelines, which outline the specific type and number of qualitative and quantitative tests that should occur.

Quality assurance procedures and qualitative testing equipment for the facility can range from $3,000 to $8,000 [64]. Qualitative tests can range from $2 to $5 per test (conducted daily), while periodic outside quantitative testing (usually conducted every month or every few months) can range from $10 to $100 per test [63]. There is a significant range in up-front costs, generally speaking, from $6,000 to $40,000, in addition to the cost of premix and quality testing (considered recurring costs). However, these estimates are highly dependent on production parameters, the type of fortification vehicle, and nutrients chosen. As a result, these numbers should be seen as gross generalizations that pertain mostly to the production of fortified flour. Each specific situation will differ.

Finally, new packaging that designates the product as fortified is required. In many cases, this simply includes the addition of the country or region's designated fortification logo.

Financial assistance to industry is sometimes provided by outside donors or government for the first year or two. However, up-front costs, in most cases, can be recouped by industry through the market advantage fortification gives producers (via consumer demand and regional fortification regulations). Additional costs may be folded into the price of the final product and either absorbed by the company or passed on to the consumer. Even when all programs costs are passed on to the consumer, the price increase tends to be only 1–2 % on top of the usual price—an amount that is less than normal market price variation [5].

References

1. World Health Organization (WHO) and United Nations Human Settlement Programme (UN-HABITAT) joint report: hidden cities: unmasking and overcoming health inequalities in urban settings. The WHO Center for Health Development, Kobe, and United Nation's Human Settlements Programme (UN-HABITAT), 2010.
2. Crush J, Frayne B, McLachlan M. Rapid urbanization and the nutrition transition in Southern Africa. Urban food security series no. 7. Queen's University and African Food Security and Urban Network (AFSUN): Kingston and Cape Town. 2011.
3. Dary O. Food fortification as a public health strategy and the contributions of A2Z. Sight Life Magazine. 2009;1:6–15.
4. Harvey P, Rambeloson Z, Dary O. The 2008 Uganda Food Consumption Survey: determining the dietary patterns of Ugandan women and children. A2Z: the USAID micronutrient and child blindness project. AED, Washington DC, 2010.
5. Allen L, de Benoist B, Dary O, Hurrel R, editors. Guidelines on food fortification with micronutrients. Geneva: World Health Organization; 2006.
6. Investing in the future: a united call to action on vitamin and mineral deficiencies, micronutrient initiative. FFI, GAIN, MI, USAID, World Bank, and UNICEF. 2009.
7. World Health Report. Geneva, World Health Organization, 2000.
8. World Health Organization (WHO) Global database on vitamin A deficiency. 2009.
9. Solomons NW. Sight and life luncheon forum on contributions of micronutrients to achieve the MDGs. Sight Life. 2011;25(3):76–80.
10. Center for Disease Control (CDC). IMMPACT Project. http://www.cdc.gov/immpact/micronutrients/index.html#Folate. Accessed 16 July 2012.
11. Dary O. The cost of food enrichment. Nutriview. 2010;1:2–4.
12. Rawe K, Jayasinghe D, Mason F, Davis A, Pizzini M, Garde M, Crosby L. A life free from hunger: tacking child malnutrition. Save the Children Fund. 2012.
13. Linus Pauling Institute. http://lpi.oregonstate.edu/infocenter/minerals/iodine/. Accessed 11 June 2012.
14. Rowe LA, Dodson DM. A knowledge-to-action approach to food fortification: guiding principles for the design of fortification programs as a means of effectively addressing micronutrient malnutrition. Health. 2012;4(10):904–9.
15. EFA Global Monitoring Report 2005. http://unesdoc.unesco.org/images/0013/001373/137333e.pdf. Accessed 12 July 2012.
16. Howson CP, Kennedy ET, Horwitz A, editors. Prevention of micronutrient deficiencies: tools for policymakers and public health workers. Institute of medicine. Washington, DC: National Academy Press; 1998. p. 17–8.

17. Badham J, Kraemer K. The link between nutrition, disease, and prosperity: preventing non-communicable diseases among women and children by tackling malnutrition. Sight Life. 2011;25(2):32–6.
18. Barker DJP. In utero programming of chronic disease. Clin Sci. 1998;95:115–28.
19. Victoria CG, Adair L, Fall C, Hallal PC, Martorell R, Richter L, Sachdev HS. Maternal and child undernutrition: consequences for adult health and human capital. Lancet. 2008;371:340–57.
20. Deshmukh US, Lubree HG, Yajnik CS. Intrauterine programming of non-communicable diseases: role of maternal micronutrients. Sight Life Magazine. 2011;25(2):16–22.
21. Leon D. Cites, urbanization and health. Int J Epidemiol. 2008;37:4–8.
22. Garcia OP, Long KZ, Rosado JL. Impact of micronutrient deficiencies on obesity. Nutr Rev. 2009;67(10):559–72.
23. Hales CN, Barker DJP. Type 2 (non-insulin dependent) diabetes mellitus: the thrifty phenotype hypothesis. In: Deshmukh US, Lubree HG, Yajnik CS, editors. Intrauterine programming of non-communicable diseases: role of maternal micronutrients. *Sight and Life Magazine.* 2011;25(2):16–22.
24. The World Bank. Repositioning nutrition as central to development: a strategy for large-scale action. 2006.
25. Horton S. The economics of nutritional interventions. In: Semba RD, Bloem MW, editors. Nutrition and health in developing countries. Totowa: Humana Press; 1999.
26. World Health Organization. Poverty and Health. http://www.who.int/hdp/poverty/en/. Accessed 1 Aug 2012.
27. Horton S, Begin F, Greig A, Lakshman A. Copenhagen Consensus best practices paper on micronutrient supplements for child survival (vitamin A and zinc) 2008. In: Investing in the future: a united call to action on vitamin and mineral deficiencies. FFI, GAIN, MI, USAID, World Bank, UNICEF. 2009.
28. Global Alliance for Improved Nutrition. Investment in food fortification yields high returns. http://www.gainhealth.org/programs/gain-national-food-fortification-program. Accessed 1 Aug 2012.
29. Codex Alimentarius. General principles for the addition of essential nutrients to foods. http://www.fao.org/docrep/w2840e/w2840e03.htm.
30. Kim SS. Developing a national food fortification program in the dominican republic. In: Pinstrup-Anderson P, Cheng F, editors. Case studies in food policy for developing countries. Ithaca: Cornell University Press; 2009. p. 57–68.
31. Linus Pauling Institute. http://lpi.oregonstate.edu/infocenter/vitamins/vitaminA/. Accessed 18 July 2012.
32. Linus Pauling Institute. http://lpi.oregonstate.edu/infocenter/minerals/iodine. Accessed 18 July 2012.
33. West KP. Interactions between nutrition and infection in the developing world. Johns Hopkins Bloomberg School of Public Health. 2007. http://ocw.jhsph.edu/courses/EpiInfectiousDisease/PDFs/EID_lec10_West.pdf. Accessed 1 August 2012.
34. Hussey GD, Klein M. A randomized, controlled trial of vitamin A in children with severe measles. In: Howson CP, Kennedy ET, Horwitz A, editors. Prevention of micronutrient deficiencies: tools for policymakers and public health workers. Institute of medicine. Washington, DC: National Academy Press; 1998. p. 17–8.
35. Sommer A, West KP. Infectious morbidity. In: Howson CP, Kennedy ET, Horwitz A, editors. Prevention of micronutrient deficiencies: tools for policymakers and public health workers. Institute of medicine. Washington, DC: National Academy Press; 1998. p. 17–8.
36. Arroyave G, Dary O. Manual for sugar fortification with Vitamin A, Parts 1, 2, and 3. In: Howson CP, Kennedy ET, Horwitz A, editors. Prevention of micronutrient deficiencies: tools for policymakers and public health workers. Institute of medicine. Washington, DC: National Academy Press; 1998. p. 17–8.
37. Smith RS, Goodman DS, Zaklama MS, Gabr MK, El Maraghy S, Patwardhan VN. Serum vitamin A, retinol-binding protein, and prealbumin concentrations in protein-calorie malnutri-

tion I. In: Howson CP, Kennedy ET, Horwitz A, editors. Prevention of micronutrient deficiencies: tools for policymakers and public health workers. Institute of medicine. Washington, DC: National Academy Press; 1998. p. 17–8.

38. Smith RF, Suskind R, Thanangkul O, Leitzmann C, Goodman DS, Olson RE. Plasma vitamin A, retinol-binding protein and prealbumin concentrations in protein-calorie malnutrition III. In: Howson CP, Kennedy ET, Horwitz A, editors. Prevention of micronutrient deficiencies: tools for policymakers and public health workers. Institute of medicine. Washington, DC: National Academy Press; 1998. p. 17–8.

39. Nestel P, Bouis HE, Meenakshi JV, Pfeiffer W. Biofortification of staple food crops. J Nutr. 2006;136:1064–7.

40. Ministerio de Salud Publica de Nicaragua. Sistema Integrado de Vigilancia de Intervenciones Nutricionales (SIVIN). Informe de Progreso 2003–2005. 2008.

41. Martinez C, Mena I, Boy E, Dary O. Evaluation of nutritional blindness in Guatemala and its association with sugar fortification and vitamin A supplementation: Retrospective study of hospital cases from 1980 to 2000. Guatemala City: PAHO/Institute of Nutrition of Central America and Panama; 2005.

42. Personal communication with Omar Dary. July 13, 2012.

43. Lotfi M, Manar MGV, Merx RJHM, Naber-van den Heuvel P. Micronutrient fortification of foods: developing a program. J Food Technol Africa. 1999;4:2–4.

44. Toolkit for developing a national flour fortification monitoring and surveillance system: a purposive and convenience sampling approach. Smarter Futures. March 12, 2011.

45. Frankenberg E, Thomas D, Beegle K. The real costs of Indonesia's economic crisis: preliminary findings from the Indonesia family life survey. In: Adams P. Fortification remains wise investment in midst of global economic woes. Flour Fortification Initiative. White Paper. http://www.sph.emory.edu/wheatflour/economicbenefit.php. Accessed 23 July 2012.

46. Micronutrient initiative. An impact study on small-scale fortification project in Lalitpur District: Feb 2009–April 2011.

47. Project Healthy Children (PHC), Imagine Lalitpur, and Micronutrient Initiative (MI) preliminary data from Nepal small-scale fortification pilot project. July 2012. Unpublished.

48. Horton S. The economics of food fortification. J Nutr. 2006;136:1068–71.

49. Copenhagen Consensus 2008 Results. http://www.copenhagenconsensus.com/Files/Filer/CC08/Presse%20%20result/CC08_results_FINAL.pdf. Accessed 16 April 2012.

50. Meenakshi JV et al. How cost effective is biofortification in combating micronutrient malnutrition? An ex-ante assessment. In: Investing in the future: a united call to action on vitamin and mineral deficiencies, micronutrient initiative. FFI, GAIN, MI, USAID, World Bank, and UNICEF. 2009.

51. Adams P. Fortification remains wise investment in midst of global economic woes. Flour fortification initiative. White Paper. http://www.sph.emory.edu/wheatflour/economicbenefit.php. Accessed 23 July 2012.

52. Mora J, Dary O, Chinchilla D, Arroyave G. Vitamin A Sugar Fortification in Central America: Experience and Lessons Learned. Washington, DC: The USAID Micronutrient Program (MOST)/ US Agency for International Development (USAID)/Instituto de Nutricion de Centro America y Panama (INCAP) / Pan American Health Organization (PAHO). 2009.

53. Gottlieb J. Center for Global Development. Case Study #16: Prevention of Neural-Tube Defects in Chile. Available from: http://www.cgdev.org/doc/millions/MS_case_16.pdf. Accessed on June 22, 2012.

54. Hertramph E, Cortes F. Folic acid fortification of wheat flour: Chile. Nutr Rev. 2004;62(6):S44–8.

55. Chen J, Zhao X, Zhang X, Yin S, Piao J, Huo J, Yu B, Qu N, Lu Q, Wang S, Chen C. Studies on the effectiveness of NaFeEDTA-fortified soy sauce in controlling iron deficiency: a population-based intervention trial. Food Nutr Bull. 2005;26:177–89.

56. Sayed A, Bourne D, Pattinson R, Nixon J, Henderson B. Decline in the prevalence of neural tube defects following folic acid fortification and its cost-benefit in South Africa. Birth Defects Res, Part A Clin Mol Terol. 2008;82:211–6.

57. Assey VD, Peterson S, Kimboka S, Ngemera D, Mgoba C, Ruhiye DM, Ndoss GD, Greiner T, Tylleskar T. Tanzania national survey on iodine deficiency: impact after twelve years of salt iodization. BMC Public Health. 2009;9:319.

58. Ray JG, Meier C, Vermeulen MJ, Boss S, Wyatt PR, Cole DEC. Association of neural tube defects and folic acid food fortification in Canada. Lancet. 2002;360:2047–8.

59. Serdula, Pena-Rosas, Maberly, Parvanta, Arbuto, Perrine, and Mei: Flour fortification with iron, vitamin B12, vitamin A, and zinc: Proceedings of the Second Technical Workshop on Wheat Flour Fortification, The United Nations University. 2010.

60. Fletcher RJ, Bell IP, Lambert JP. Public health aspects of food fortification: a question of balance. Proc Nutr Soc. 2004;63:605–14.

61. Fortification Rapid Assessment Tool & Guidelines Micronutrient Initiative & PATH Canada, 2000.

62. Food and Agricultural Organization (FAO). Preventing micronutrient malnutrition: A guide to food-based approaches. http://www.fao.org/docrep/x0245e/x0245e02.htm#P220_21819. Accessed 11 July 2012.

63. Emory University School of Public Health. Flour Miller's Tool Kit on Fortification. Presentation. March 2011.

64. Johnson Q, Mannar V, Ranum P. Fortification Handbook. Vitamin and mineral fortification of wheat flour and maize meal. The Micronutrient Initiative. June 2004.

65. ECSA Manual for Internal Monitoring of Fortified Maize Flour. First edition. 2007.

66. Dary O. Mass food fortification programs as public health nutrition interventions. In: Dary O. The importance and limitations of food fortification for the management of nutritional anemia. In: Kraemer K, Zimmerman MB (eds) Nutritional Anemia. 2007. Basel: Sight and Life. pp. 315–36.

67. Serlemitsos JA, Fusco H. Vitamin A Fortification of Sugar in Zambia 1998–2001. The USAID Micronutrient Program (MOST). 2001.

68. USAID Micronutrient Project (MOST)/UNICEF/CDC/The National Food and Nutrition Commission of Zambia. Report of the national survey to evaluate the impact of vitamin A interventions in Zambia. 2003.

69. Hurrel R, Ranum P, de Pee S, Biebinger R, Hulthen L, Johnson Q, Lynch S. Revised recommendations for iron fortification of wheat flour and an evaluation of the expected impact of current national wheat flour fortification programs. Food Nutr Bull. 2010;31:S7–S21.

70. Flour Fortification Initiative. Economic Benefits. http://www.sph.emory.edu/wheatflour/economicbenefit.php . Accessed on 23 July 2012.

Part II
Innovations to Address Specific
Urbanization-Related Threats to Health

Chapter 4
Innovations in Anti-Trafficking Efforts: Implications for Urbanization and Health

Roy Ahn, Genevieve Purcell, Anita M. McGahan, Hanni Stoklosa,
Thomas F. Burke, Kathryn Conn, Hannah L. Harp, Emily de Redon,
Griffin Flannery, and Wendy Macias-Konstantopoulos

Introduction to Human Trafficking

Human trafficking is a significant human rights violation and emerging global health problem that has been estimated to involve nearly 21 million victims worldwide [1]. As defined by the United Nations *Protocol to Prevent, Suppress and Punish Trafficking in Persons, especially Women and Children*, trafficking is:

> The recruitment, transportation, transfer, harbouring or receipt of persons, by means of the threat or use of force or other forms of coercion, of abduction, of fraud, of deception, of the abuse of power or of a position of vulnerability or the giving or receiving of payments or benefits to achieve the consent of a person having control over another person, for the purpose of exploitation. Exploitation shall include, at a minimum, the exploitation of the prostitution of others or other forms of sexual exploitation, forced labour or services, slavery or practices similar to slavery, servitude or the removal of organs [2].

R. Ahn, M.P.H., Sc.D, (✉) • H. Stoklosa, M.D. • T.F. Burke, M.D., F.A.C.E.P., F.R.S.M.
W. Macias-Konstantopoulos, M.D., M.P.H.
Division of Global Health and Human Rights, Department of Emergency Medicine,
Massachusetts General Hospital, Zero Emerson Place Suite 104, Boston, MA 02114, USA

Harvard Medical School, Boston, MA, USA
e-mail: RAHN@mgh.harvard.edu

G. Purcell, B.A. • K. Conn, B.A. • E. de Redon, B.A. • G. Flannery, B.A.
Division of Global Health and Human Rights, Department of Emergency Medicine,
Massachusetts General Hospital, Zero Emerson Place Suite 104, Boston, MA 02114, USA

A.M. McGahan, Ph.D.
Rotman School of Management, University of Toronto, 105 St. George Street, Toronto,
ON, Canada M553E6

H.L. Harp, B.A.
Division of Global Health and Human Rights, Department of Emergency Medicine,
Massachusetts General Hospital, Zero Emerson Place Suite 104, Boston, MA 02114, USA

Boston University School of Medicine, Boston, MA, USA

© Springer New York 2015
R. Ahn et al. (eds.), *Innovating for Healthy Urbanization*,
DOI 10.1007/978-1-4899-7597-3_4

Trafficking encompasses a wide spectrum of coercive activities, such as debt bondage, involuntary domestic servitude, recruitment of child soldiers, child sex trafficking, and organ trafficking. It occurs internationally (and within national borders) in all regions of the world where individuals are made vulnerable by environments of poverty, unemployment, war, natural disaster, and desperation [3]. Our increasingly globalized world has given rise to an ecosystem that supports the traffic of human beings for all these purposes. With globalization has come the growth of cities as increased numbers of people migrate from rural to urban areas. Urbanization itself is a major facilitator of human trafficking. The International Labour Organization (ILO) notes the importance of understanding, for example, sex trafficking as enabled by migration:

> The reality is that human trafficking is not just an issue of sexual exploitation but a social development problem closely related to the economies and labour markets…and the exploitation of vulnerable people confronted with these realities. It is, in many cases, linked to deeply rooted habits relating to work and the movement of people [4].

While the ILO describes this phenomenon in the specific cases of Southeast Asia and the Greater Mekong Subregion, others describe its applicability worldwide. As Shelley (2001) suggests, the growth in disparities between "developed" and "developing" countries has created both supply and demand for human trafficking, and this phenomenon is exacerbated by the existence of numerous interrelated and cyclical factors, such as the feminization of poverty and marginalization of rural communities, that affect the lives of many vulnerable people in the developing world [5, 6]. Combined, these factors create an environment in which human trafficking can flourish as individuals from more rural, impoverished communities seek opportunity in urban centers.

Chapter Overview

This chapter describes the nexus of urbanization, human trafficking, and public health and identifies promising innovations to address global human trafficking. First, we briefly describe why human trafficking is an urban health concern. Second, we provide a brief overview of the social determinants of human trafficking. Third, we highlight innovative anti-trafficking efforts, including public awareness campaigns, vocational training, community education, and victim identification while supporting initiatives that target these social determinants. Finally, we summarize the implications of these anti-trafficking interventions on urbanization and global health.

Human Trafficking as an Urban Health Concern

The health and demographic significance of human trafficking are significant. Human trafficking—whether sex, labor, or organ trafficking—is linked to myriad physical and mental health conditions that specifically arise from the abuse and deprivation that victims experience [7]. Concerns exist about the potential for

Table 4.1 Summary of the health risks and consequences of being trafficked

Health risks	Potential consequences
Physical abuse, deprivation	Physical health problems, including death, contusions, cuts, burns, broken bones
Threats, intimidation, abuse	Mental health problems including suicidal ideation and attempts, depression, anxiety, hostility, flashbacks, and reexperiencing symptoms
Sexual abuse	Sexually transmitted infections (including HIV), pelvic inflammatory disease, infertility, vaginal fistula, unwanted pregnancy, unsafe abortion, poor reproductive health
Substance misuse Drugs (legal and illegal), alcohol	Overdose, drug of alcohol addiction
Social restrictions and manipulation and emotional abuse	Psychological distress, inability to access care
Economic exploitation Debt bondage, deceptive accounting	Insufficient food or liquid, climate control, poor hygiene, risk-taking to repay debts, insufficient funds to pay for care
Legal insecurity Forced illegal activities, confiscation of documents	Restriction from or hesitancy to access services resulting in deterioration of health and exacerbation of conditions
Occupational hazards Dangerous working conditions, poor training or equipment, exposure to chemical, bacterial or physical dangers	Dehydration, physical injury, bacterial infections, heat or cold overexposure cut, or amputated limbs
Marginalization Structural and social barriers, including isolation, discrimination, linguistic and cultural barriers, difficult logistics, e.g., transport systems, administrative procedures	Unattended injuries or infections, debilitating conditions, psychosocial health problems

Adapted from Page 17, Caring for trafficked persons: guidance for health providers. Geneva, Switzerland: International Organization for Migration; 2009

trafficking—specifically sex trafficking—to fuel the spread of sexually transmitted infections, including HIV, in urban centers [8]. Macias Konstantopoulos and colleagues' study of sex trafficking in eight cities of the USA, the UK, Brazil, the Philippines, and India found a wide range of reported health problems among trafficking victims—from sexually transmitted infections to depression [9]. Additional studies on human trafficking have documented health problems among victims, such as drug/alcohol addiction; dehydration or malnutrition resulting from insufficient food or liquid; and psychological distress resulting from threats, intimidation, and abuse by traffickers [7, 10]. Notably, victims experience a compendium of health problems during various "stages" of their trafficking experience (e.g., in transit to their trafficking location, during their captivity, post-rescue (if applicable)) [10].

The International Organization for Migration's *Caring for Trafficked Persons* provides a synopsis of the health issues of human trafficking victims (Table 4.1) [7].

Social Determinants of Human Trafficking

Numerous factors fuel the human trafficking trade. Individuals may be "pushed" into urban migration and become vulnerable to trafficking by economic disparities associated with a lack of employment opportunities [3, 5, 7, 11–14].

The centralization of educational and employment opportunities that occurs with urbanization has dramatic economic effects [15]. As the United Nations Population Fund (UNFPA) describes, changes brought on by urbanization have resulted in the "transformation of national economies, with growing numbers of people moving away from employment in agriculture and into industries and service sectors, and in the process increasing their productivity" [16]. These changes disrupt traditional livelihoods and influence individuals' migration decisions. For example, citizens of the Philippines have found it difficult to maintain a sustainable livelihood through traditional agriculture and fishing practices, largely due to environmental degradation and restrictive policies. Such circumstances often result in forced migration, as individuals who find themselves "pushed" to urban areas seek better economic opportunities [7].

Chuang states that women's "vulnerability is exacerbated by well-entrenched discriminatory practices that relegate women to employment in informal economic sectors and further limit their avenues for legal migration" [10]. With reduced legal migration options, individuals are more likely to turn through informal channels to brokers, recruiters, or pimps for economic opportunity and are therefore at higher risk of being trafficked [4]. Finally, experts identify political instability, civil unrest, armed conflict, and natural disasters as conditions that stimulate migration [5, 7, 10, 17]. Bales, for example, notes that the "[d]estabilization and displacement of populations increase their vulnerability to exploitation and abuse" [12].

Complementary forces "pull" individuals into human trafficking. The high demand for workers, and particularly for migrant labor, in destination areas continues to drive trafficking. Chuang describes the unmet labor demands that exist in wealthier destination countries because of aging populations, particularly in positions she describes as "3D" jobs (dirty, dangerous, or difficult). These countries often rely on migrant labor to fill these positions [10]. In addition, Nogales, Shelley, and Chuang describe a phenomenon in which the demand for migrants' "foreignness" is often a factor in the sex or domestic service industries because foreign migrants are seen as more vulnerable, flexible, cooperative, and malleable [5, 9, 10]. In the case of organ trafficking, the high demand for kidneys in developed countries (due to long waiting lists for kidney transplants) means that individuals from lower-income countries may fall prey to organ traffickers, who promise—but fail to deliver—to pay these vulnerable individuals once their organs have been removed.

These push and pull factors result in a "culture of migration," as social and economic disparities combine to create a supply of and demand for individuals seeking to migrate to cities.

Innovative Anti-trafficking Efforts Around the World

This section provides a typology of selected, promising anti-trafficking initiatives from around the world initiated by a wide variety of stakeholders, including governments, civil society organizations, and multinational corporations.[1] Some are designed to increase the number of trafficking victims identified and assisted; others focus on instigating community responses to trafficking. Some initiatives focus on addressing the push factors in rural areas that serve as a source of trafficking victims, while others try to mitigate the pull factors in urban areas that create demand for trafficking. Among these profiled initiatives, there is a strong emphasis on addressing the root causes of trafficking. Furthermore, many harness the power of modern technology (e.g., mobile devices, new media) to effect change on a large scale. Overall, these initiatives affect public health in direct and indirect ways (i.e., given the association between trafficking and health).

Public Awareness Campaigns

Public awareness campaigns remain one of the most widely used tactics in addressing the root causes of human trafficking. Public awareness campaigns convey the following types of information [18]:

- Describe the existence and scope of human trafficking.
- Garner public support for anti-trafficking campaigns.
- Reduce stereotypes and stigma of trafficking victims.
- Educate at-risk groups on how to safely migrate [19].
- Educate on how to identify and report a suspected case of human trafficking [14].
- Increase advocacy and inform policy-makers with the aim to introduce human trafficking as a human rights issue or to advocate legislation [14].

Contemporary awareness-raising campaigns increasingly incorporate new technologies, such as social media and advertising that deliver a specific message to a targeted group [13]. The following informational campaigns promote messages that aim to prevent human trafficking through the use of creative dissemination strategies.

MTV EXIT (End Exploitation and Trafficking) Campaign

The MTV EXIT campaign targets youth in low-income countries—using celebrity-powered documentaries and concert tours with popular musicians to promote cautionary messages and tips on safe migration. The MTV EXIT campaign aims to increase general awareness and prevention of human trafficking by promoting safe

---

[1] Many of these initiatives have not been rigorously evaluated; thus we label them as "promising," but the lack of sound evaluation data is a gap that the anti-trafficking field needs to address.

migration in countries with reportedly high levels of human trafficking with messages such as:

"Don't rush to migrate" [20]
"Verify jobs with 3 different individuals and a NGO" [15]
"Retain your personal documents" [15]

The campaign also describes potential dangers, realities, and consequences of life in a destination country after migration. By debunking the illusion of a better life, it aims to encourage at-risk youth to undertake various precautions while deciding whether to travel and/or work abroad (i.e., check whether a recruitment agency is reliable, and properly proceed with visas, passports, embassies, tickets, and other forms of documentation). MTV EXIT has produced several celebrity-narrated documentaries, short films, television shows, music videos with popular bands, online content in 14 languages, and, uniquely, live concert events all over the world. Local anti-trafficking organizations are invited to distribute trafficking awareness and prevention information. The concerts have proven to be widely popular—800,000 concert goers to date—and have amassed support for anti-trafficking activities worldwide [15]. MTV also notes that more than 80 million people have visited the MTV EXIT website [15].

Project for the Prevention of Adolescent Trafficking in Latvia (PPAT)

The Project for the Prevention of Adolescent Trafficking (PPAT) was developed by the International Organization for Adolescents (IOFA) as the first comprehensive human trafficking prevention initiative for youth and adolescents in Latvia and Eastern Europe. Included in this program is a nationwide information campaign throughout Latvia that specifically targets youth (14–25 years) at high risk for human trafficking (i.e., homeless, disabled, runaway/throwaway, sexually exploited, and orphans) [14]. Similar to MTV EXIT, PPAT delivers messages around how to migrate safely by teaching youth how to verify whether a job opportunity is legitimate, increasing awareness around current recruitment schemes of traffickers, who the traffickers are, and where and how to find protection if they are trafficked. The campaign utilizes traditional information dissemination strategies (i.e., public service announcements, magazine articles, brochures, and posters) as well as movie trailers, chats on Latvian Internet sites, and free screenings of *Smooth Flight*—a 30-min documentary on the experiences of migration of Latvian youth—organized for orphans in five sites across the country [14].

At the conclusion of their campaign, PPAT collected data from 348 youth who were planning to work abroad in the next 6 months. They demonstrated that youth who had been exposed to three or more sources of information were 37 % more likely to take a safe migration precaution [14]. In these sessions, a counselor helps clients determine if they are making an informed decision about traveling to a specific country, reviews the client's employment contract, and offers a viewing of *Smooth Flight* to learn more about the risks of trafficking.

Men Can Stop Rape

The *Men Can Stop Rape* initiative operates a trafficking-related program that engages young men to create a culture free of violence, especially men's violence against women. The organization has created two public awareness campaigns that show men role modeling healthy choices and behaviors that "associate strength with character and integrity" [21]. Specifically, the *Where Do You Stand?* campaign addresses issues of consent to help prevent sexism and sexual assault. The Strength Campaign, including its youth development programs—the *Men of Strength Club* and *Campus Men of Strength Club*—promotes messages around gender-based harassment, teasing, bullying, and cyber harassing through public service announcements and posters that teach boys and teens how to intervene in situations of harassment at an early age [22]. Social media materials have been distributed in "all 50 states and 20 foreign countries, totaling over 100,000 items sold" and have appeared in several publications including *The Washington Post*, *Chicago Sun Times*, and *O Magazine* [23]. *Men Can Stop Rape* brings together community-based training activities that provide men with tools to challenge sexual assault with information campaigns that saturate the environment with messages that aim to prevent and fight not only violence but also the devaluation and low status of women and girls in society, all of which are determinants of human trafficking [24].

Vocational Training, Microcredit, and Social Enterprise Programs

Vocational training, microcredit, and social enterprise programs are community-level interventions that aim to address the lack of education/skills development and income-generating opportunities that often exist in regions that serve as "supply" areas for human trafficking. The ILO's International Program on the Elimination of Child Labor also describes the effect of microfinance and vocational training on the elimination of migration push factors: generating income for families so that children can remain in school and creating employment opportunities at home so that individuals are not required to migrate for jobs [4]. In addition, microfinance provides savings and emergency loans to buffer against financial emergencies such as family illness or crop failures, and offers people affordable credit options [25].

Vocational training and microcredit activities can take a variety of forms, and they are often bundled together into combined programs that provide skills as well as credit. Below we describe several initiatives that aim to improve livelihoods through these types of community-level interventions.

SWEEP, Uganda

Implemented by Century Entrepreneurship Development Agency (CEDA) International and funded by the UN Youth Habitat Fund, the Slum Women Economic Empowerment Project (SWEEP) is a program specifically designed to protect women living in Ugandan slum areas against the threat of human trafficking and sexual exploitation. The program is a multifaceted, 12-month training program for young women on entrepreneurial skills (i.e., develop business ideas and attain financial literacy). SWEEP trains single mothers, aged 15–32, living in the Kawempe slum in the capital city, Kampala. Upon "graduating" from this intensive program, "…the young women will be supported to join employment through internship with selected partners and those interested in entrepreneurship will be connected to incubation programs to actualize their ideas. The mentored women will form mentoring clubs and become peer mentors each required to mentor two other women in their community and the two will mentor four to grow the factor tree. They will also form savings and Investment [sic] clubs as a source of future financing" [26].

Young Women in Enterprise, Kenya

The Young Women in Enterprise program in Kenya combines efforts that economically and socially empower women, thereby addressing two different determinants of human trafficking. Run by US-based nonprofit TechnoServe and sponsored by a grant from Nike, the urban antipoverty program targets young women ages 15–22 years and aims to help them launch "employment-generating, women-owned businesses that support Kenya's communities" [27]. Three thousand women have participated in the YWE initiative since 2005 [21].

According to the program's website:

> The YWE program comprises four components: training on using tools to plan, implement, and manage a small business; links to financing, with an emphasis on the importance of savings; mentorship guided by leading women entrepreneurs, among others; and mini-business plan competitions, which identify promising business ideas and enable talented entrepreneurs to further advance their businesses [21].

One notable aspect of the program is the Enterprise Club Competitions, in which young women present their business plans to a local panel of judges, receive feedback, and compete for prizes and/or cash. The most promising business plans are presented to new regional judging panels, and young women can win up to 500,000 KSH (approximately 6,000 USD) for their enterprise ideas. Prize winners may be qualified to seek funding for their businesses from the Youth Enterprise Development Fund through the Ministry of State for Youth Affairs [21]. Additionally, the program provides life skills training and education, particularly around the issue of HIV/AIDS. TechnoServe hopes that this combination of interventions will "[help] them avoid the vulnerability that too often leads girls to become child brides or at risk for HIV/AIDS" [21].

GoodWeave International (GWI)

GoodWeave International is an international nonprofit organization that addresses root causes of child labor in the "weaving communities" of Afghanistan, India, and Nepal, and consumer countries of Germany, the UK, and the US through a corporate certification and schooling program for "rescued" children. The GWI Child Labor Free certification program licenses rug importers and exporters who sign a legally binding contract ensuring that child labor will not be used to make rugs. Importers must agree "to source only from GoodWeave certified exporters in India and Nepal and any other country in which GoodWeave rugs are available." Only licensed importers are permitted to sell GoodWeave label carpets [28].

Exporters (looms) undergo unannounced, random inspections by local inspectors [22]. If they find children working, manufactures lose their GoodWeave certification, and children working for these manufacturers are subsequently offered a fully sponsored education. After reunification with their families, GoodWeave will match the child with an educational program that includes intensive literacy and math training. This program leads to more formal education that incorporates language, social studies, math, science, and other extracurricular activities, such as music and art. The child has the opportunity to enter a vocational training program at age 14. GoodWeave also provides day care, early childhood education, and school sponsorship for children of adult weavers as well as adult literacy programs and health clinics in weaving communities [29]. To help support GoodWeave in its commitment to provide rehabilitation and schooling for all "rescued children," exporters pay 0.25 % of the export value of each rug and importers pay a licensing fee of 1.75 % of the shipment value [22].

GoodWeave is working to further address root causes of child labor by expanding its standard and by working with producers to include criteria that ensure employees work under safe conditions for a "reasonable wage" [22].

Not for Sale Rebbl Tonic

Not for Sale (NFS) is a US-based nonprofit organization that addresses human trafficking by "creating enterprise opportunities for vulnerable communities, offering social services to survivors and those at risk for human trafficking, and evaluating the use of forced labor in mainstream supply chains" [30]. NFS addresses key economic determinants for trafficking, namely, access to economic opportunity and access to education, via social enterprises. Currently, NFS produces Rebbl Tonic, an herbal tonic sourced from the Peruvian Amazon—a region that is reportedly the site of 50 % of Peru's forced labor [31]. By sourcing key ingredients for the drink from indigenous communities located in the region, Rebbl hopes to stimulate economic development in the area and generate revenue back into NFS field activities. In addition to creating sustainable employment for the providers of ingredients, 2.5 % of proceeds are donated back to the Not For Sale Campaign and reinvested into the community in the form of improvements in the education, nutrition, and transportation infrastructure [32].

LAO/021 Village Development Fund, Laos

Microfinance initiatives are prevalent throughout the world and are designed to empower individuals economically, thus providing a buffer against poverty—a major trafficking determinant. A village banking program called the Village Development Fund, or "VDF," established by the Bolikhamxay Livelihood Improvement and Governance Project utilizes an innovative approach to microfinance—built on the principle that in order to borrow money, one must save money as well. This method "displac[es] loan sharks and their high-interest loans and instill[s] a culture of savings and planning" [4]. The VDF savings-based approach to rural finance is coupled with vocational and business management training. The approach is particularly important for women in Laos, who own most of the registered small businesses in the country but who often have limited access to technical training, financial services, and information about the local market [4].

A nonprofit called the Lao Sustainable Community Development Promotion Association helped communities adapt to the new VDFs. Guidelines established included the requirement of maintaining a minimum amount of savings for at least 3 months prior to taking out a loan from the bank; this guideline increased participants' personal investment in the bank's success. Another requirement was the inclusion of both men and women on the bank's managing committee. The ILO notes: "Village fund savings average more than 1,000 USD and loan repayments are now 100 % [19]. Well over 100 villages are now participating and the Government and its institutions have pledged to continue the programme and indeed expand it" [4].

Targeted Community Education

The public awareness campaigns discussed previously address a broad audience and seek to establish basic knowledge about human trafficking. By comparison, community education programs can provide more in-depth and *targeted information* to affected or at-risk populations and other stakeholders who may come into contact with trafficking (e.g., groups that assist victims and survivors, men who solicit sexual services).

Community Education Programs for Adolescent Girls

Programs such as Thai Women of Tomorrow use traditional pedagogical techniques to raise awareness about labor trafficking and the sex trade. Thai Women of Tomorrow functions primarily in rural northern Thailand, where 80 % of all migration is directed to the metropolitan Bangkok area [33]. This organization provides education about sex trafficking and supports secondary education for young women who otherwise would remain at risk for trafficking.

Training of Key Responders to Human Trafficking

Community-based responses extend to the training of professionals in fields relevant to trafficking. The Joint Knowledge Online (JKO) is the US Department of Defense's (DoD) online training program for government departmental employees. This program takes an innovative approach by training DoD employees through a mobile application accessible via smartphone. One of the many required courses of the military and civilian DoD employees, Combating Trafficking in Persons (CTIP), includes six sections, each followed by a short quiz. There is also a final posttest to demonstrate mastery of the material. Successful completion of the training is verified by JKO, and proof of completion is required by those mandated to complete the training. This particular form of training, which is easy to update and correct, allows employees of the DoD to access this important training remotely and complete it on their own time. The accessibility allows the DoD to disseminate appropriate training materials to the people in their employ who are best suited to address human trafficking [34].

Similarly, the nonprofit Polaris Project, which operates the US National Human Trafficking Resource Center, maintains a website of online training modules and webinars for anti-trafficking stakeholders. The training topics address a wide array of professional audiences; titles on this website include, "Human Trafficking: An Introduction to Military, Civilians, and Contractors," "Human Trafficking and Traveling Sales Crews," and "Building a Local Crisis Response to Human Trafficking" [35].

Training programs for law enforcement and social service professionals abound, but there has been a recent increase in training programs for professional communities such as health care. In 2011, Zimmerman et al. published a conceptual model for involving the healthcare community in the fight against trafficking, and a recent review of anti-trafficking resources for health-care workers notes that "because of trafficking victims' increased risk of experiencing acute and chronic health effects, healthcare professionals may be in a unique position to identify, interact with, and support victims" [9]. The Florida Medical Association has developed a continuing medical education module on "domestic violence with an emphasis on human trafficking" that is mandatory for physician relicensing in the state of Florida [36]. The Human Trafficking Initiative (HTI) at the Massachusetts General Hospital's Division of Global Health and Human Rights[2] conducts training aimed at enlisting healthcare workers in the identification, treatment, and referral of labor and sex trafficking victims. The training focuses on trafficking definitions, epidemiology, risk factors for trafficking, principles of trauma-informed care in screening, response and referral, and collaborations with service providers and law enforcement. Thus far, training sessions have taken place across the USA as well as in Kenya and the Caribbean—in both urban and rural settings [37]. In addition, in 2014, the HTI

---

[2] The authors of this chapter are all affiliated with the Human Trafficking Initiative, Massachusetts General Hospital Division of Global Health and Human Rights, Department of Emergency Medicine.

opened a novel academic hospital-based clinic (called the MGH Freedom Clinic) that provides trauma-informed, comprehensive health care to survivors of human trafficking; this clinic also allows researchers to better understand the physical and mental health needs of survivors.

Targeting Demand

A community-based approach also can address the demand side of trafficking. The so-called john schools—educational and community service programs required of convicted customers of sex workers—aim to prevent trafficking by educating potential customers about the significant presence of trafficking victims in the sex worker community. The Red Zone program is such a diversion program for purchasers of sex in Indianapolis, Indiana. Red Zone is unique among john schools for its emphasis on community: participants meet residents of the community in which they were arrested and discuss how the presence of sex trafficking is detrimental to that neighborhood. Participants also interact with each other, discussing their own neighborhoods and children while drawing parallels to the damage that they may be fostering in other neighborhoods. One of the key messages emphasized by Red Zone is that "men who buy sex seldom buy in the neighborhood in which they live" [38]. Rather than serve as a platform for education about the sex trade—including sex trafficking—Red Zone takes the extra step of making that information relevant to the participants, taking advantage of the power of participatory community action.

Similarly, an independent, scientific evaluation of the San Francisco "john school" program demonstrated a significant reduction in recidivism among men— i.e., rearrest for solicitation. This program, called the First Offender Prostitution Program (FOPP), gave men arrested for solicitation an opportunity to avoid prosecution by attending a one-day education course on the harmful consequences of sex trafficking [39].

Initiatives to Improve Victim Identification and/or Disruption of Trafficking Rings

Educating Businesses and Their Workers

Communities that come in contact with trafficking victims in transit have become involved in efforts to prevent new cases of trafficking through early identification of victims and detection of human trafficking rings. The US Department of Homeland Security (DHS) and Department of Transportation (DOT) established the Blue Lightning Initiative, which provides training materials to airline workers about the warning signs of human trafficking—and how to report suspected cases to the US government [40]. The US DHS has also partnered with Amtrak to train upwards of

8,000 Amtrak police officers to recognize the signs of human trafficking and intervene on behalf of the victims [41]. Both of these operations fall under the umbrella of the Blue Campaign, which is an initiative led by the DHS aimed at forming partnerships between government agencies, nongovernmental organizations, and private companies to help fight human trafficking. The tourism industry has also been identified as an arena in which workers are more likely to encounter sex traffickers and sex-trafficking victims. "Thecode.org" is a website run by ECPAT-USA, which provides information on trafficking, and registers corporations to provide voluntary trainings for their employees to help recognize human trafficking and intervene on behalf of the victims [42]. In a similar vein, Truckers Against Trafficking trains truck drivers and employees of travel plazas to recognize and report suspected cases of sex trafficking. Truckers Against Trafficking leverages the interactions truckers have as potential customers of sex trafficking victims to identify and dissolve trafficking rings.

UN.GIFT, the United Nations' anti-trafficking program, and the End Human Trafficking Now! campaign (EHTN) have created an e-learning tool and training manual for business leaders, managers, and employees to identify the risks of human trafficking in their supply chains and take action to mitigate these risks [43]. The tool is targeted toward a business audience and draws on information from case studies completed by and within the business community, such as human trafficking in the production of sporting goods, cosmetics, and textiles, as well as in the air travel, tourism, and hospitality markets [37].

Mobile Smartphone Applications for Early Identification and/or Assistance for Survivors

Two new mobile applications for smartphones, created by Redlight Traffic and Orphan Secure, aim to crowdsource the identification of individuals in trafficking situations and streamline the process of reporting potential incidents of human trafficking. Both applications provide user-friendly forms to report a case of suspected trafficking, while the built-in location services of the users' mobile phones provide exact locations to the organization that manages the information, which then communicates with local law enforcement agencies [44, 45]. Orphan Secure's "FREEDOM!" app is available in 12 different languages, and Redlight Traffic enables user photographs to be attached to the reports [38, 39].

Mobile applications are also under development on the victim services side. For example, the application SafeNight (Fig. 4.1) will crowdsource funding for short-term housing to provide emergency shelter for human trafficking victims. As the SafeNight founders state, "By creating a mechanism that engages individual donors to fund emergency, on-demand hotel placements SafeNight will increase the availability of emergency shelter for human trafficking survivors; provide an opportunity for additional services and support to be offered by case managers; and provide data for the field, as a whole, on the real needs for shelter" [46].

Fig. 4.1 Caravan Studio's
SafeNight App [40]

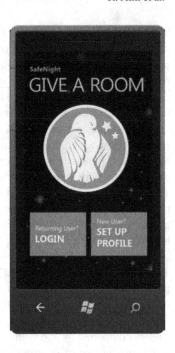

Information Technologies to Identify Criminal Rings Involved in Global Trafficking

Novel information technology is being utilized to disrupt child pornography rings in the USA and throughout the world. Microsoft Corporation's PhotoDNA image recognition technology, which "creates a unique signature for a digital image, something like a fingerprint, which can be compared with the signatures of other images to find copies of that image," is being used by law enforcement agencies to identify child victims through image matching [47]. Social media companies such as Facebook are using this technology to scan all images posted by users and to collaborate with the National Center for Missing & Exploited Children (USA) to flag any images suspected to be child pornography. Furthermore, the technology is being used by the Child Exploitation Tracking System (CETS), a transnational network of law enforcement (e.g., Brazil, the US, the UK) to help track suspected child pornographers [48].

Discussion

Trafficking in persons is a criminal activity that has severe repercussions for individuals' physical and mental health. Furthermore, the population health consequences of this crime (e.g., spread of sexually transmitted infections across populations) are profound. The innovative anti-trafficking initiatives described in this chapter are diverse; some directly target trafficking, while others address one or more social determinants of human trafficking. Some initiatives specifically target trafficking in urban settings, while others address trafficking in rural and/ or urban locales.

From slum-based economic training programs for young women in Kenya and Uganda to "john schools" in San Francisco, these interventions work to address multiple levels of society. At the societal level, public awareness campaigns aim to change gender norms, eliminate violence against women, and promote safe migration. At the community level, training and social enterprise programs create job opportunities and promote awareness of trafficking in "origin" areas. Educational initiatives aim to eliminate trafficking within certain industries and train nontraditional professionals to respond early to human trafficking cases. At the individual level, programs provide skills, business opportunities, and education to vulnerable populations and aim to improve girls' self-esteem.

Technology and "new media," including mobile applications and social networking sites, are beginning to play a more significant role in global anti-trafficking efforts. Human traffickers have been adept at using the Internet and other information technologies to exploit vulnerable individuals. The increased use of information technology by anti-trafficking stakeholders to neutralize and ultimately defeat traffickers is a promising development as such reliance potentially exposes traffickers to scrutiny. Much work is needed to take up this opportunity to advance the anti-trafficking field. For example, as Marshall describes in his article on trafficking behavior theory, shortcomings of current prevention efforts include "the limited evidence on which many interventions are based; insufficiently clear objectives; limited evaluation of outcomes and impacts; and the fact that many prevention activities have been isolated rather than part of a strategic package of interventions" [49].

Overall, eliminating human trafficking is a complex task, especially as urbanization continues its unabated course. The role of innovations in addressing human trafficking cannot be overstated—as a catalyst of ideas for durable interventions and enhancer of multi-sectoral solutions to this global problem. The examples of innovations in anti-trafficking in this chapter have the potential to improve urban health—both directly, by improving health-care access for victims and survivors in cities, and indirectly, by addressing urban poverty, which is a key determinant of trafficking. The health-care community has a particular role to play in anti-trafficking innovations. For instance, the prospect of integrating efforts to combat trafficking into health-care protocols carries particular promise. Prevention, diagnosis, and treatment of trafficking victims demand innovation that accounts for the social embeddedness of exploitation. By focusing attention particularly on the processes of migration, the health-care community can dramatically improve population health in cities and combat the heinous violation of the rights of vulnerable persons.

References

1. International Labour Organization. ILO global estimate of forced labour: results and methodology. Geneva: ILO; 2012. http://www.ilo.org/wcmsp5/groups/public/---ed_norm/---declaration/documents/publication/wcms_182004.pdf.
2. United Nations Office of Drugs and Crime. Protocol to prevent, suppress and punish trafficking in persons, especially women and children, supplementing the United Nations convention against transnational organized crime, 2000. http://www.uncjin.org.
3. US Department of State. Trafficking in Persons Report. 2012. http://www.state.gov/j/tip/rls/tiprpt/2012/.
4. International Labour Organization. Meeting the challenge: proven practices for human trafficking prevention in the Greater Mekong sub-region/Mekong sub-regional project to combat trafficking in children and women, International programme on the elimination of child labour. 2008. http://www.ilo.org/dyn/migpractice/docs/59/2008_traff_meetingthechallenge_mekong_en.pdf.
5. Shelley L. Human trafficking: a global perspective. Cambridge: Cambridge University Press; 2010.
6. Samarasinghe V, Burton B. Strategizing prevention: a critical review of local initiatives to prevent female sex trafficking. Development Practice. 2007;17(1):51–64.
7. International Organization for Migration. Caring for trafficked persons: guidance for health providers. Geneva: International Organization for Migration; 2009.
8. Gupta J, Raj A, Decker MR, Reed E, Silverman JG. HIV vulnerabilities of sex-trafficked Indian women and girls. Int J Gynaecol Obstet. 2009;107(1):30–4.
9. Macias Konstantopoulos W, Ahn R, Alpert EJ, et al. An international comparative public health analysis of sex trafficking of women and girls in eight cities: achieving a more effective health sector response. J Urban Health. 2013;90(6):1194–204.
10. Zimmerman C, Yun K, Shvab I, Watts C, Trappolin L, Treppete M, Bimbi F, Adams B, Jiraporn S, Beci L, Albrecht M, Bindel J, Regan L. The health risks and consequences of trafficking in women and adolescents. Findings from a European study. London: London School of Hygiene & Tropical Medicine (LSHTM); 2003.
11. Nogales A. Human trafficking: sexual slavery—an online course. Zur Institute, Sonoma; 2011. www.zurinstitute.com/human_trafficking_course.html.
12. Williams TP, Alpert EJ, Ahn R, et al. Sex trafficking and health care in metro Manila: identifying social determinants to inform an effective health system response. Health Hum Rights. 2010;12(2):135–47.
13. Huda S. Sex trafficking in South Asia. Int J Gynaecol Obstet. 2006;94(3):374–81.
14. Chuang J. Beyond a snapshot: preventing human trafficking in the global economy. Indiana J Global Legal Studies. 2006;13(1) Article 5:137–63.
15. Wheaton EM, Schauer EJ, Galli TV. Economics of human trafficking. Int Migration. 2010;48:114–41.
16. Tacoli C. Urbanization, gender and urban poverty: paid work and unpaid carework in the city. UNFPA/IIED. 2012. http://pubs.iied.org/pdfs/10614IIED.pdf.
17. United Nations Office on Drugs and Crime. Toolkit to combat trafficking in persons: addressing the root causes. Global programme against trafficking in human beings. 2008. http://www.unodc.org/documents/human-trafficking/HT_Toolkit08_English.pdf.
18. Warnath S. Best practices in trafficking prevention in Europe & Eurasia. Washington, DC: United States Agency for International Development, Creative Associates International, Inc., & Aguirre Division of JBS International. 2009. http://www.nexusinstitute.net/publications/pdfs/Prevention.pdf.
19. Boak A, Boldosser A, Biu O. Smooth flight: a guide to preventing youth trafficking. Project for the prevention of adolescent trafficking. 2003. http://www.childtrafficking.com/Docs/ppat_2003_smooth_flight_guide_prevent_youth_trafficking.pdf.
20. MTV EXIT: join the fight to end human trafficking & modern slavery. 2013. http://mtvexit.org.

21. Men Can Stop Rape: Public Education. 2011. http://files.meetup.com/1337582/MenCanStop Rape.pdf.
22. Men Can Stop Rape: The [YMOST] Campaign. 2011. http://www.mencanstoprape.org/Strength-Media-Portfolio/ymost.html.
23. Men Can Stop Rape: Public Awareness. 2011. http://www.mencanstoprape.org/Public-Awareness/.
24. Men Can Stop Rape: Our Mission & History. 2011. http://www.mencanstoprape.org/Our-Mission-History/.
25. Zhang D. Human trafficking an microfinance: the Lao village development funds. 2007. International Programme on the Elimination of Child and Labour International Labour Organization. http://www.ilo.org/public/english/region/asro/bangkok/child/trafficking/downloads/microfinance-laos.pdf.
26. Century Entrepreneurship Development Agency International: Sweep. 2014. http://ceda-uganda.org/programs/sweep/.
27. TechnoServe: Young Women in Kenya Learn Entrepreneurial Skills. 2014. http://www.technoserve.org/our-work/stories/young-women-in-kenya.
28. GoodWeave: Child-labor-free Certification. 2009. https://www.goodweave.org/about/child_labor_free_rugs.
29. GoodWeave: Schools and Opportunities. 2009. https://www.goodweave.org/about/schools_education_opportunities.
30. More Than Sport: Project Details. 2014. http://www.morethansport.org/partner/185.
31. Not for Sale: Peru Archives. 2013. http://www.notforsalecampaign.org/stories/categories/peru/page/2/.
32. Rebbl Tonic: Sustainability. https://rebbltonic.com/#sustainability.
33. Amare M, Hohfeld L, Waibel H. Finding quality employment through rural urban migration: a case study from Thailand. Proceedings of the German Development Economics Conference, Berlin 2011, No. 4.
34. Breeden J. GCN: Training for combating human trafficking goes mobile. 2013. http://gcn.com/articles/2013/08/26/human-trafficking-app.aspx.
35. Polaris Project. Online Training. http://www.polarisproject.org/what-we-do/national-human-trafficking-hotline/access-training/online-training. Accessed 8 Aug 2014.
36. Domestic violence in Florida: special focus on human trafficking. Florida Medical Association. http://www.dcf.state.fl.us/programs/humantrafficking/docs/DVandVOT.pdf.
37. Massachusetts General Hospital, Division of Global Health & Human Rights, Department of Emergency Medicine: Human Trafficking Initiative. 2014. http://www.massgeneral.org/emergencymedicineglobalhealth/initiatives/Initiative_to_End_Slavery(IES).aspx.
38. Shively M. An overview of the "Red Zone" program, Marion County & Indianapolis. National Institute of Justice & Abt Associates. 2012. http://www.demandforum.net/wp-content/uploads/2012/01/Overview-of-Indianapolis-Red-Zone-Program.pdf.
39. Bell E, Ring M. The sage project: first offender prostitution program. 2013. http://sagesf.org/first-offender-prostitution-program-fopp.
40. Blue Lighting. U.S. Customs and Border Protection. 2014. http://www.cbp.gov/border-security/human-trafficking/blue-lightning.
41. DHS, DOT and Amtrak Announce New Partnership to Combat Human Trafficking. 2013. http://www.dhs.gov/news/2012/10/04/dhs-dot-and-amtrak-announce-new-partnership-combat-human-trafficking.
42. The Code: About. 2012. http://www.thecode.org/about/.
43. Human trafficking and business: an eLearning course on how to prevent and combat human trafficking. United Nations Global Initiative to Fight Human Trafficking. http://www.ungift.org/doc/knowledgehub/resource-centre/GIFT_EHTN_elearning_tool_training_handbook.pdf.
44. Orphan Secure: The Freedom! App Android and iPhone. 2013. http://www.orphansecure.com/orphan_secure_mobile.php.
45. Redlight Traffic: Programs. 2013. http://www.redlighttraffic.org/app/index.html.

46. Caravan Studios: Press. http://www.caravanstudios.org/#!press/cee5.
47. Net clean: Microsoft and NetClean provide PhotoDNA technology to help law enforcement fight online child sexual exploitation. 2012. https://www.netclean.com/en/press/microsoft-and-netclean-provide-photodna-technology-to-help-law-enforcement-fight-online-child-sexual-exploitation/.
48. Microsoft in Public Safety and National Security: Child Exploitation Crimes. 2013. http://www.microsoft.com/government/ww/safety-defense/initiatives/Pages/dcu-child-exploitation.aspx.
49. Marshall P. Rethinking trafficking prevention: a guide to applying behavior theory. United Nations Interagency Project on Human Trafficking and Asian Development Bank. 2011. http://www.ungift.org/doc/knowledgehub/resource-centre/rethinking_Trafficking_Prevention.pdf.

Chapter 5
Securing Cities: Innovations for the Prevention of Civic Violence

Horacio R. Trujillo, Elena Siegel, Malcolm Clayton, Gabe Shapiro, and David Elam

Introduction

The character of large-scale deadly violence around the world is changing. Since World War II, wars between nation states have declined in both number and deadliness. And while it is commonly perceived that wars within states have risen in place of wars among them, intrastate wars have also declined since the end of the Cold War.[1] Nevertheless, as interstate and intrastate wars decline, large-scale violence is increasing in a different form—endemic and oftentimes warlike civic violence or *reactive* and *recurrent* violent expressions of grievances among citizens, individuals, and groups that can range from spontaneous protests to gang warfare to even

---

[1] Human Security Centre, *Human Security Report 2005. War and Peace in the 21st Century*, Oxford University Press (Oxford), December 2005; Edward Newman, "Conflict Research and the 'Decline' of Civil War," *Civil Wars* 11(3), 2009, pp. 255–78. The misstatement regarding the trend in intrastate wars was reported by the International Commission on Intervention and State Sovereignty (ICISS) in its report, *The Responsibility to Protect*, published in 2001 by the International Development Research Centre (Ottawa).

H.R. Trujillo, M.Phil., M.B.A., Ph.D. (✉)
Departments of Politics and of Diplomacy and World Affairs, Occidental College,
Los Angeles, CA, USA
e-mail: htrujillo@oxy.edu

E. Siegel, B.A. • M. Clayton, B.A.
Department of Diplomacy and World Affairs, Occidental College, Los Angeles, CA, USA

G. Shapiro, M.P.D.
University of Southern California, Los Angeles, CA, USA

D. Elam, M.I.A.
Johns Hopkins School for Advanced International Studies, Washington, DC, USA

© Springer New York 2015
R. Ahn et al. (eds.), *Innovating for Healthy Urbanization*,
DOI 10.1007/978-1-4899-7597-3_5

intentional mass violence by the state against its citizenry.[2] Importantly, such violence is largely particular to rapidly growing cities in the developing world, leading to observations that "urban zones are fast-becoming new territories of conflict and violence."[3] In addition, the development of military and humanitarian doctrine is beginning to reflect a more primary concern with the violent city.[4] With this type of endemic and increasingly large-scale urban civic violence representing one of the growing threats to human security around the world, it is critical to outline a research agenda for identifying effective approaches for addressing this threat.

This chapter is an effort to call for and develop one approach to inform a research program on urbanization and violence: the identification of notable innovations to address large-scale civic violence that is associated with the growing challenge of managing heretofore unrealized levels and rates of urbanization. This approach is particularly useful for identifying promising solutions to such large-scale civic violence, because this phenomenon, which is largely urban in character, is still becoming more recognized and understood as urbanization. Even more so, because of the relative novelty of the unprecedented levels of urbanization, even efforts that appear to be effective have largely not yet been subject to more formal empirical analysis. As such, the effort to identify examples of innovative approaches to addressing this type of violence that are more robustly acknowledged to be effective by a variety of sources can help to advance a research agenda in at least three ways—(1) for policymakers, beginning a cataloguing of "good practice" from which others can learn and to spur a careful conversation about what constitutes good practice in these efforts; (2) for researchers, identifying a number of cases to be more carefully evaluated from empirical perspectives to deepen our collective understanding of causal relationships between urbanization and large-scale collective violence, as well as interventions undertaken to address this violence; and (3) for policymakers and researchers, suggesting common phenomena and relationships among these model programs that could be investigated further in an effort to develop the theoretical understanding of this emergent, critical field.

---

[2] On the rise of a new type of urban violence, see both Jo Beall, Dennis Rodgers, and Tom Goodfellow, "Cities, Terrorism and Urban Wars of the 21st Century," *Crisis States Working Papers Series 2*, 85, London School of Economics (London), January 2011, and Robert Muggah with Kevin Savage, "Urban Violence and Humanitarian Action: Engaging the Fragile City," *The Journal of Humanitarian Assistance*, January 19, 2012. The definition of "civic violence," drawn from Beall et al., and its analytical value will be further clarified later in the chapter.

[3] Elena Lucchi, "Between War and Peace: Humanitarian Assistance in Violent Urban Settings," *Disasters* 34:4, October 2010, p. 973.

[4] According to the World Health Organization, in 2004 the approximate number of deaths due to interpersonal violence was nearly 600,000, representing an increase nearly 20 % from 500,000 in 2002. In comparison, the number of deaths in 2004 due to war was approximately 170,000, less than 10 % increase from 182,000 2 years earlier; from World Health Organization, *Cause of Death Estimates: Death by Violence*, World Health Organization (Geneva), 2004. Sean Fox and Christian Hoelscher, "The Political Economy of Social Violence: Theory and Evidence from a Cross-Country Study," *Crisis States Working Papers Series* 2, 72, London School of Economics (London), April 2010. See Alexandre Cautravers, "Military Operations in Urban Areas," *International Review of the Red Cross* 92:878, June 2010, on urbanization's influence on the importance of cities as sites of military and humanitarian operations.

With these objectives in mind, we have reviewed the literature on urban violence, urbanization and violence, and efforts to address urban violence, in order to identify those cases that we felt could be presented as examples of promising innovations to address specifically endemic, large-scale, and collective violence related to urbanization. We focused our attention on this type of violence because of the lesser degree of attention paid to this phenomenon than to urban violence more generally — whether on testing the causal relationship between violence and urbanization, per se, or on identifying good practice in addressing urban violence broadly, which can focus on more individualized even if endemic violence — as well as the potential difference in character of this type of violence, which has generally been understudied.[5]

Case Studies of Addressing Urban Violence

Given the intentionally narrow focus on larger-scale, endemic, and collective violence in urban settings, as well as our effort to identify cases for which we could ascertain some degree of effectiveness, we narrowed our selection down to six cases. These six cases include: a) three programs focused on addressing particularly endemic, large-scale, and collective forms of violent crime in the cities of Diadema, Brazil; Lagos, Nigeria; and Boston, U.S.A.; b) one focused on broad efforts to prevent a recurrence of primarily urban, large-scale electoral violence in Kenya; and c) two focused on inuring urban environments against the risk of endemic urban violence through urban upgrading in Khayelitsha, South Africa, and Women's Safety Audits in various communities.

Together, these cases illustrate three broad lessons for efforts to protect cities from larger-scale, endemic urban violence in particular. The most important of these is not simply a restatement that the causes of violence are myriad and thus a variety of approaches are needed to address it, but rather that endemic, large-scale, and collective violence in urban areas is particularly complex and cannot be effectively addressed as only a problem unto itself. Instead, this violence must be viewed as the ultimate manifestation of other challenges of urbanization that are addressed in this book, ranging from those of the health of individuals and their communities to those related to environmental conditions of cities. Correspondent with this first lesson, a second is that the search for solutions to endemic, large-scale, and collective violence in cities can benefit greatly from an augmented use of a public health approach for

---

[5] See, for example, Halvard Buhaug and Henrik Urdal, "An Urbanization Bomb? Population Growth and Social Disorder in Cities," *Global Environmental Change*, 23:1, February 2013, pp. 1–10; Alessandra Heinemann and Dorte Verner, "Crime and violence in development: A literature review of Latin America and the Caribbean," *World Bank Policy Research Working Paper* 4041, 2006; Brennan-Galvin, Ellen, "Crime and violence in an urbanizing world," Columbia University Journal of International Affairs, 56:1, 2002, pp. 123–46; Caroline O.N. Moser, "Urban violence and insecurity: an introductory roadmap," *Environment & Urbanization*, 16:2 October 2004; Peter Gizewski and Thomas F. Homer-Dixon, "Urban Growth and Violence: Will the Future Resemble the Past?" *American Association for the Advancement of Science*, 1995.

analysis and program design. Because of the increasing potential for such violence to flare up in the face of unprecedented urbanization and yet still be limited to a small number of cases, as well as the variation among these cases, it is not likely that we will be able to rely on broad empirical analysis of a large number of interventions to better establish clear evidence of universal best practice. Instead, we are more likely to have to rely on continual innovation in the face of emerging conditions, matched by more careful evaluation of the effectiveness of these interventions, documentation of the results of these efforts, and increased sharing of this understanding. This brings up the third lesson, again drawing from the public health field: to move us ahead in the efforts not only to intervene to stop this form of violence but even more so to prevent it from arising in the first place requires more careful data collection and evaluation regarding the effects of these various innovations. These efforts will provide more cases from which we can draw strong lessons and will prevent us from relying on models that we can only hold up as promising.

Urbanization and Endemic, Large-Scale Violence

While the relationship between violence and urbanization is colored by the character of the urbanization—with violence being more strongly associated with growth in inequality and other factors than simply growth in the geographic expanse, population size or population density of cities—it is nonetheless the case that many cities, especially larger cities in Latin America and Africa, have experienced dramatic increases in the levels of violence affecting their populations.[6] It should not be overlooked that if the pace of urbanization is taken into account, there is a stronger association between urbanization, per se, and violence, with higher rates of violence seen in more rapidly urbanizing environments, particularly urban agglomerations.[7] Moreover, as Gizweski and Homer-Dixon note, studies that find little causality from urbanization to growth are looking at levels of urbanization that pale in comparison to the levels we look to face in the not-too-distant future, and oftentimes use a limited number of theories that do not take into careful consideration urbanization as an influence that can catalyze other causal factors rather than being a uniquely causal factor in itself.[8]

To this point, the dynamic relationship between urbanization and violence can itself sow the seeds of greater violence. For example, in some cases, the entire neighborhoods, or even larger areas of cities, particularly poorer areas, can become so violent that the climate of fear and distrust created by chronic violence gets entrenched, such that it engenders additional violence justified as defense. In some

---

[6] Beall, Rodgers and Goodfellow, *op cit.*

[7] World Bank Social Development Department Conflict, Crime and Violence Team, *Violence in the City*, The International Bank for Reconstruction and Development/The World Bank, April 2011, pp. 18–19.

[8] Among the factors that can contribute to large-scale violence and which urbanization could potentially catalyze, Gizewski and Thomas F. Homer-Dixon, *op cit*, identify economic crisis, deteriorated social capital due to communalism or criminality, democratization, and the availability of arms.

of these cases, such areas can become effectively "no-go zones" into which public safety officials will not venture, trapping the already marginalized populations in a mutually reinforcing cycle of insecurity, violence, and poverty. In other cases, governments can take more forceful actions to reassert control that undermine the governance of the city or even the broader country, such as in the case of heightened violence in capital cities, again unintentionally fostering conditions that put societies at higher risk of such violence. Even in countries where most of the population is rural, such as in Guatemala, and in regions with relatively lower levels of urban violence, such as in the Middle East or Western Europe, urban violence can often-times still be significantly higher than violence outside of cities.[9]

The Impacts of Urban Violence

In economic terms, the costs of urban violence are found in both a direct loss of gross national income and, even more significantly, in the reduction of growth rates, contrib-uting to worsened socioeconomic prospects over the long run. At a microlevel, violence, and even the fear of it, deters and constrains individuals from investing to improve future prospects. It can prevent citizens from furthering their own education, saving financial capital, or developing businesses and even from seeking efficient and improved employment opportunities due to the risk of intracity travel. At a macro level, violence erodes trust among persons, limiting the formation and even distorting both civil and governmental social capital critical to effective collective action and governance.[10] Various studies have attempted to quantify the overall economic cost of violence in rapidly urbanizing regions, suggesting that the direct costs of urban crime and violence can amount to significant percentages of GDP and stunt growth rates. For example, the UN Office on Drugs and Crime (UNODC) and the World Bank report that in Guatemala, violence concentrated primarily in the capital city cost the country $2.4 billion or 7.3 % of GDP in 2005 alone. Given the higher risk for violence that is associated with lower levels of economic development, the need to curtail violence is a critical objective in breaking the poverty-violence trap.[11]

Worse, this challenge is likely to be aggravated as cities in the developing world that are already home to half of the world's population continue to grow rapidly over the next 25 years, ultimately absorbing almost all of the new population growth expected during this time.[12] While the development of cities has been key to economic growth and improved life opportunities for millions of persons in these countries,

---

[9] World Bank Social Development Department Conflict, Crime and Violence Team, *op cit*; Oliver Jütersonke et al. "Gangs and Violence Reduction in Central America," *Security Dialogue* 40, October 2009; UN-HABITAT, *Global Report on Human Settlements 2007: Enhancing Urban Safety and Security*, Earthscan (London), 2007.

[10] World Bank Social Development Department Conflict, Crime and Violence Team, *op cit.*

[11] World Bank, *World Development Report 2011: Conflict, Security and Development*; Paul Collier, *Breaking the conflict trap: Civil war and development policy*, Oxford University Press, 2003.

[12] UN-HABITAT, *op cit.*

especially over the past several decades, many urban areas are now themselves sites of increasing poverty, driven both by their absorption of more of the rural poor and dramatic rises in economic inequality. As a result, today more than one-quarter of all urban residents around the world live in slums.[13] The collection of global trends thus unfortunately exemplifies a commonly accepted understanding of the dynamics of urban violence—as cities grow larger, different social conditions are manifest, including lower probabilities of being recognized and punished, which influence the preferences of individuals, criminality, and the rise of violence. The growth of slums that accompanies particularly rapid growth of cities exacerbates this permissiveness because of the characteristically weaker governance of these spaces.[14]

New Levels of Violence and Novel Approaches

While the sketch above outlines the critical challenge of urban violence broadly, we focus our attention in this chapter on innovations that present promising models for addressing endemic and larger-scale civic violence that has the potential for becoming mass violence. We have identified this focus, both to explore a specific aspect of the problem of urban violence and to suggest a new direction for further development of the field, given the trends reviewed above that indicate that the risk of larger-scale civic violence in cities may be rising.[15] Our approach builds upon the argument of Beall, Rodgers, and Goodfellow, who themselves suggest that while cities have historically been seen as critical elements in the process of political consolidation due to their concentration of economic and political power, they are increasingly becoming primary sites of state erosion across much of the developing world.[16] The passages below explore the political theory of conflicts and changing conceptions of the relationship between urbanization, politics, and violence, before focusing on theoretical concepts from work on civic conflicts and "collective efficacy" to support a new direction for analysis developed in the case studies.

Why the change in the role of cities from bulwarks of political consolidation, as was the case in the development of Europe, to loci of political disintegration in today's rapidly urbanizing countries? A critical difference, according to Beall and Fox, is that cities in the developing world, particularly in fragile regions, have had a tendency, due to patterns inherent in both colonialism and decolonization, to grow rapidly without the concurrent emergence of an industrial working class or an

[13] UN-HABITAT, *op cit*; see David Mayer, *Urbanization as a Fundamental Cause of Development*, Centro de Investigación y Docencia Económicas, División de Economía (Mexico), 2010, for a recent study on the contribution of urbanization to development.

[14] Edward L. Glaeser and Bruce Sacerdote, "Why is There More Crime in Cities?" *NBER Working Paper*, w5430, January 1996; Mayra Buvinić and Andrew R. Morrison, "Living in a More Violent World," *Foreign Policy*, 118 Spring 2000, pp. 58–72; Joseph L. Derdzinski, *Rapid Urban Settlement, Violence, and the Democratizing State: Toward an Understanding*, United States Air Force Academy Institute for National Security Studies, 2006.

[15] Gizewski and Homer-Dixon, *op cit*.

[16] Beall et al., 2011, *op cit*.

autonomous urban capitalist class that can undergird the state.[17] A related factor is that this previously seen relationship between political authority and urban productive classes that supported nation-building is weaker today when political authorities are able to seek resources for state consolidation from external sources, in the form of not only foreign investment but also official development assistance. Ironically, this externally-sourced financing of the state can even serve to help the state quell generative political contestation that can advance nation-building.[18] This work builds on Beall's observation that cities have historically been sites and sources of such generative political contestation, but today such conflict can also turn violent due to various factors, ranging from the influence of international terrorism to the model of governments using violence against their own citizens.[19] In his own work, Rodgers similarly explores the political character of violence typically considered to be only "social," such as violence among gangs and associated with organized crime.[20]

As such, in defining the focus of our study, we borrow from Beall, Rodgers and Goodfellow's exploration of the changing forms of violent conflict in fragile settings and especially how these forms of conflict relate to cities in their useful framework for categorizing conflict. In their framework, they move past previous efforts to categorize conflict as "political, social, or economic" or "interstate or intrastate" and instead classify conflict as "sovereign," "civil," and "civic." *Sovereign conflicts* are those situations in which international actors are directly and explicitly involved, and thus the sovereignty of at least one state's territory is challenged. While cities are involved in sovereign conflicts, because they are sites of political and economic power considered important to capture and control, this paper does not address this particular form of urban violence, as it tends to be extraordinary. *Civil conflicts*, in comparison, are violent conflicts in which organized, non-state, military groups with political objectives for the territory and the ability to resist the state for a sustained period of time challenge the monopoly of violence typically held by the state.[21]

---

[17] Jo Beall and Sean Fox, *Cities and Development,* Routledge (London), 2009.

[18] See Mick Moore, "Revenues, State Formation, and the Quality of Governance in Developing Countries," *International Political Science Review*, 25(3), 2004, pp. 297–319; Mick Moore, Democratic Governance and Poverty Reduction, Working Paper, University of Sussex Institute of Development Studies Centre for the Future State, 2004; Mick Moore, "Political Underdevelopment. What Causes Bad Governance?" *Public Management Review* 3(3), 2001, pp. 385–418.

[19] See Jo Beall, Cities, Terrorism and Urban Wars of the 21st Century, *Crisis States Working Papers Series 2*, 9, February 2007, London School of Economics (London).

[20] See Dennis Rodgers, "Urban violence is not (necessarily) a way of life: towards a political economy of conflict in cities," *UNU-WIDER Working Paper* 2010/20, March 2010 UNU-WIDER (Helskinki); Dennis Rodgers, "Slum Wars of the 21st Century: Gangs, *Mano Dura* and the New Urban Geography of Conflict in Central America," *Development and Change* 40(5), September 2009, pp. 949–76; and Dennis Rodgers, "Slum Wars of the 21st Century: the new geography of conflict in Central America," *Crisis States Working Papers Series 2*, 10, February 2007 London School of Economics (London).

[21] This definition largely coincides with that of Melvin Small and J. David Singer from their *Resort to Arms: International and Civil War, 1816–1980*, 1982 Sage (Beverly Hills). See Richard Sambanis, "What is Civil War? Conceptual and Empirical Complexities of an Operational Definition," *Journal of Conflict Resolution* 48(6), December 2004, pp. 814–58, for a recent discussion of the debate over the methodology for distinguishing "civil wars" from other forms of organized, collective violence, particularly interstate and extrastate wars.

Beall, Rodgers, and Goodfellow further suggest that the relationship between civil conflict and urban areas is more complicated. This complexity is due in part to a difference in tactics used, as parties in civil wars can undertake efforts to destabilize social and economic structures, generate fear among noncombatants, and even target particular groups of persons, such as ethnic/racial, religious, or political minorities.[22] While cities have historically not been seen as central in civil conflict, because rebel and minority groups tend to strategically militarize by basing themselves in rural areas or holding fast to their homelands outside of urban centers to avoid the reach of the state, Staniland offers a corrective to this interpretation in his identification of several civil conflicts characterized primarily by urban insurgency.[23]

Civic conflicts, in contrast to sovereign and civil conflicts, are *reactive* and *recurrent* violent expressions of grievances—be they social, political, or economic—among citizens, individuals, and groups, including the state. These conflicts can range from spontaneous protests or communal riots to organized violent crime or gang warfare, and even to terrorism and intentional persecution of the state against its citizenry.[24] Civic conflicts generally occur in cities, which offer physical and social characteristics for mass mobilization, including high population density, diversity, and compressed inequality, and are oftentimes spurred specifically by the state's inadequacy in properly providing the infrastructure for security, growth, and welfare of urban populations. Civic conflicts can overlap with civil conflict and even sovereign conflict; however, unlike these other conflicts, civic conflicts may be isolated expressive events or connected by a sustained set of political demands, but they do not have goals of seizing or permanently altering formal structures of power. Because civic conflicts are thus less characterized by "indivisible" goals that require an "all or nothing" settlement, they are more amenable to resolution.

This definition of the subject of our study as civic violence also corresponds with the observation of the World Bank that current policy approaches that treat social, political, and economic violence separately can be found lacking in power, given that the lines between these different expressions of violence are blurry.[25] As such, in its study, the World Bank leans heavily on the theory of Robert Sampson, in which he proposes a theory of violence prevention as a product of "collective efficacy" that is necessary for communities to maintain public order. According to Sampson,

---

[22] Jo Beall, Dennis Rodgers, and Tom Goodfellow, op cit, and Stathis Kalyvas, *The Logic of Violence in Civil War*, Working Paper presented at the Laboratory in Comparative Ethnic Processes (LiCEP-1) at Duke University, March 2000.

[23] Paul Staniland, "Cities on Fire: Social Mobilization, State Policy and Urban Insurgency," *Comparative Political Studies* 43(12), December 2010, pp. 1623–49.

[24] Beall, Rodgers and Goodfellow, *op cit*, emphasize the link with the state and the association with citizenship that leads them to use the term "civic conflict" rather than social, economic, or political violence, although what we consider under the rubric of civic conflict has also been described in these terms.

[25] World Bank Social Development Department Conflict, Crime and Violence Team, *Violence in the City*, The International Bank for Reconstruction and Development/The World Bank, April 2011.

communities need more than networks and social ties to effectively maintain public order; collective efficacy, defined as "social control enacted under conditions of social trust," is itself a product of shared expectations for action with working trust. According to this theory, despite weak ties among community members, the existence of shared values and expectations can enable enough trust for the community to achieve common goals. Sampson's "collective efficacy" theory thus offers a more robust framework through which we can identify and understand the potential for innovative interventions to address civic violence.

Without relying on the theoretical conclusions of Beall, Rodgers, and Goodfellow or the World Bank and Sampson, we utilized their concepts of civic violence and collective efficacy to guide both our selection of case studies and the lessons we draw from them. We turn now to reviewing these cases studies individually before pulling together common lessons and, in particular, restating our suggestions for further research in our conclusion. We begin first with the case studies focused on city-level efforts to address endemic civic violence in Diadema, Brazil; Lagos, Nigeria; and Boston, USA, before moving on to the particularly contemporary example of civic violence associated with national elections in Kenya. Finally, we look to a case study focused on a particular methodology employed in multiple cities: Women's Safety Audits.

Case Studies

Case 1: Diadema, Brazil

The city of Diadema, Brazil, rapidly grew in population between 1950 and 1980, making it the second most densely populated location in Brazil. By 1999, Diadema's murder rates ranked among the highest in the world, reaching 141 per 100,000 persons. As suggested in the 2007 *Enhancing Urban Safety and Security: Global Report on Human Settlements*, this level of large-scale violence was significant enough to culminate in near anarchy and a complete collapse of law and order.[26] To address the high incidence of violence, the municipal government in Diadema enacted a multi-sectoral, mixed-model approach for violence reduction, including a cost-effective preventive measure restricting alcohol sales. This approach presents a useful model for cities experiencing high rates of crime, particularly due to its emphasis on local actors, risk factors, and prevention policies.

A diverse group of political actors in Diadema, including the mayor, city council, military and police chiefs, businesses, and religious and community leaders, created a holistic approach to intervene and prevent violence.[27] The monthly town meetings

---

[26] UN-HABITAT, *Global Report on Human Settlements 2007, op cit.*, p. 94.

[27] World Bank Poverty Reduction and Economic Management Sector Unit Latin America and the Caribbean Region, *Crime, Violence, and Economic Development in Brazil: Elements for Effective Public Policy*, The International Bank for Reconstruction and Development/The World Bank, June 2006, p. 58.

resulted in a strategy with security, health, education, and urban development policy implications.[28] While the variety of policy interventions resulted in a mixed-model approach, a simple yet significant element of the strategy was the "Last Call" law that closed bars in Diadema between 11:00 pm and 6:00 am. The law was motivated by the municipal government's tracking of violence, which revealed that two of every three homicides in Diadema were alcohol related and that nearly the same proportion occurred between these hours.[29] Prior to its implementation, public education programs and alcohol retailer education occurred, garnering public support for the policies. After implementation, the municipal national guard and the state police forces partnered to engage in daily monitoring to ensure compliance and enforcement. This rather simple adjustment of policy alone contributed to a reduction in the number of homicides by more than 100 per year.[30]

It is important to note that the multi-sectoral strategy came into fruition during a period of slum reurbanization, which began in 1983 to address poor health and education systems and infrastructure.[31] The municipal government in Diadema implemented the "Last Call" law after the overall trends in violence began decreasing after 1999, and thus, while its impact is a factor, the law should be considered in the context of other interventions.[32] Additionally, demographic shifts in Brazil over time are another important factor in the decrease in homicide rates.

Nonetheless, the case of Diadema demonstrates one essential factor to consider in the construction of public health approaches to urban violent crime: local governments are best equipped to evaluate the protection and risk factors in their communities. While resource scarcity may present challenges to the creation of prevention policies at the municipal level, political resistance can be overcome through the implementation of preventive policies that have short-term results, such as the model adopted in Diadema.[33] Prevention measures are less costly than reactive interventions and can lead to both short- and long-term goals in violence prevention. The case of Diadema demonstrates both how a multi-sectoral, integrated response can diminish violence, and how one particular policy applied in the appropriate context can lead to great strides in violence reduction and prevention. Diadema also presents an opportunity for researchers to revisit and renew data collection and monitoring efforts while

---

[28] Shelley de Botton, "Diadema's historic plunging homicide rate, when government and civil society join forces," Comunidad Segura (www.comunidadsegura.org), October 10, 2006.

[29] Sergio Duailibi, et al., "The Effect of Restricting Opening Hours," *American Journal of Public Health* 97:12, December 2007.

[30] Ibid.

[31] Jose de Felipi, "Diadema, SP, Brazil: Housing, Urban Design, and Citizenship," *ReVista: Harvard Review of Latin America*, Spring/Summer 2010.

[32] Joao M. De Mello and Alexandre Schneider, "Assessing São Paulo's Large Drop in Homicides: The Role of Demography and Policy Interventions" in Rafael Di Tella et al., *The Economics of Crime: Lessons for and from Latin America*, University of Chicago Press (Chicago), 2010, p. 209.

[33] World Bank Conflict, Crime, and Violence Team, *Violence in the City: Understanding and Supporting Community Responses to Urban Violence,* April 2011; World Bank Poverty Reduction and Economic Management Sector Unit Latin America and the Caribbean Region, *op cit,* p. 62.

further evaluating the complex causal relationships between reurbanization, demographic shifts, and levels of large-scale collective violence, as well as the interventions undertaken to address them.

Case 2: Lagos, Nigeria

Lagos, Nigeria, has sustained high growth in population, recently becoming the largest "megacity" in Africa.[34] However, the city was marked not just by a high level of violence but also by a breakdown in social trust in part due to the perceived inadequacy of police responses to crime.[35] In 1999, the newly reinstituted civilian government began to create reforms to diminish crime rates and increase perceived citizen security.[36] Within these reforms, public-private partnerships were created to fund the security sector and improve relations between civilians and police forces. While the confluence of reforms is responsible for the period of reduced crime rates, the approach in Lagos demonstrates the utility of public-private partnerships in rapidly urbanizing cities to improve and expand access to funds.

In Lagos, rapid urbanization has weakened infrastructure and contributed to larger resource deficits.[37] Furthermore, inequality within the civilian population has led to an "architecture of fear" that causes the wealthy to create elaborate security buffers, leading to the fragmentation of public space.[38] A 2004 survey of Lagos indicated that sixty-nine percent of respondents feared being victims of crimes, with eighty-nine percent of these respondents suggesting they feared in particular the loss of their own lives.[39] Indeed, in the first 5 years following the implementation of reforms, perceived rates of crime remained high.[40] To address the pervasive effect of large-scale violence on social trust, the Lagos state government began a multifaceted

---

[34] John Campbell, "This is Africa's New Biggest City: Lagos, Nigeria, Population 21 Million," *The Atlantic*, July 10, 2012.

[35] Fola Arthur-Worrey and Innocent Chukwuma, "The Lagos State Crime and Safety Survey, Challenges and Outcome" in Margaret Shaw and Vivien Carli (eds), *Practical Approaches to Urban Crime Prevention: Proceeding of the Workshop held at the 12th UN Congress on Crime Prevention and Criminal Justice, Salvador, Brazil, April 12–19, 2010*, pp. 51–58.

[36] Michael O. Filani, *A City in Transition: Vision, Reform, and Growth in Lagos, Nigeria*, unpublished monograph, nd (ca 2010–2011), p. 64.

[37] Arthur-Worrey and Innocent Chukwuma, *op cit*, p. 51.

[38] Tunde Agbola, *The Architecture of Fear: Urban Design and Construction Response to Urban Violence in Lagos, Nigeria*, Institut français de recherche en Afrique, 1997, accessed in June 2013 via OpenEdition Books at http://books.openedition.org/ifra/485

[39] E.O. Alemika and I.C. Chukwuma (2005) *Criminal Victimization and Fear of Crime in Lagos Metropolis, Nigeria*, Cleen Foundations Monograph Series No. 1, accessed in June 2013 at http://www.cleen.org/LAGOS%20CRIME%20SURVEY.pdf

[40] 44 % of survey respondents answered that crime had increased between 1999 and 2004, while 38 % answered that it had decreased. Source: Alemika and Chukwuma, *op cit*, p. 23.

approach that included security and safety reforms, social and environmental development, and government-community dialogue.

Interventions to improve security in Lagos include the creation of a central security surveillance system and an emergency call center, the expansion of the state's Rapid Response Squad, and the amplification of complementary community security outfits and a community security assembly.[41] Within the context of these initiatives, a state security committee gave its recommendations to the government, indicating that deficient resources greatly inhibited police forces in decreasing rates of crime.[42]

To address the concern of underfunded security forces, one important initiative was the creation of the Lagos State Security Trust Fund (LSSTF) in 2007. The LSSTF mobilizes resources from the government, private sector, and citizens to sustain and improve security operations in Lagos. In its first 2 years alone, the LSSTF raised twenty-seven million US dollars in voluntary contributions to direct to efforts including the provision of direct support to security forces in the form of equipment supplies; training and development for local patrolling capacity; and underwriting community assemblies and town hall meetings to foster constrictive interaction between security forces and Lagos residents.[43] In the years immediately following the creation of LSSTF, reported rates of both murder and armed robbery incidents fell and perceived rates of crime decreased.[44,45] Though crime rates have recently increased again in Lagos, the relative peaceful state experienced for multiple consecutive years after reforms were implemented indicates that providing resources for security forces contributed to quelled crime and violence.[46]

It is clear that rapidly urbanizing cities will need to improve and expand security forces to maintain citizen safety and security, while struggling to attain available funds. By adopting innovative funding models similar to the Lagos State Security Fund, governments can gain access to more resources for more effective security forces to decrease violence, while realizing better resource management, greater transparency, and improved accountability. Furthermore, the Lagos public-private partnership model should also be considered for areas outside of security. As rapid urbanization continues, an increasing population will need to rely on proper infrastructure and government institutions with limited resources. In this way, the Lagos model for public-private partnerships to fund government entities should be implemented to better provide for citizens of growing cities in other areas of governance that will become increasingly important due to rapid urbanization.

---

[41] Filani, *op cit*, pp. 64–5.

[42] Lagos State Security Trust Fund, "About us…" *Lagos State Security Trust Fund* website accessed in June 2013 at http://www.lagosstatesecuritytrustfund.org/profile

[43] Arthur-Worrey and Innocent Chukwuma, *op cit*, pp. 51–3.

[44] Arthur-Worrey and Innocent Chukwuma, *op cit*, p. 57, and Alemika and Omotosho, *op cit*, p. 47.

[45] Arthur-Worrey and Innocent Chukwuma, *op cit*, p. 57.

[46] Arthur-Worrey and Innocent Chukwuma, *op cit*, p. 58; and Comfort Oseghale. "Mixed Feelings in Lagos Over Crime Rate," *Punch Magazine* (Nigeria), July 14, 2012, accessed in June 2013 at http://www.punchng.com/feature/crime-digest/mixed-feelings-in-lagos-over-crime-rate/

Case #3: Boston, USA

Although not applied in a rapidly urbanizing location, Operation Cease Fire, the problem-oriented policing model applied in Boston from 1996–1999, provides an example of an innovative midterm approach for addressing violence in the city.[47] In the midst of the crack cocaine epidemic and more lucrative trade for Boston gangs, youth homicide rates in Boston increased sharply, with homicide victimization rates doubling for young white males and tripling for young black males between 1987 and 1990.[48] The Cease Fire model combines data analysis, centralization and coordination of enforcement responses, and innovative communication practices to reduce youth homicides resulting from gang violence. In Boston, the program reduced youth homicides by two-thirds over a 4-year period.[49]

At the suggestion of a group of criminologists, a working group was formed with assistance from the Boston Police Department's (BPD) gang unit that included members from across a wide swath of government agencies. The working group served as a centralizing body to direct, not simply coordinate, enforcement action toward reducing lethal violence by and against youth. Academics in the group conducted research and analysis that enabled development of an enforcement approach specific to the communities, types of weapons, agents of violence, and victims of violence. Four key findings arose from the analysis: First, a geographic mapping of homicides narrowed problem areas. Second, clear data on the source and types of guns used in the homicides was collected. Third, analysis showed that a majority of the youth offenders had been arraigned at least once in the past, and a significant portion had been in social services, on probation, or previously on probation. Fourth, the violence was highly concentrated among gang members. Three percent of the youth in the problem neighborhoods were in gangs, but they accounted for 60 % of the youth homicides.[50] This analysis challenged some previously held assumptions and

[47] Michael S. Scott, "Problem-Oriented Policing: Reflections on the First 20 Years." Office of Community-Oriented Policing Services, U.S. Department of Justice. October 2000. Problem-oriented policing is a framework developed by Herman Goldstein that calls upon police to address the underlying conditions of problems and then address them with a broader tool set than traditionally applied, specifically to apply a community-oriented approach that considers methods beyond improving normal enforcement and procedural tools to expanding resources and networks to addressing a specific problem.

[48] Anthony Braga, et al., "Reducing Gun Violence: The Boston Gun Project's Operation Ceasefire." U.S. Department of Justice Office of Justice Programs/National Institute of Justice, NCJ 188741, September 2001. According to Braga, et al., minority of men suffered in particular due to a combination of stressors including street drug activity, structural social and economic difficulties, and a concentration of violence in their communities.

[49] Boston Police Department, "Operation Cease Fire: Deterring Youth Firearm Violence," Submission for the Herman Goldstein Award, Center for Problem–Oriented Policing website, accessed in June 2013 at http://www.popcenter.org/library/awards/goldstein/1998/98-08(W).pdf

[50] Anthony Braga, et al., "Problem-Oriented Policing, Deterrence, and Youth Violence: An Evaluation of Boston's Operation Ceasefire," *Journal of Research in Crime and Delinquency* 38:3, August 2001, p. 196.

reinforced others, allowing for more effective design of the program than one based on existing conventional logic.

Though a crackdown on gun trafficking was included as part of the program, the bulk of the enforcement operation was the "pulling levers" strategy, developed to greatly increase the costs of violence to gangs. The strategy was implemented by applying a response that was "certain, rapid, and whatever range of severity the working group felt appropriate" only to the gangs that committed violence. If a gang engaged in violence, the working group would, within days, organize a crackdown on that gang's activities by calling in outstanding warrants, disrupting drug activity, imposing stricter parole and probation arrangements, and bringing in federal authorities, thereby increasing the costs of business for that specific gang.[51]

The innovation of direct communication of the working group to the gangs is credited with the success of the program. The working group communicated via "forums," wherein known gang members with probation or parole obligations were forced to attend. Here the working group laid out expectations, provided explanations of why certain gangs were targeted, provided handouts, and made the cause and effect mechanism explicitly clear: that the enforcement was a penalty directly tied to engagement in violence. The forums were reinforced through one-on-one communication of social service workers, beat cops, and parole officers to identified youth and their families. This message to stop the violence was also greatly supported by black churches in coordination with the operation.[52]

This communications project amplified the power of the agencies. Constrained by resources, the operation could only organize a crackdown on a few gangs at any given time. By leveraging credible threat and community legitimacy, the deterrence capabilities never had to be tested on a major scale.

The importance of the communication channels is evidenced by the resurgence of violence in the early 2000s. When the operation ceased, violence resurged in familiar gun violence "hot spots."[53] A shifting of personnel led to a discontinuation of the communication program, signaling the end of the operation.[54] This led to fraying of community contacts, in particular with the churches. Once rates of youth violence grew again, a broad and un-targeted application of police presence in communities exacerbated the strained relations with communities, and a subsequent weakening of police legitimacy followed.[55]

This case shows that partnership between academics and law enforcement officials directed at solving a specific problem is a viable undertaking. Furthermore, the Boston case presents an opportunity for researchers to explore data collection

---

[51] Boston Police Department, p. 5.

[52] Anthony Braga et al., "Losing Faith? Police, Black Churches, and the Resurgence of Youth Violence in Boston," *Ohio State Journal of Criminal Law*, Vol. 6, Fall 2008, p. 141, 136.

[53] Michael Buerger et al., "Hot Spots of Predatory Crime: Routine Activities and the Criminology of Place," *Criminology*, 27: 1, February 1989, pp. 27–56.

[54] Esther Scott, "Revisiting Gang Violence in Boston," Kennedy School of Government Case #1887.0, 2007, p. 20.

[55] Braga et al. (2008), *op cit.*, p. 185.

methods surrounding causal links between large-scale collective violence and interventions involving partnership between academics and law enforcement officials, which in turn may provoke innovative methods for future evaluation from empirical perspectives. Additionally, clear, direct communication of law enforcement goals through various and coordinated channels can provide needed leverage when resources are limited to prevent gangs from engaging in outright violence.

Case #4: Nairobi, Kenya

The violence that followed the 2007 presidential election crisis in Kenya was concentrated largely in Nairobi and other urban environments, and is one of the most vivid examples of civic violence in recent global memory. More than one thousand persons were killed in the violence, with an estimated six hundred thousand additional persons displaced from their homes and communities. The shadow of the violence was so large that as the 2013 presidential elections neared, concerns about a recurrence of such violence—and potentially even worse violence—were high, not only in Kenya but across the globe. This concern, however, was matched, and arguably even surpassed, by widespread efforts, particularly by civil society actors, to innovate effective means by which to prevent such violence.

The conflict centered on allegations of electoral manipulation by incumbent President Mwai Kibaki by his opponent Raila Odinga. The violence fell largely along ethnic divides, with acute effects of the violence in impoverished regions. Early efforts at mediation failed and protests began to increase in intensity, frequency, and attendance. Eventually, a mediation led by UN Secretary General Kofi Annan developed a tenuous power-sharing agreement called the National Accord and Reconciliation Act, establishing an office of Prime Minister and creating a coalition government. Kibaki retained his presidency and Odinga became the new Prime Minister.

The violence that emerged in Kenya after the elections was not solely the result of perceived vote rigging, but reflected a deeper malaise within the population; widespread unemployment (especially among the youth), the lack of ability to vote for a large percentage of the population (only 69 % of eligible voters were registered to vote), and public frustration with the government set the stage for the crisis. Ethnic tension was another factor; the Council on Foreign Relations indicates that the country is divided among 5 ethnic groups. Much support for the incumbent Kibaki was drawn from the Kikuya, which is the largest ethnic group. Given the ethnic divisions, it is perhaps unsurprising that the largest contributing factor to the violence has been identified as the caustic rhetoric of the politicians themselves, disseminated via mobile phones (especially text messages). Additional methods of dissemination included more public mediums, such as ethnic radio talk shows. It is important to note that for Kenyans, these are the two dominant forms of mass communication.[56]

[56] Joel D. Barkan, "Electoral Violence in Kenya, Contingency Planning Memorandum No. 17," *Council on Foreign Relations*, January 2013.

Radio broadcasts are easy to monitor and shut down; mobile phone communication, on the other hand, represents a serious challenge of control. Unless monitors have access and control to the network itself, monitoring becomes an impossible task. Not to be overlooked is the manner of the violence itself, which was characterized by its brutality; much of the violence was undertaken with crude weapons, such as machetes, clubs, and even bows and arrows.[57,58] The police force in Kenya was (and still is) ill-equipped in personnel and training to deal with the level of unrest that followed the 2007 elections, and it lacks legitimacy as a separate civil service entity. Criminal gangs, which sensed opportunity in the unrest, were noted to have taken advantage of the confusion to commit crimes and killings unrelated to the politics of the crisis.[59]

In the face of these challenges, a new Kenyan constitution and various structural reforms have been adopted to address the threat of election-related violence.[60] A ban on hate speech is now in place, with broadcasters held responsible for the propagation of any such messages and all radio stations equipped with technology to broadcast on delay so that hate speech can be identified and blocked. Structural reforms to the election itself may also play a role in mitigating violence related to a two-candidate runoff situation. A complex election system has created roles for 384 members of a new legislature, including 47 governors. In addition, introduction of a new county system of subnational government structures might serve to mitigate ethnic violence by changing the nature of representation within the election process for different groups.

Structural top-down changes were necessary. However, bottom-up, unique, and innovative responses to the crisis are particularly encouraging, because they seek to involve greater swaths of the population. The most celebrated of these responses has been a new form of mobile crowd-sourcing technology from the nonprofit Ushahidi. The technology creates citizen reporters out of those who have mobile devices and allows them to report intimidation or crimes anonymously. The data is directly uploaded to a virtual map, where authorities, civil service organizations, and international watchdog groups can witness and monitor what is happening and where. Ushahidi ("testimony" in Swahili) has also launched a new project specific to the 2013 elections called Uchaguzi ("elections"). The service has been specifically tailored to enable citizens to monitor the electoral process and includes categories for hate speech and polling clerk bias.[61] Uchaguzi is different from Ushahidi in that it will include a verification process (utilizing over 200 volunteers) before sending

---

[57] Gray Phombeah, "Can Kenya avoid election bloodshed?" *BBC News* online (www.bbcnews.co.uk), October 16, 2012, accessed in June 2013 at http://www.bbc.co.uk/news/world-africa-19948429

[58] Ryan Cummings, "Kenya's 2013 election: Will History Repeat Itself?" *Think Africa Press* online (www.thinkafricapress.com), November 8, 2012, accessed in May 2013 at http://thinkafricapress.com/kenya/projections-upcoming-2013-elections

[59] Joel D. Barkan, *op cit.*

[60] Ibid.

[61] Sara Jerving, "Can Technology and 'Testimony' Prevent Violence in Kenyan Elections?" *TechPresident*/Personal Democracy Media (www.techpresident.com), February 6, 2013.

the reports to electoral authorities or security personnel on the ground to respond. This technology's innovation is twofold: one is its aggregation of user responses into a single, discernible resource available to all, and the other is its increasing social leverage to scale with the penetration of mobile devices. In 2007, Kenya had 8 million mobile phone subscribers; today they boast a subscriber base of over 30 million.[62] These numbers do not just indicate the penetration of devices but also how ubiquitous those devices are to the daily lives of Kenyans. The creation of a system for reporting voter fraud and criminal activity so closely tied to everyday experience takes full advantage of the technology available to people and organizations wishing to avoid conflict. Of particularly interesting note here is the level of outreach that Uchaguzi has been pursuing with civil service organizations, radio stations, marketing campaigns, street graffiti, and comic books to educate the populace on how to use the technology.

In addition to technology monitoring instances of corruption or violence on the ground, Ushahidi has also created Umati, a digital language filter designed to sift through social media, blogs, and comment sections to identify and report hate speech.[63] The Kenyan Ministry of Information and Communication seems to be in close partnership with the Umati project, announcing stiff financial penalties and imprisonment for hate speech. Interestingly enough, the KMIC reached out to Internet service providers (ISPs) in the country to warn them that they would be held accountable for violations of the hate speech law. This model of government control over the ISPs seems to be inherited from the United States, which has similar laws regarding violations.

In Kenya, innovation in reporting has been coupled with innovation in networking, consensus building, and information delivery. The development of online spaces like SODNET (Social Development Network) or Google's Kenya Elections Hub established places for local groups or causes to facilitate conversation and action related to political issues.[64] However, not all initiatives are based on technology: the most successful persuasion is person-to-person, undertaken by projects like the Alternatives to Violence Project taking place in Kapyemit (a hot spot of postelection violence), which trains members of communities across Kenya to promote a peaceful election process and become citizen reporters.

Given the relative absence of violence during and following the 2013 elections, it is difficult to deny that these various innovations had some effect. This seeming success, however, does not actually demonstrate the effectiveness of these programs

---

[62] Ibid.

[63] Ibid.

[64] Dave Mayers, "Kenyans use technology to help avoid electoral violence," *Smart Planet* online (www.smartplanetcom), January 22, 2013, accessed in May 2013 at http://www.smartplanet.com/blog/global-observer/kenyans-use-technology-to-help-avoid-electoral-violence/8851; Fred Oluoch. "Kenya on the Spot for Not Abiding by AU Rules," *The East African Online* (Nairobi, Kenya), July 12, 2010, accessed in May 2013 at http://www.theeastafrican.co.ke/news/Kenya-on-the-spot-for-not-abiding-by-AU-rules/-/2558/955838/-/8i7ppd/-/index.html

or indicate their transferability to other settings. For this to be done, more careful evaluation is still needed, as well as more detailed documentation of good practices stemming from the considerable efforts undertaken. The case remains an area for researchers to evaluate from empirical perspectives, potentially utilizing data outputs from the technologies employed to prevent violence, to elaborate our knowledge of important causal relationships between urbanization and such large-scale civic violence. Nevertheless, it is undeniable that the spectrum of efforts undertaken to prevent the recurrence of widespread civic violence around the elections offers an effective model for policymakers addressing similar risks of civic violence.

Case #5: Khayelitsha, South Africa

Urban upgrading as a mechanism for violence prevention centers on social, situational, and institutional crime prevention. Combining community engagement, enhancement of the physical and spatial environment, and the improvement of local governance,[65] urban upgrading has been looked to as a critical approach to addressing the risk of violent crime in communities characterized by endemic crime and in particular a propensity for violent crime, ranging from San Salvador, El Salvador, and Bogota, Colombia, to Cape Town, South Africa. In El Salvador, a nongovernmental organization has implemented slum rehabilitation programs, which focus on improving local self-help and cooperation potential. Projects target specific neighborhoods and include assisting families with understanding land tenure legislation and credit schemes or focusing on refurbishment of community space. In Colombia, the creation of municipal infrastructure for preventive work with youth has provided an alternative to criminal activity. And in South Africa, the City of Cape Town, with the support of the German Federal Ministry for Economic Cooperation and Development, launched in 2006 a $55.6 million development program to comprehensively pursue violence prevention through urban upgrading. Each of these projects illustrates the importance of innovating public space in urban environments for the mitigation of violence, through improving general living and housing conditions, building the capacities of local governments, and emphasizing the importance of local stakeholders to development, including enabling marginalized communities to engage in self-help programs.

Looking more carefully at the case of Khayelitsha, South Africa, violence prevention through urban upgrading is considered to be a meaningful factor in decreasing violent crime rates. The urban upgrading program came at a crucial juncture during

---

[65] Bettina Bauer, *Violence Prevention Through Urban Upgrading: Experiences from Financial Cooperation*, Kf W Bankengruppe, Frankfurt, March 2010.

which 430 murders were committed in Khayelitsha from April 2006 to March 2007. This resulted in a murder rate of 106 incidents per 100,000 people, more than two and a half times the South African average of 41 murders per 100,000 people, which was already twenty times the murder rate of Western Europe.[66] Therefore, Khayelitsha faced very significant levels of civic violence at the outset of its urban upgrading projects. Since the inception of the urban upgrading program in 2006, police statistics identified a decrease in overall crime by two-thirds from 2004–2010, to the extent that one Cape Town news outlet declared the township had transformed from "Rape Capital to Safe Capital."[67]

Reflecting these notable achievements in the reduction of crime and particularly violence, the Violence Prevention Through Urban Upgrading (VPUU) program was initiated in 2006 to address the high rates of violent crime in Khayelitsha. Of particular concern were social and environmental risk factors, such as high rates of poverty and unemployment resulting in part from the unanticipated and rapid growth of the township, which was originally planned to house 250,000 residents when established in 1983 but grew to nearly 1.5 million residents by the early 2000s.[68,69] Violence prevention in South Africa has had a unique recent history. While the efforts to address crime and violence in South Africa have been similar to those of other countries, policies were retarded by the country's apartheid-related isolation until 1994. Correspondingly, crime rates rose dramatically in South Africa from 1985 until 1994, after which they stabilized. However, homicide accounted for nearly half of all nonnatural deaths (46 %), and gun violence was the leading cause of nonnatural death in the age group 15–65 years.[70] It should be noted that although these statistics are shocking, they fail to show the marked disparities that continue

---

[66] Ndodana Nleya and Lisa Thompson, "Survey Methodology in Violence-prone Khayelitsha, Cape Town, South Africa," *IDS Bulletin* 22:3, May 2009, p. 53.

[67] Fadela Slamdien, "Crime in Khayelitsha for April to March 2003/2004–2011–2012" and "From Rape Capital to Safe Capital." *West Cape News.* May 17, 2010, accessed in May 2013 at http://westcapenews.com/?p=1456

[68] "Crime in Khayelitsha for April to March 2003/2004–2011–2012." *Crime Research and Statistics— South African Police Service* accessed in June 2013 at http://www.saps.gov.za/statistics/reports/crimestats/2012/provinces/w_cape/pdf/khayelitsha.pdf; Frank Bliss and Luise Zagst, "Investing in People: Violence Prevention and Empowerment through Urban Upgrading in the Township of Khayelitsha South Africa," KfW Development Bank (Urban Upgrading in South Africa (BMZ/KfW) POVNET Task Team on Empowerment), 2011, accessed in June 2013 at https://www.kfw-entwicklungsbank.de/migration/Entwicklungsbank-Startseite/Entwicklungsfinanzierung/L%C3%A4nder-und-Programme/Subsahara-Afrika/S%C3%BCdafrika/Storyline-Khayelitsha.pdf

[69] Khayelitsha Community Trust, "Khayelitsha," Khayelitsha Community Trust website, accessed in February 2013 at http://www.kctrust.org/about-us/khayelitsha/

[70] Alexander Butchart, *A Profile of Fatal Injuries in South Africa 1999: First Annual Report of the NIMSS*, National Injury Mortality Surveillance System (NIMSS), Cape Town, South Africa, November 2000.

to characterize crime in South African society. Those most vulnerable to crime are the poorer sectors of society, which are still predominantly black.[71,72]

Central to the VPUU project are the principles of surveillance and visibility, territoriality, defined access and movement, image and aesthetics, physical barriers, and maintenance and management. Each of these principles applies to the creation and maintenance of community-owned public space, which is designed to improve the Khayelitsha urban environment. The VPUU project emphasizes monitoring and evaluation, which began well before a formal program was established. In 2001, a pre-feasibility study was conducted to identify possible settlement upgrading projects for crime prevention. In 2006, baseline, business, and household surveys were conducted for monitoring and evaluation of the VPUU program. To track developments, photographic change detection and crime maps were created in 2007 and have been updated throughout the project.

---

[71] In her analysis, Palmery cites both the South African Department of Safety and Security's *In Service of Safety: White Paper on Safety and Security 1999–2004*, 1998 Government of South Africa (Pretoria), and Alexander Butchart's *A Profile of Fatal Injuries in South Africa 1999*. 1999 A. Butchart (Cape Town). Regarding the unequal concentration of crime in South Africa, Palmery refers to the South African Government's White Paper on Safety and Security 1999–2004, noting that during the apartheid era, the system of policing strongly focused on political control rather than on crime prevention, with the role of the police being minimal even in formerly "white" areas in which 74 % of police stations were located. Palmery further cites the South African Government's *National Crime Prevention Strategy* for the year 1996 in noting that this legacy led to various challenges in implementing new approaches to crime prevention even after apartheid, including limited accountability for dealing with local communities' safety priorities, collaboration with other departments or organizations, and monitoring and research of crime and capacity for an information-based approach to crime prevention, all contributing to a generally poor understanding of and capacity for identifying effective strategy for crime *prevention*, especially those incorporating and social crime prevention.

[72] Ingrid Palmery, *Social Crime Prevention in South Africa's Major Cities*, City Safety Project at the Centre for the Study of Violence and Reconciliation (South Africa), June 2001. In her analysis, Palmery cites both the South African Department of Safety and Security's *In Service of Safety: White Paper on Safety and Security 1999–2004*, Government of South Africa (Pretoria), 1998, and Alexander Butchart's *A Profile of Fatal Injuries in South Africa 1999*. *A Profile of Fatal Injuries in South Africa 1999: First Annual Report of the NIMSS*, National Injury Mortality Surveillance System (NIMSS), Cape Town, South Africa, November 2000. Regarding the unequal concentration of crime in South Africa, Palmery refers to the South African Government's White Paper on Safety and Security 1999–2004, noting that during the apartheid era, the system of policing strongly focused on political control rather than on crime prevention, with the role of the police being minimal even in formerly "white" areas in which 74 % of police stations were located. Palmery further cites the South African Government's *National Crime Prevention Strategy* for the year 1996 in noting that this legacy led to various challenges in implementing new approaches to crime prevention even after apartheid, including limited accountability for dealing with local communities' safety priorities, collaboration with other departments or organizations, and monitoring and research of crime and capacity for an information-based approach to crime prevention, all contributing to a generally poor understanding of and capacity for identifying effective strategy for crime *prevention*, especially those incorporating and social crime prevention.

One key element of the VPUU project is the creation of safe area nodes. Community members, through a lengthy consultation process combining workshops and public meetings, decided the specific elements of each safe area node based on community needs.[73] This consultation process took 3 years, and in 2009 the first safe area nodes were constructed. These nodes are multiuse public spaces, designed to cater to 50,000 people. The use of public space is designed based on community needs (for use as youth centers, sports centers, or trading). Live-work units have also been installed, to provide previously informal trading a space for work. Additionally, the safe area nodes have Active Boxes, which are well-lit buildings with a 24-hour caretaker, located in areas that were previously "crime hot spots."

Khayelitsha is therefore a notable case for policymakers and researchers. The broad engagement of the VPUU project with the physical urban environment represents a striking innovation to address large-scale civic violence. Additionally, the VPUU project's emphasis on monitoring and evaluation should provide a rich basis for researchers to more carefully evaluate the case empirically and for policymakers to catalogue good practices arising from the intervention. Most importantly, innovative community engagements that informed efforts to reshape the physical environment of Khayelitsha seemed to have a positive effect on building a larger sense of social trust and collective efficacy, ultimately reducing violence in the period highlighted.

Case #6: Women's Safety Audits (Various Cities)

Safety audits, in which citizens are consulted to identify issues that make them feel unsafe, are a component of various urban upgrading efforts. An innovative approach to this type of effort that has been replicated globally with recognized success is the use of safety audits undertaken specifically by women. In these cases, the mechanics are relatively straightforward yet flexible: "using a checklist, a group of women users of a particular urban or community space walk around that space, noting factors that make those users feel unsafe or safe in that space."[74] In fact, Women's Safety Audits were identified in the 2007 Global Assessment on Women's Safety as the most frequently used international tool to address women's security.[75]

First developed in Canada following the recommendations of a 1989 report on violence against women, the Women's Safety Audit approach has further been developed by UN-HABITAT and others in various communities across the globe—from Cote d'Ivoire, Kenya, South Africa, and Tanzania to India and even

---

[73] Violence Prevention Through Urban Upgrading in Khayelitsha, "Community Participation." Violence Prevention Through Urban Upgrading in Khayelitsha (Cape Town, South Africa) website, accessed in February 2013 at http://www.vpuu.org.za/page.php?page=8

[74] Carolyn Whitzman et al., "The effectiveness of women's safety audits," *Security Journal* 22:3, July 2009, p. 206.

[75] Women in Cities International, *Women's Safety Audits: What Works and Where?*, UN-Habitat Safer Cities Programme (Nairobi, Kenya), 2008.

Poland and the United Kingdom.[76] These audits help to address the gendered experiences of violence. It is well known that men are the victims of fatal violence more, at roughly twice the rates for women. Men are also responsible for committing the majority of violent crimes. However, men are only slightly less likely than women to be victimized by nonfatal violence.[77] As such, Women's Safety Audits can help users and decision-makers to understand how men and women experience the urban environment in different manners and to fill the gap between attention to lethal violence and endemic violence more broadly. Similarly, Women's Safety Audits are tools that can increase awareness of violence against vulnerable groups more generally. These are valuable outcomes in themselves, but are also critical to reducing the risk of lethal violence, given the ever-worsening spiral that can result from endemic violence. Lastly, the nature of these audits is such that they can be readily tailored to local contexts, as highlighted by Women in Cities International and UN-HABITAT in their review of the effectiveness of these audits across the world, and exemplified in the diversity of cases analyzed by Whitzman et al. in their case studies of selected audit efforts in Africa, Asia, and Europe. Three of these case studies from Whitzman et al. are briefly summarized, below, to illustrate the diversity of applications of such safety audits.

Sample Questions from Women's Safety Audits[78]

- *Lighting*—Are the street lights working? Are they distributed evenly? Do they light the streets? Mark on maps lights that are not working. How long does it take to repair the lights?
- *Entrapment areas and unused land*—Are there any recessed doorways, alleys, and demolished or unfinished buildings which could be unsafe? What is the condition of vacant/unused land?
- *Social usage of space*—Are there people on the streets? Note if men are more than women. What are they doing? Observe the location of cigarette and liquor shops.
- *Formal surveillance*—Is there any visible policing?
- *Informal surveillance*—Do surrounding buildings provide informal surveillance?
- *Priority improvements*—Among all recommendations and corrective measures you suggested improving the situation, which ones are priorities?

---

[76] Ibid.

[77] Alexander Butchart et al., *Preventing Violence and Reducing Its Impact: How Development Agencies Can Help*, World Health Organization (Geneva, Switzerland), 2008.

[78] Adapted from Surabhi Tandon Mehrotra, *A Handbook on Women's Safety Audits in Low-Income Urban Neighbourhoods: A Focus on Essential Services*, Jagori (New Delhi, India), November 2010, and United Nations Human Settlements Programme, *Women's Safety Audits For a Safer Urban Design*, United Nations Human Settlements Programme (Warsaw, Poland), August, 2007.

In Tanzania, Women's Safety Audits were piloted in Manzese, an informal settlement of Dar es Salaam with particularly high rates of violence. These Women's Safety Audits in Manzese are credited with having led to critical alterations to the physical space that contributed to decreasing the crime rate and expanding and improving the economic and social opportunities for residents. Notably, however, the value of such audits might not be recognized in the case of Manzese if only the first experience with them was reviewed, as no improvements to the settlement's physical space were implemented following an audit in 2000, due to a lack of funding. Two years later, however, with support from UN-HABITAT and other donors, another audit led to improvements ranging from improved street lighting (funded by residents in the form of lighting for exterior porches on houses) to better transportation resulting from the local government's clearing and improving of commonly used paths and roads that had become blocked or deteriorated. And again, 4 years later, in 2006, the audits were key to securing World Bank support to further improve and pave roadways, install additional street lighting and particularly public lighting, and enhance the job creation program that had started as a result of the previous audit. An example of the effects of the audit cited by the coordinator is the job creation program's spurring of the transition of women engaged in high-risk income-generating activities, such as prostitution, to less risky income-generating activities, such as vending food, charcoal, and second-hand clothing.

In India, Women's Safety Audits identified needed improvements related to the transportation systems. In Mumbai, the audits led to specific improvements in lighting in and around train stations, and in Delhi, audits led to the municipal transportation commission's creation of a gender sensitization and women's safety awareness campaign in which over 1,000 drivers and conductors within the city were trained. The South Delhi Auto Union members also displayed and distributed printed materials promoting women's safety and women's rights to safety. In Petrozavodsk, Russia, Women's Safety Audits undertaken from 2003 onwards are credited for contributing to improvements in housing and neighborhood design, reported decreases in crime rates (including domestic violence, even though this issue was not the focus of the public space-focused audits), as well as increased awareness generally on both gender and safety issues.

Lastly, in the United Kingdom, Women's Safety Audits were incorporated into urban revitalization programs in the early 2000s in three cities—London, Bristol, and Manchester. While many specific recommendations from the audits were implemented, Whitzman et al. note that the more important result of the audits might be that the consistent rate of acceptance of the recommendations by local authorities is a critical signal of legitimation of women's concerns regarding safety.

Regardless of whether any alterations of urban space actually result directly from Women's Safety Audits, in each of the cases reviewed by Whitzman et al., the audits contribute to the raising of awareness of safety as a concern in the communities. These audits also promote the development of the social network among community members and entities, and they result in greater sharing of values and expectations with regard to safety through more frequent and meaningful engagements among residents, intentional education campaigns, and local media coverage.

Considering the role of "collective efficacy" in violence prevention, a la Robert Sampson as introduced earlier, the example of Women's Safety Audits can be seen even more readily as not only critical to addressing the particular safety concerns of women but as models of building collective efficacy and thus inuring urban environments to the potential of large-scale civic violence.

Case studies and selected characteristics

City	Violence	Interventions	Innovation
Diadema, Brazil	• High murder rate of 141 per 100,000 persons • Near anarchy, collapse of law and order • Process of reurbanization	• Multi-sectoral, mixed-model approach for violence reduction • Preventive measures restricting alcohol sales ("Last Call" Law)	• Local government spurred multi-sectoral, mixed-model approach to intervene and prevent violence • Diverse group of local political actors
Lagos, Nigeria	• High crime rates • Perceived civilian insecurity • Inadequate police response	• Community trust fund for support of security efforts (Lagos State Security Trust Fund) • Centralization and expansion of state and private security outfits	• Innovative funding for multifaceted security and safety reforms • Social and environmental development • Government–community dialogue
Boston, USA	• Spike in youth homicide rates from 22–73 victims per year • Crack cocaine epidemic • Gang rivalries	• Working group of criminologists and Boston Police Department to address violence (Operation Cease Fire)	• Data analysis • Centralization and coordination of enforcement responses • Direct communication with gangs • Severe and rapid response to violent gangs
Nairobi, Kenya	• More than 1,000 killed in electoral violence • Estimated 600,00 displaced persons • Increased opportunistic gang-associated killings	• Technology-based monitoring of violence and corruption (Ushahidi and Uchaguzi) • Development of online spaces for political organization (SODNET)	• Widespread, crowd-sourced efforts through technology to witness, monitor, verify, and aggregate instances of hate speech, intimidation, and crimes • Online and person-to-person promotion of peaceful election processes
Khayelitsha, South Africa	• 106 murders per 100,000 people in 2006–2007 • High rates of unemployment and poverty • Rapid growth of townships	• Urban upgrading • Community engagement • Enhancement of physical and spatial environment • Improvement of local governance	• Creation and maintenance of community-owned public space with community engagement for collective efficacy • Safe area multiuse public spaces catering to 50,000 people (nodes)

(continued)

City	Violence	Interventions	Innovation
Various cities	• High rates of violence • Fear of violence and victimization • Gendered violence	• Safety audits consult citizens in order to identify issues that make them feel unsafe (safety audit)	• Checklist to engage women users of an urban space; list allows women to note factors that make them feel unsafe or safe in that space

Conclusion

In this chapter, we have presented a selection of case studies of promising innovations to address endemic and large scale violence associated with urbanization. The availability of such examples is still limited, so we cannot offer authoritative guidance for policy. We present this survey as a model for further research to identify and interrogate such efforts in order to better inform the development of more effective policies for addressing violence related to increasing urbanization. In this manner, we are suggesting that the issue of rising and increasingly threatening civic violence is particularly amenable and even requires the employment of a public health approach to identify solutions. As numerous others have already identified, the relationship between urbanization and violence is not clear—and yet it is also unquestionable. Urbanization might not lead directly to violence and increasingly harmful levels and types of violence, but urbanization very likely exacerbates the risks of violence and those associated with violence. And because of both the complexity and the urgency of the relationship, we cannot approach the issue from a perspective of removed academic inquiry but need to undertake the best efforts possible, informed by a careful understanding of the complex causal relationships. We must then carefully reflect on the results of these efforts and rapidly improve upon them; this is the epitome of the public health approach. The public health approach also underscores the importance of both more attention to the careful monitoring and evaluation of the influence of efforts, which have up until now not been as well documented and are subject mostly to retrospective and anecdotal documentation. An openness to the appropriate and necessary innovation of methods to monitor and evaluate these efforts is also required, since they are unlikely to be as amenable to more traditional methods of inquiry, due to their complexity.

Beyond this higher level intention of this chapter and the previous statement that we are far from identifying any clear guidance for policy, we can nonetheless identify some important, even if not entirely novel, lessons to be drawn from these case studies to inform efforts to address endemic and large-scale urban violence. First and foremost of these is that violence is largely a symptom of many other challenges related to urbanization. And while violence can certainly interact with these other challenges—such as those related to health, environment, and economic opportunities—efforts to reduce violence will always have a floor if adequate progress is not made on addressing these other challenges. While all of the cases represent this multidimensionality of the causes and necessary efforts to address civic violence, the cases of Diadema, Lagos, and Boston in particular, highlight the importance of comprehensive approaches to address the challenges of urbanization that underlie violence.

Similarly, while many of the cases illustrate the promise of technology to assist in more carefully identifying and delivering information both to improve violence prevention policies and as violence prevention efforts in themselves, this can be most clearly seen in the cases of the data-informed efforts to change behavior in Boston and the SMS-messaging efforts to shape behavior in Kenya. While technology is never a panacea in itself, these two cases demonstrate the increasing potential of technology—and particularly information communication and analysis technology—to play a critical role in strategies to address the endemic structural drivers of violence.

Finally, all of the cases illustrate the importance of engaging with the breadth of stakeholders that have influence on the factors that contribute to the risk of civic violence, but two in particular most exemplify this practice—the cases focused on urban upgrading and on Women's Safety Audits. In both of these cases, the engagement of the populations with the local government authorities not only helped to identify particular factors that could be addressed to reduce violence, improve safety, and increase residents' sense of safety. Arguably more importantly, these efforts—one focused on the reshaping of the built environment and the other on engaging the population in identifying particular issues to be addressed—engendered a greater sense of social trust and collective efficacy that may be ultimately necessary for inuring urban communities from violence.

Returning to our idea most simply stated in our introduction, as the potential for such violence to flare up increases in the face of unprecedented urbanization, and as we will continue to still be limited to a small number of cases as well as signification variation among these cases, it is not likely that we will be able to rely on broad empirical analysis of a large number of interventions to better establish clear evidence of universal best practice. Instead, the search for solutions to endemic, large-scale, and collective violence in cities can benefit greatly from an augmented use of a public health approach for analysis and program design.

Chapter 6
Disaster Preparedness and Response Innovations: Implications for Urbanization and Health

Laura Janneck and Paul Biddinger

Background

Although there are many challenges facing modern cities, the response to natural and man-made disasters after catastrophe strikes often receives some of the most intense retrospective worldwide scrutiny. This is particularly true for cities in developing countries. Delays in communication, mobilization, and/or response are routinely criticized when cities show deficient response to calamitous events. Further, while nearly every city struggles with its efforts to improve and promote health for its citizens every day, their hard-fought efforts to improve outcomes can be thrown into disarray in an instant when disaster strikes. Health systems can be set back years or even decades in the aftermath of a disaster. The impact of disasters on urban areas is, of course, not a new phenomenon. Since ancient times, with events such as the 1138 C.E. earthquake that struck Aleppo [1] and countless others, the devastating effects of extreme natural events on urban human settlements have been known and feared. However, in recent decades, there have been both increasing numbers of disasters and disproportionate increases in the number of people being affected by disaster [3].

The world population is rapidly urbanizing. As more people move into urban settings where they live and work together in tightly clustered spaces, the human impact of disasters increases. According to the United Nations, the world population became more urban than rural between 2007 and 2008 [11]. The urban centers of low- and

L. Janneck, M.D., M.P.H. (✉)
Cambridge Health Alliance, 1493 Cambridge Street, Cambridge, MA 02139, USA

Harvard Medical School, Boston, MA, USA
e-mail: laura.janneck@gmail.com

P. Biddinger, M.D., F.A.C.E.P.
Department of Emergency Medicine, Massachusetts General Hospital, 45 Fruit Street, Boston, MA 02114, USA

Harvard Medical School, Boston, MA, USA

© Springer New York 2015
R. Ahn et al. (eds.), *Innovating for Healthy Urbanization*,
DOI 10.1007/978-1-4899-7597-3_6

middle-income countries will house most of the world's population growth over the next several decades, and many of these cities are located in low-lying coastal zones or other areas at risk of flooding and extreme weather [16]. Within these cities, approximately one billion people are thought to live in slums, also known as informal settlements, with many of these areas at risk of flooding or landslides [16], and the number of people living in these settlements is expected to double by 2030 [22].

As with most environmental factors on human health, when disasters strike, those most negatively impacted are vulnerable populations. This includes women, who may be physically less capable of self-protection if pregnant, carrying infants, or caring for small children. Likewise, the elderly and young children may not be as mobile or as able to physically withstand the forces of disaster. People living in poverty are more likely to spend their time in inadequate buildings unable to withstand extreme forces of nature, have limited access to stores of food and safe water after disaster, and may be unable to travel away from impending threats. Additionally, the poor, migrants, and refugees frequently have fewer social and systemic supports upon which to rely.

Disasters can, of course, be caused by forces of nature or man-made. Man-made disasters are often the result of armed conflicts involving urban areas and can cause large population displacements to or from cities—the war in Afghanistan drove refugees from Kabul; the Somali Civil War pushed refugees from Mogadishu to Nairobi; and the Iraqi insurgency precipitated a large migration to various cities in the Middle East. Other man-made causes of disaster include terrorist attacks and efforts to mitigate climate change, such as dam construction that leads to the flooding of towns. This chapter will primarily focus on preparation for, mitigation of, response to, and recovery from natural disasters. However, many of the innovative methods and concepts used to plan for natural disasters can also be applied to those that are human-made.

Because of the need for resilience in the face of disaster and because of increasing visibility of the importance of disaster planning, leaders in global cities as well as health and humanitarian experts around the world are focusing increasing attention on disaster preparedness as an activity where there is great need for improvement and much opportunity for innovation. Limiting the negative consequences of disasters on urban areas requires improved awareness, research, and innovation in each of the four phases of disaster preparedness, from planning and mitigation to response and recovery. In this chapter, we will explore some of the latest advances in disaster preparedness and response in each of these four phases.

Planning

Risk Assessments

One of the first activities required when beginning to plan for disasters is to perform a formal and structured assessment of risk. This risk assessment allows city planners to combine analyses of both the most likely and the most severe potential hazards.

A structured risk assessment also takes into account existing plans and response capabilities; therefore, it enables a rational approach to the use of constrained resources. This critical step of carefully analyzing risk and existing preparedness involves gathering a great deal of data necessary for effective disaster mitigation, response, and recovery.

Some of the data that needs to be gathered for a risk assessment relates to the likelihood of certain potential hazards. For example, planners need to know the relative likelihood of a typhoon, a landslide, or an earthquake of magnitude 7.0 or greater. Other important data used in planning is detailed demographic information that describes both the population and the environment in which they live: how many people are in a given area, where do they live, and what are their ages? Also important is data about the built structures in which people spend their time. What are the construction materials used in houses and buildings; are they able to withstand earthquakes, floods, or high winds? Similarly, disaster planners need to know many details about the resources available to the local community in the event of a disaster—and how available those resources will be after a disaster. Planners must know not only the locations of hospitals, fire stations, schools, and community centers that can act as shelters but also know their strengths and vulnerabilities to know if they can be relied upon when disaster strikes. They also need to know data on the resilience of basic community services to know if they can be expected to function in an emergency. Planners must understand the likelihood of water and power system disruptions, how durable the waste management systems are, and how basic food chains may be vulnerable to disruption. This data can be used during and after a disaster for a range of tasks, from predicting the spread of infectious diseases and providing accurate maps for search and rescue to identifying gaps in service delivery [9].

In cities of more-developed countries, much of this data is readily available. Although it needs to be updated regularly, the data can be organized so as to be useful when a disaster hits. In less-developed cities, however, the task of collecting even the most basic data can be a colossal task. Many urban slums are not recognized by the local government; therefore, the census does not count the people in these settlements, let alone describe the structures, systems, or neighborhoods in which they live.

Fortunately, many city governments and municipalities are beginning to take the lead in organizing and performing more accurate assessments of difficult-to-document populations and neighborhoods. For example, the World Health Organization (WHO) Kobe Centre developed the Urban Health Equity Assessment and Response Tool [24], a tool that analyzes and tracks health inequalities in order to identify populations vulnerable to natural disasters [14]. The Urban HEART tool has been implemented in dozens of cities around the world, including Tehran, Iran; Nakuru, Kenya; and Parañaque City, Philippines [24]. Although the Urban HEART tool was intended for use in reducing health inequalities, its structures and data are easily adapted to support improved risk assessment and planning.

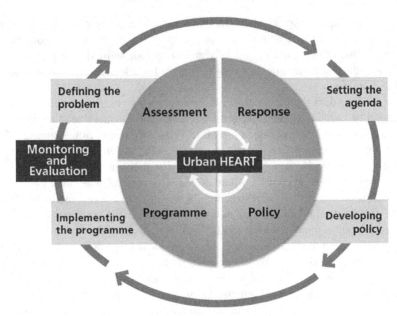

Source: WHO, Urban HEART, 2013

While local surveys and risk assessments can provide invaluable information for emergency planners, it is important to recognize that such data gathering and investigation can be viewed by vulnerable populations as intrusive and threatening. Many slums in poor cities are unofficial settlements, and the people living in the slums do not own the land they occupy. Historically, many slums have been partially or completely demolished by city officials to make way for new urban developments. Slum residents, aware of these circumstances, are often suspicious of any government-led efforts to count them or survey the area. Therefore, there is a need for political bodies to provide assurance that the surveys will not be used to the detriment of the residents.

As with all urban health initiatives, thoughtful engagement of the community provides potential solutions. Compared to an externally imposed survey by an academic or governmental body, data gathering by community-based organizations can be more effective. In some cities, local groups such as slum dweller associations are developing community-managed enumerations and surveys [16]. Local residents can draw on their own knowledge of the layout of a slum—socially and physically—that has never been officially mapped, and simply mapping informal settlements can be a major first step in assessing risks. One example is Cuttack, India, where digital maps were created by community members for city authorities with assistance from NGOs [26]. In slums and urban areas at large, this information is then able to be utilized when disasters occur so that responders know where to focus their efforts.

Collaboration

Since a disaster, by definition, overwhelms the local capacity to respond, and perhaps because the local municipalities are more aware of their own resource limitations, disaster planning in the developing world often encourages involvement from a broad array of partners who come from outside the local and regional governments. NGOs are heavily involved in particular cities around the world, and, in some cases, act as consultants to urban disaster planners. For example, after the Yogyakarta earthquake in Indonesia, the World Bank and Iranian Red Crescent were able to gather data from the government and various NGOs to produce a common base map [11]. Alternatively, in Kabul, CARE instituted a program that identified shelter opportunities from a land usage survey and then used community councils to select beneficiaries in clusters [11].

Private companies have also taken on leadership roles, particularly in cities where they are based and have a large investment in human resources. Maintaining continuity of operations, supporting rapid local economic recovery, and reestablishing local markets greatly improve the livelihood of local populations affected by disaster [11]. The World Food Program's food-for-work programs target women and are coupled with child care services [11]; they are an innovative approach that simultaneously addresses the need to create an economy while providing food relief. Another successful example of this intertwining of goals: In Jakarta, after the El Nino of 1998, NGOs worked quickly to supply wheat from international suppliers to Indonesian mills. From that point on, the established private sector food production chain of Indonesian mills, noodle production factories, and distribution was able to stem part of the food insecurity in Jakarta [11]. Also, in India, the Gujarat Urban Development Company (GUDC) was established by the government to implement urban development projects [11]. After the 2001 Bhuj earthquake, the government designated the GDUC as the implementing agency for overseeing recovery plans and outsourced many tasks to consultants [11]. By doing so, it facilitated investment in infrastructure and services as part of the recovery process [11]. Collaborations, such as these between private businesses and relief organizations, are increasingly seen as critical to rebuilding the local economy after disaster.

Mapping

Much of the data collected by municipal authorities and local community organizations can be spatially related. Beyond knowing the numbers and demographic details of people living in a certain neighborhood, it is extremely useful to know how many of those people live on a flood plain or how far away they live from storm shelters. To answer these questions, spatial data is gaining increasing attention in disaster planning and response, and with it comes a variety of innovative methods to collect and analyze such data. The creation of accurate and current maps at a local level, often by the indigenous population, can help in disaster recovery. In Bhuj, India, after an earthquake in 2001, the Atlas for Post-Disaster Reconstruction was created, which included publicly made and publicly shared maps that guided the reconstruction process [11]. In Kabul, CARE worked with the local community to make maps to guide the construction of shelters, drains, roads, and wells [11].

One area of innovative technology that is being used in disaster preparedness is remote sensing. Remote sensing uses satellite data to create maps of urban areas and can spatially map out factors that are not easily measured on the ground. For example, remote sensors are able to detect electromagnetic radiation, which includes a much wider range of energy waves than visible light. Electromagnetic data enables mappers to track a wide range of features, including land use, urban area growth, arrangement of green space in a city, farmland use, and heat islands. In addition, spatial data in many areas is becoming open source, with organizations such as OpenStreetMap allowing global collaborators to share data [12]. Another organization, the Satellite Sentinel Project [15], combines satellite imagery analysis and field reports with Google's Map Maker to deter the resumption of full-scale civil war between North and South Sudan. The mappers for this group have used satellite imagery to find mass graves, movement of tanks, and bombed villages, and their data have been thought to be influencing the progression of the conflict in the region.

Closer to the earth, local disaster planners have also begun to use GIS data to facilitate and enhance risk assessment models. With the advent of widespread GIS technology, particularly with GIS data available from the cell phones that are ever more densely distributed around the globe, the opportunities for researchers, surveyors, and disaster planners to use GIS data in disaster planning are growing at a fast pace. Many types of GIS data can support emergency planners' and others' efforts to assist airports, community centers, fire and other emergency services, hospitals, transportation services, telecommunication services, power generators, and schools [9]. GIS can be used in a variety of other ways, including estimating risks, estimating populations in hazard zones, mapping vulnerable populations, predicting demand for services in known emergencies, evaluating emergency response, and performing risk and vulnerability assessments [9].

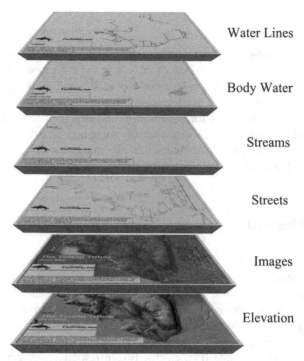

Water Lines

Body Water

Streams

Streets

Images

Elevation

Source: Tulip Tribes GIS Center, 2013

In a successful application of GIS technologies, one study combined crowdsourcing data and GIS data to creatively track population movements after the 2010 Haiti earthquake [2]. Researchers followed the daily positions of SIM cards using mobile phone towers and tracked cards that made calls before and after the earthquake. In Port-au-Prince, there were an estimated 3.2 persons per SIM card followed. Using this data, the authors were able to extrapolate that an estimated 630,000 people who were in Port-au-Prince on the day of the earthquake had left the city within 19 days, corresponding to 20 % of the pre-earthquake population, and they identified the areas that received the largest outflow of internally displaced persons. The authors then utilized such data in helping to track population movements after a cholera outbreak, in order to identify other regions where new outbreaks might occur. The authors demonstrated the feasibility of using this method to do rapid estimates by producing reports on SIM card movement from a cholera outbreak area at the outbreak's immediate onset and within 12 hours of receiving data.

Potential downsides of relying too heavily on this method in the future include the possibility that certain vulnerable populations have low cell-phone use (including children and the elderly) and considerations that power for charging cell phones may be limited or mobile towers may be damaged. However, potential future uses of this data include estimates of mortality from non-responding SIMs, estimations of buried but alive persons, more valid needs assessments, and the ability to send information to users' cell phones [2].

Mitigation

The second phase of disaster management is mitigation. Mitigation describes the set of actions taken to decrease the effects of a disaster, and mitigation efforts have the potential to significantly lessen or prevent loss of life and property following a disaster event. In many cities of the developing world, city leaders are better recognizing patterns in vulnerability for certain areas and targeting their efforts to limit the effects of disasters on those who predictably are at highest risk. When planning and assessment identify potential future hazards, mitigation efforts can have an enormous effect on reducing the impacts of disasters when they do occur.

Early Warning Systems

One notable area where the benefits of mitigation are evident is with development and deployment of early warning systems. Early warning systems are communication networks whereby, when a disaster is expected, warning can be given to the local population with associated instructions for steps to take to protect themselves. Many of these systems—like storm, flood, and tornado warnings—were pioneered in developed countries; therefore, many rely on expensive equipment or resources that are not always available (i.e., electricity). In resource-poor countries, early warning systems must be adapted to the circumstances of the population. Radio warnings will not be effective if most of the population does not own a radio. Sirens are not effective unless they are paired with an educational program so the population knows what the sirens signify. Messages to the public should be clear, concise, and credible, with information about expected hazards, actions to take, where to go, and what to bring [9]. In addition, an understanding of local knowledge and resources is essential to an effective early warning system. During cyclone Sidr in Bangladesh, the National Disaster Management Prevention Strategy's early warning system included not only alerting the population of the threat but also distributing cash, rice, and house-building grants before the cyclone struck to increase resilience [26]. In another example, in one of the slums of Jakarta, an early warning system for floods was developed and sent SMS messages to residents' mobile phones but also broadcasted from the minarets of the local mosques [26].

The most prominent example of a well-implemented early warning system is the Indian Ocean Tsunami Warning System. After the 2004 tsunami, the governments around the Indian Ocean developed an Indian Ocean Tsunami Warning System [8]. This effort was led by the United Nations Education, Scientific, and Cultural Organization (UNESCO) Intergovernmental Oceanographic Commission [20]. By 2006, 26 of 28 possible national tsunami information centers had been established, each capable of receiving and distributing tsunami warnings around the clock [21]. Twenty five new seismographic detection stations were built and linked to analysis centers, and three new deep-ocean sensors were established [21]. UNESCO now runs regular drills to evaluate the early warning system, but the system was tested by an actual event in April of 2012 when an earthquake occurred off the western coast of Sumatra, not far from the epicenter of the 2004 earthquake that triggered the historic tsunami. Within minutes of the earthquake, the Indian Ocean Regional Tsunami Service Providers of Australia, India, and Indonesia had issued detailed bulletins, and national bulletins were issued within 10 minutes of the event [19]. In some locations, precautionary evacuations were ordered. In some areas, people also self-evacuated, reflecting the success of public education on tsunamis [19]. As the sea-level monitoring network of deep sea buoys confirmed that a large tsunami had thankfully not been generated, bulletins and forecasts were updated, and reassurances were disseminated to the population [19]. Though the 2012 earthquake did not itself create a large tsunami, it did demonstrate the effectiveness of the Indian Ocean tsunami early warning system.

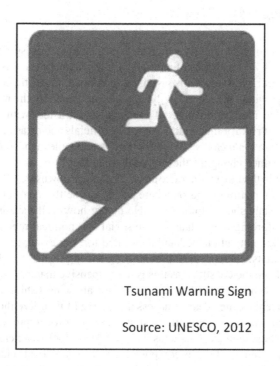

Tsunami Warning Sign

Source: UNESCO, 2012

Building Codes

Another crucial form of disaster mitigation that is beginning to take hold in some parts of the developing world is the development and enforcement of building codes. In order to adequately begin to prepare for expected disasters, local governments must at least proclaim that buildings be built to withstand likely climatologic impacts. While such policy proclamations are of value, much greater value can come from the actual implementation and enforcement of building codes, which is inconsistent at best. For example, after the 2008 Sichuan earthquake, the Chinese government began to investigate why over 7,000 schools collapsed, despite many nearby buildings remaining intact [25]. They concluded that building codes for schools in that area were particularly weak and unenforced and responded with an amendment to improve construction standards for primary and middle schools in rural areas [25]. In addition to refurbishing buildings to withstand earthquakes and other environmental threats, communities should also have structurally sound large structures available for emergency shelter in the event of widespread building collapse [17].

Urban Planning

Disaster planners can often identify which areas of a city are most susceptible to the damaging effects of various forms of natural disasters. Sometimes, this information is gathered through risk assessments, as discussed above. Other times, it becomes apparent after a previous disaster. Low-lying areas are generally the most at risk in floods, coastal areas may be in danger of tsunamis, and hillsides with unstable surface soil are most at risk for mudslides. Some city officials and disaster planners are implementing mitigation measures to reduce the risk to people in these areas through urban planning, either changing the physical topography of an area or limiting human settlement in the most vulnerable areas. The major downside of this approach is, however, that it puts limitations on where people can settle and often requires the relocation of preestablished communities. No matter how well-meaning the urban planners are in enforcing these changes, the social and political repercussions can be severe if they are not anticipated and accounted for. For example, one option in preparing for future tsunamis is to restrict housing developments from building less than 300 meters from the coastline, as this is less expensive than building dikes [8]. However, this must be done with attention toward allowing fishing communities and others dependent on the ocean to access the source of their livelihood.

In dense urban areas, and particularly slums, the need for improved infrastructure is extreme. Constraints in slum areas include a lack of all-weather roads, drainage, and electricity, and all of this is compounded by a lack of legal status of the area itself that disincentivizes investments in infrastructure [16]. Despite these limitations, in some places, local people and groups have devised successful mitigation strategies. In Indore, India, households and small businesses raised platform levels, paved courtyards, used materials resistant to flooding and furniture less likely to be washed away, and put electricity and shelves high up [16]. Many households in the area also have suitcases at the ready and detachable roofing [16]. In Nairobi, residents of informal settlements mitigate their flood risks by developing strategies to move children, bail out water from flooding houses, dig trenches around houses, construct temporary dikes, and use sandbags [16].

Policies of urban planning that have been effective in disaster preparation in wealthier countries include increasingly sophisticated building codes, land subdivision regulation, restrictions on buildings in high-risk areas, and special provisions for extreme events [16]. The cities of Manizales, Colombia, and Ilo, Peru, for example, have implemented plans converting high-risk areas into parks or acquiring land from the poor to prevent them from settling in the high-risk areas [16]. Policies are particularly effective when they include tangible new benefits for the community as well. Jakarta has developed a plan for disaster risk reduction, incorporating long-term planning for the area, including restoring mangrove forests, improving mass transit, refining building regulations, and reserving open spaces to absorb rainfall [26]. After the Bam earthquake, the Housing Federation in Iran led the process of home rebuilding with community consultation, allowing the process to take into account the importance of land ownership and date trees [11].

Response

Even with excellent efforts toward disaster planning and mitigation, disasters will most certainly occur, be difficult to predict, and be challenging to respond to. Currently, climate change appears to be causing significant changes in the frequency and intensity of severe weather events, such as hurricanes, cold snaps, and heat waves, making forecasting such events difficult. Complicating matters further, the urban population is booming, and in a short time, surveys of the population will become out dated. Cities swell and shrink with greater speed because of increasingly expansive rapid transit systems, and therefore, remarkably, disasters can have widely variable effects on a city depending on the time of day the event occurs. As an example, the 1989 Loma Prieta earthquake occurred during the warm-up of the World Series between the two Bay Area baseball teams, the Oakland Athletics and the San Francisco Giants. Because of the game, many people had either left work early or had stayed out late to watch the game, and therefore the usual afternoon rush hour was particularly light. Disaster specialists attribute the low death toll of the earthquake in large part to the fact that very few people were on the roads at the time. Thus, because disaster events themselves remain somewhat unpredictable, disaster response must be dynamic and flexible. In the cities of poor countries, a variety of innovations are improving the quality of this immediate disaster response from both local communities and international responders.

Crowdsourcing

The ability of local responders to organize and assist in a disaster setting is largely reliant on their ability to assess events as they happen. One innovative tool that is being utilized in disaster response is crowdsourcing. This is a technology platform by which local people can report, via phone call, text message, or email, in real time about events as they occur. These reports are compiled and mapped by a central processing server, and the data is generally made open source so that disaster responders can utilize the data in their efforts. Crowdsourcing in this capacity was initially developed by an organization called Ushahidi, which developed a crowdsourcing platform during the violence following the 2008 Kenyan elections [23]. The Ushahidi website was used to map incidents of violence throughout Kenya based on reports submitted via the internet and mobile phones [23]. Since then, Ushahidi has expanded to become an open-source platform that can be used by groups around the world and can provide both new insights into events happening in real time and publicity to events not well-covered in the mainstream media [23].

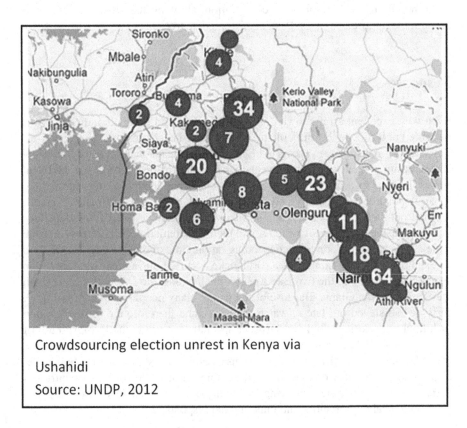

Crowdsourcing election unrest in Kenya via
Ushahidi
Source: UNDP, 2012

Sphere Standards

In disaster response, particularly in resource-poor cities, the response of local public safety officials and spontaneous volunteers is often followed by the response of the international humanitarian community. International humanitarian response is an increasingly complex and rapidly developing field, as well as a growing industry, with global humanitarian assistance reaching approximately US$15.1 billion in 2009 [5]. Humanitarian responders are continually increasing in their sophistication and learning from the humanitarian emergencies in which they operate, and have developed many innovations in disaster planning and response. One development is the creation of the Sphere Standards [18]. These comprise a handbook that outlines both quantitative and qualitative measures of what a consensus group of humanitarian agencies thought should be minimum standards in disaster response. These standards allow for measurable goals for urban disaster responders and are generally accepted as the minimum necessary for quality of life and dignity. Most humanitarian agencies operating in the field reference the Sphere Standards in their work, and many provide formal training to their responders. With the increased prevalence of urban refugees and disasters affecting urban areas, however, humanitarian agencies are finding that in some aspects, the Sphere Standards are untenable or not entirely applicable to urban settlements (rather than the prototypical rural refugee camps for which they were developed). Of note, many of the quantifiable Sphere Standards are not met by many urban slums at baseline [6]. Therefore, the humanitarian community is in the early phases of determining how the Sphere Standards should be modified or replaced in the urban setting [6].

Cluster System

While international humanitarian assistance frequently follows major disasters around the world, and while such assistance is frequently invaluable to the victims of catastrophe, such assistance has also been plagued in the past by a lack of coordination on the ground amongst the various responders. Therefore, the international disaster response community has developed a system by which organizations can specialize in the various aspects of humanitarian response and coordinate their actions and efforts with other similarly oriented organizations. This system, developed by the UN's Inter-Agency Standing Committee (IASC), is called the Cluster System. There are 11 clusters—groups of UN agencies, NGOs, and other organizations specialized in a sector of humanitarian assistance—each led by one agency during any given disaster response. The clusters are Protection, Camp Coordination and Management, Water Sanitation and Hygiene, Health, Emergency Shelter, Nutrition, Emergency Telecommunications, Logistics, Early Recovery, and Education and Agriculture [10]. While the cluster system is still developing, it is creating streamlined mechanisms to refine responding agencies' efforts. While the system has its critics, it represents a laudable high-level effort to organize widely disparate responders to global disasters and attempt to eliminate redundancy and waste in humanitarian response.

How are disaster relief efforts organised?

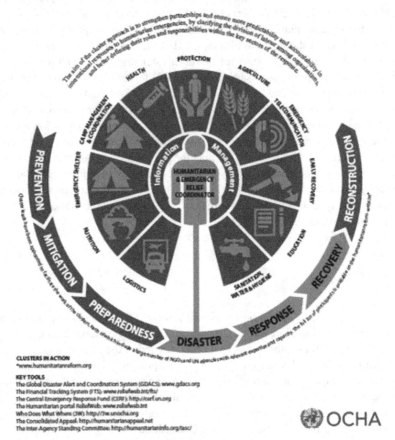

Source: business.UN.org, 2013

Recovery

While the acute disaster response phase invariably gets the greatest global media attention and scrutiny, most experts would agree that it is the recovery phase of disaster response where the most long-term impact is made. Although the transition from acute response to recovery is not always dramatic or clear, recovery is generally considered the period of rebuilding and recreating the infrastructure that was damaged or destroyed during the disaster. At times, the recovery phase offers opportunities to change the overall infrastructure of an urban environment, which can affect both economic and human capital. Indeed, many aspects of recovery planning are also considered aspects of planning and mitigation for future disasters as well, with this perspective being particularly pertinent in cities affected by cyclic disasters.

One major aspect of innovations in recovery is to involve the people affected by disaster as much as possible in the rebuilding of their own communities. Historically, many disaster recovery processes were organized top-down from government officials and international NGOs; therefore, the local people had little say in the details of the recovery efforts. In more recent disasters, however, responders have been more keen to involve the beneficiaries of their actions in the planning and decision-making, as doing so allows for more subtle, fair, and effective recovery. For example, after the 2004 Indian Ocean tsunami, the communities in Aceh actively joined in the decision-making around reconstruction. Because of their involvement, earlier plans for tough zoning, mandatory setbacks from the sea, and relocation of local markets were not pursued, and instead livelihoods were rehabilitated through multipronged approaches, including restoration of the agricultural and fishing sectors, rebuilding ports, replacing lost fishing boats, and offering microfinance programs, employment programs (such as cash for work), and training programs [7]. Such public consultation and involvement is very helpful to ensure public ownership of the recovery and to anticipate critical issues before decisions are made [11]. As mentioned above, urban communities have great opportunities for reestablishing local economies and livelihoods after a disaster and can do so more quickly if the local communities are involved in recovery efforts. Working with local citizens, disaster responders can rapidly assess preexisting markets and supply chains and work to reestablish markets that deliver products and services that underpin development. Food security can be established by reopening local food markets and allowing people to return to buying and cooking their food themselves, rather than relying on predetermined handouts [11].

In addition, NGOs can partner successfully with local leaders and the local population to assist with recovery efforts as well as planning and response efforts. The 2009 earthquake in Haiti was a case of a devastating natural disaster in a country that was considered by many to have a chronic humanitarian emergency before the earthquake [4]. Multiple NGOs had established a long-term presence in Haiti well before the earthquake struck, and many found themselves, by necessity, needing to reassess their development goals and mission in the setting of an acute disaster event. One organization in this situation was Partners in Health (PIH). Within two weeks of the earthquake, PIH had amended and expanded their health clinic capacities to be able to serve over 100,000 displaced people in the settlement camps around Port-au-Prince [13]. As PIH had already established a primary health system through which to provide comprehensive primary care, including maternal and child health, HIV and TB testing, mental health care, and malnutrition treatment, its task was a scaling up of these services, rather than establishing them anew [13]. Thus, PIH was able to assist with the disaster response acutely, and it continues to play a substantial role in the recovery of the nation's health system.

Conclusions

The field of disaster preparedness and response is dynamic and continually evolving. Many leaders in global cities as well as health and humanitarian experts are creating innovative new approaches to old problems around the world, particularly in low-income countries. As the world's population becomes ever more urban, and the climate becomes more extreme, the impact of disasters on global cities remains one of the greatest threats to human health and stability. As in all nascent fields, much research and discovery is yet to be done. As city officials and academics alike turn their attention to the threats of disasters in global cities, they must raise critical questions and seek to sort out the answers. The safety and security of our cities depend on it.

References

1. Aleppo Earthquake of 1138. Encyclopedia Britannica. http://www.britannica.com/EBchecked/topic/1462744/Aleppo-earthquake-of-1138. Accessed 12 July 2013.
2. Bengtsson L, Lu X, Thorson A, Garfield R, von Schreeb J. Improved response to disasters and outbreaks by tracking population movements with mobile phone network data: a post-earthquake geospatial study in Haiti. PLoS Med. 2011;8(8):e1001083.
3. EM-DAT: The OFDA/CRED International Disaster Database. Université Catholique de Louvain, Brussels, Belgium. www.emdat.be. http://www.emdat.be/natural-disasters-trends. Accessed 7/12/13.
4. European Commission. Haiti before the earthquake. 2010. http://ec.europa.eu/echo/files/aid/countries/Haiti_paper_01102010.pdf. Accessed 12 July 2013.
5. Global Humanitarian Assistance: a development initiative. Graphs and charts. http://www.globalhumanitarianassistance.org/data-guides/graphs-charts. Accessed 12 July 2013.
6. Urbanization and Humanitarian Access Working Group, Janneck LM, Patel R, Rouhani SA, Burkle FM. Urbanization and Humanitarian Access Working Group: toward guidelines for humanitarian standards and operations in urban settings. Prehosp Disaster Med. 2011;26(6):464–9.
7. Jayasuriya S, Peter M. The Asian tsunami: aid and reconstruction after a disaster. Cheltenham: Edward Elgar Publishing; 2010.
8. Karan PP, Subbiah S, editors. The Indian Ocean tsunami: the global response to a natural disaster. Lexington: University Press of Kentucky; 2011.
9. Landesman LY. Public health management of disasters: the practice guide. Washington, DC: American Public Health Association; 2005.
10. OCHA. Cluster coordination. http://www.unocha.org/what-we-do/coordination-tools/cluster-coordination. Accessed 12 July 2013.
11. O'Donnell I, Smart K, Ramalingam B. Responding to urban disasters: learning from previous relief and recovery operations. Alnap lessons.
12. Open Street Map. http://openstreetmap.org/. Accessed 12 July 2013.
13. Partners in Health. Annual report highlights: Haiti earthquake response. 2010. http://www.pih.org/annual-report/entry/annual-report-haiti-earthquake/. Accessed 12 July 2013.
14. Rouhani SA, Patel RB, Janneck LM, Prasad A, Lapitan J, Burkle FM. Urbanization and humanitarian access working group: a blueprint for the development of prevention and preparedness indicators for urban humanitarian crises. Prehosp Disaster Med. 2011;26(6):460–3.

15. Satellite Sentinel Project. http://www.satsentinel.org/. Accessed 12 July 2013.
16. Satterthwaite D, Huq S, Pelling M, Reid H, Lankao PR. Adapting to climate change in urban areas: the possibilities and constraints in low- and middle-income nations. Human Settlements Group and the Climate Change Group at the International Institute for Environment and Development (IIED). 2007.
17. Singh RB. Disaster management. Jaipur: Rawat Publications; 2000.
18. The Sphere Project: humanitarian charter and minimum standards in humanitarian response. 2011. http://www.sphereproject.org/
19. UNESCO IOC. Indian Ocean Tsunami Warning System performed well, detailed assessment underway. 2012. http://www.unesco.org/new/en/natural-sciences/ioc-oceans/single-view-oceans/news/indian_ocean_wide_tsunami_watch/. Accessed 12 July 2013.
20. UNESCO IOC. Protecting people from marine hazards, including tsunamis. http://www.unesco.org/new/en/natural-sciences/ioc-oceans/sections-and-programmes/tsunami/. Accessed 12 July 2013.
21. UNESCOPress. Indian Ocean Tsunami Warning System up and running. 2006. http://portal.unesco.org/en/ev.php-
22. UN-HABITAT. Harmonious cities: state of the world's cities 2008/9. London: Earthscan Publications Ltd.; 2008.
23. Ushahidi. http://ushahidi.com/. Accessed 12 July 2013.
24. WHO. Implementation of urban HEART. http://www.who.int/kobe_centre/measuring/urban-heart/implementation/en/index.html. Accessed 12 July 2013.
25. Wong E. A Chinese school, shored up by its principal, survived where others fell. New York Times. 2008.
26. World Bank. Climate change, disaster risk, and the urban poor: cities building resilience for a changing world. 2011. URL_ID=33442&URL_DO=DO_TOPIC&URL_SECTION=201.html. Accessed 12 July 2013.

Chapter 7
Innovations to Address Global Drug Counterfeiting: Implications for Urbanization and Health

Kendra Amico, Emily Aaronson, and Howard Zucker

Introduction

The recent rise in counterfeits has now extended from basic consumer goods and electronics to pharmaceuticals, jeopardizing the health of millions across the globe.

Estimates suggest that the counterfeit industry is now $75 billion and will grow by 20 % per year, making it one of the fastest growing public health risks [1]. Counterfeit medications, comprising more than 30 % of medications in parts of Asia, Africa, and Latin America, have only recently gained recognition by the general public and mainstream media. Although the burden of disease lies largely with the world's most vulnerable populations, Western countries are not insulated from this problem [2]. With the rapid growth of online pharmacies, the currently quoted 1 % prevalence of counterfeit medications in the United States will quickly rise [3]. The Internet, which boasts up to 50 % prevalence of counterfeit pharmaceuticals, has introduced medications such as blood pressure control, lifestyle medications, and pain modulators to the list of counterfeited medications.

The traditional definition of counterfeit medications, including both generic and brand name, is medications *deliberately and fraudulently mislabeled with respect to identity and/or source* [4]. In some instances, counterfeiting involves manufacturing a drug without its active ingredient—with chalk, starch, flour, or talcum powder in

K. Amico, M.D., M.Phil. • E. Aaronson, M.D. (✉)
Harvard Affiliated Emergency Medicine Residency at Brigham and Women's
Hospital/Massachusetts General Hospital, Boston, MA, USA

Harvard Medical School, Boston, MA, USA
e-mail: eaaronson@partners.org

H. Zucker, M.D., J.D.
Division of Global Health and Human Rights, Department of Emergency Medicine,
Massachusetts General Hospital, Boston, MA, USA

Albert Einstein College of Medicine of Yeshiva University, Bronx, NY, USA

© Springer New York 2015
R. Ahn et al. (eds.), *Innovating for Healthy Urbanization*,
DOI 10.1007/978-1-4899-7597-3_7

place of any active compound. Although less harmful than some of the more menacing manufacturing techniques, this approach puts patients at risk of morbidity and mortality from otherwise treatable diseases. In a more sinister approach, these formulations can be made with substitute medications providing relief of symptoms but not treatment of disease, for example, filling an antimalarial with acetaminophen, which will lower the fever of malaria but will not treat the underlying parasite. Other medications may have active ingredients but at nontherapeutic doses. This "up marketing" of medications runs the risk of creating resistance in the partially-treated host. These substandard medications subject patients to treatment failures and create drug-resistant organisms. Lastly, and perhaps the most publicized aspect of this issue, is the inclusion of noxious chemicals in medications marketed as therapeutic pharmaceuticals. Most notoriously, in place of the glycerin normally used in cough syrup, the toxic substance diethylene glycol has been used because of its similar taste, color, consistency, and lower cost.

Counterfeit pharmaceuticals thus have significant public health consequences beyond their individual-level effects. These falsified medications jeopardize the primary care environment by undermining people's faith in their physicians and making them question the integrity of the pharmaceutical supply chain.

This chapter will provide an overview of drug counterfeiting globally, describe its potential impact for urbanization and health, and discuss various mechanisms to address this problem.

A Global Problem

Drug counterfeiting was first identified almost 70 years ago when diethylene glycol was found in cough syrup in the United States. As a result of this incident, which caused 100 deaths, the federal government established the Food and Drug Administration (FDA). Strong regulatory standards presently monitored by the FDA limit the exposure of Americans to counterfeit pharmaceutical and biomedical products. However, in other countries with less stringent oversight, people routinely fall victim to similar attacks. One of the most publicized cases was that of a string of intentionally falsified barrels of diethylene glycol (again masquerading as glycerin) originating in China. These barrels ended up in the unknowing hands of the Panamanian government, who unwittingly mixed the lethal chemical into 260,000 bottles of cough syrup. When these were then distributed to hospitals and pharmacies throughout the country, an epidemic of progressive paralysis and respiratory collapse ensued—and resulted in the deaths of over 365 people [5].

Similar stories involving counterfeit products have occurred in many other countries. In 1995, 88 children, nearly half under 2 years old, were killed in Haiti, again from tainted glycerin reportedly manufactured in China [6]. The falsely labeled glycerin was sent to Port-au-Prince, where it was mixed into hundreds of bottles of fever medication and then given to children, almost all of whom subsequently died of kidney failure. The same year, 50,000 Nigerians were inoculated with a counterfeit meningitis vaccine, later causing 2,500 deaths from the disease [7]. Nigeria again fell victim 13 years later when 84 children died after using a tainted teething formula made by a Lagos-based pharmaceutical [2]. Similar mass poisonings have since been reported in Bangladesh, Argentina, and India. Specific reports of counterfeits have surfaced in dozens of countries, and this problem is now considered to be truly universal.

In addition to cough syrup and vaccines, malaria medications have been a prime target for falsification, with the most recent data suggesting that more than 36 % of malaria medications in Southeast Asia and 20 % in Sub-Saharan Africa are intentionally falsified [8].

Behind these tragic tales of unsuspecting victims are often complex webs of illegal networks. The initial act of forging the medicine is often followed by the arrangement of concealed shipments and falsified documents, which ultimately leads to distribution to the public. Interestingly, by the time these medicines reach the hands of distributors, they are often unaware that the medicines they are peddling are false, which only further complicates the issue of accountability and enforcement.

Inciting Factors

The reasons for the continued growth and evolution of drug counterfeiting are multifactorial. Often, patients in poorer countries buy their medications out-of-pocket, even when hospitalized. Expensive medications, in either original or generic forms, can be an insurmountable barrier. Thus, patients are persuaded to buy medications from unregulated vendors [3]. This scenario creates demand for cheaper medications and makes poorer populations particularly vulnerable to counterfeits that are less expensive than authentic pharmaceuticals [9]. Consumers who abuse controlled substances, such as narcotics, and utilize unregulated markets, are another target population susceptible to counterfeiters [10]. Similarly, consumers who are too embarrassed to ask for a prescription for lifestyle medications (e.g., those targeted at impotence or baldness) and utilize Internet retailers are vulnerable targets of counterfeiters.

From an economic perspective, the business of counterfeiting offers high profit margins. Though the true cost is hard to determine, estimates suggest that counterfeiting brought in US$70 billion in profits in 2010 [11]. Many apprehended counterfeiters had simply constructed operations in their homes, backyards, or in small industry settings, all environments in which production costs remained low [3]. These "cottage industries" are not held to the same safety and regulatory standards as legitimate pharmaceuticals, further increasing their profits [3]. Urban environments allow for even easier fraud and abuse of medications, while those same settings are simultaneously fostering increased incidence of certain ailments from triggers, such as overcrowding and pollution.

Underdeveloped regulatory systems in many countries cannot reliably or efficiently detect breeches in their manufacturing and distribution pathways; thus, it is quite difficult to identify the problem, let alone trace it back to instigators [3, 9]. Medicines typically pass through the hands of numerous parties crossing into several countries, each of which has its specific customs and trading regulations. Given this fragmented and at times corrupt system, it is easy to imagine how counterfeit pharmaceuticals can slip into the system undetected [3]. And one must remember that an episode of counterfeiting does not involve just one pill; rather, it is a batch of thousands of counterfeit pills. Thus, there is great complexity and difficulty in containing this problem.

Even when counterfeiters are apprehended, there is ongoing debate on how to handle this crime or even if it should be considered a true criminal offense. Lack of stringent enforcement and adequate punishment creates a favorable environment for counterfeiters to operate. Illustrating this perfect storm, in 2004, toxic ingredients substituted for iron resulted in liver failure and death in a 22-year-old Argentinian girl undergoing treatment for anemia. The official national investigation was hampered by falsified paperwork, inability to identify all parties involved, and uncertainty over how to proceed with suspected offenders, rendering it powerless in preventing subsequent deaths and ill effects from the same counterfeit medications [3].

As a result of these factors, efforts to combat counterfeiting remain unchecked and provide fertile ground for counterfeiters to prey on vulnerable and often quite ill people. Though numerous stakeholders have attempted to resolve this problem, coordination remains a Herculean task. Multiple distractions contribute to failure in troubleshooting the counterfeit medicines problem. Most notable among these factors is the debate over the intellectual property rights of pharmaceuticals. Specifically, should anticounterfeiting measures focus solely on the content, production, safety, and efficacy profile of pharmaceuticals, or should they also address the right to manufacture generics? Concern abounds that the fight against counterfeit pharmaceuticals would infringe on the development and trade of generics, thus having a stronger detrimental effect on developing countries [9]. Failure to agree promotes discord and draws attention away from the core issue, namely, stopping counterfeit activities [9]. In addition, many countries fail to recognize the benefits of prioritizing the fight against counterfeit medicines or choose not to invest capital into troubleshooting efforts [3]. Achieving consensus on the definition of the crime and the extent of punishment is imperative if public health experts, policymakers, law enforcement, and regulatory agencies want to combat drug counterfeiting.

Drug counterfeiting is extremely difficult to monitor, as information is amassed from multiple sources and is often incomplete in some regard. Developing countries lack regulatory systems to identify and collect counterfeiting data, so reporting from them is even more infrequent and fragmented; efficiently distributing resources without an accurate accounting of drug counterfeiting activity is problematic.

Based on available data, counterfeiting is thought to be less than 1 % of market value in industrialized countries, including Australia, Canada, Japan, United States, and most nations within the European Union. This estimate excludes Internet purchases, which are estimated to be counterfeits in up to 50 % of cases where the address of the originator is not provided. Countries with weak regulatory systems

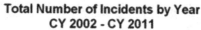

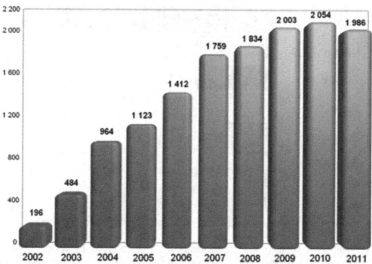

Fig. 7.1 Total number of counterfeit drug incidents by year identified worldwide by the Pharmaceutical Security Institute (PSI) [12]

are at greater risk: Counterfeit estimates approach 20 % in the former Soviet Union and 30 % in some regions of Africa, Asia, and Latin America [3].

The Pharmaceutical Security Institute (PSI), now comprised of 25 pharmaceutical companies, has created a dynamic system over the past decade for identifying counterfeit drug incidents and alerting the appropriate authorities. In 2011, they reported 1,986 verified incidents (Fig. 7.1) [12]. These incidents involved 532 different pharmaceutical products; the top three drug categories were genitourinary, anti-infective, and cardiovascular. The majority of arrests occurred in Asia (Figs. 7.1, 7.2, and 7.3).

Given the breadth of the drug counterfeiting problem and its increasing infiltration of the drug market, success in combating this problem requires a multifaceted approach. Efforts are already underway and include national legislation, improved regulation for manufacturers and distributors, communication, and collaboration among stakeholders, public education, and the necessary technologies to detect counterfeits. The following sections will highlight the challenges, lessons learned, and best practices among these different aspects while looking ahead to future needs. Specifically, legislative and regulatory efforts, enforcement measures, technology developments, and communication networks will be discussed as they pertain to fighting counterfeit medicines.

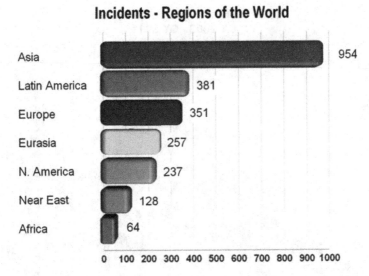

Fig. 7.2 Number of counterfeit drug incidents in 2011 recorded by region from by the Pharmaceutical Security Institute (PSI). A region is included if it is the "origin, point of seizure or transit, or destination" of illegal pharmaceuticals [12]

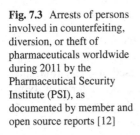

Fig. 7.3 Arrests of persons involved in counterfeiting, diversion, or theft of pharmaceuticals worldwide during 2011 by the Pharmaceutical Security Institute (PSI), as documented by member and open source reports [12]

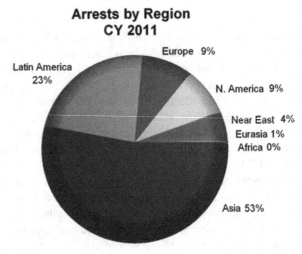

Legislation

International and national efforts to overcome the challenge of counterfeit medications begin with effective legislative reform. Although efforts to combat counterfeits to date have largely revolved around identification, detection, and seizures, there have also been some important steps taken toward creating a better foundation to deter or prevent the creation of these pharmaceuticals in the first place. Efforts that have centered on multi-group involvement, engaging stakeholders from the government, the pharmaceutical industry, drug suppliers, importers, distributors, and the public sector, have set the benchmark for effective action. This legislative landscape, however, is complicated by debates surrounding the definition of a counterfeit, fear of infringement on generic medications and pharmaceutical sales, and the need to navigate the complex waters of transnational jurisdictions. As counterfeit drug sales continue to climb, with an estimated 90 % increase in sales from 2005 to 2010, this will be an issue that governments will increasingly have to face at a legislative level [8]. The ability to create strong, international policies on the issue of counterfeit medications hinges on the ability to come up with a standardized definition. Increasingly, organizations have adopted the WHO definition:

> The term counterfeit medical product describes a product with a false representation (a) of its identity (b) and/or source (c). This applies to the product, its container or other packaging or labeling information. Counterfeiting can apply to both branded and generic products. Counterfeits may include products with correct ingredients/components (d), with wrong ingredients/components, without active ingredients, with incorrect amounts of active ingredients, or with fake packaging. Violations or disputes concerning patents must not be confused with counterfeiting of medical products. Medical products (whether generic or branded) that are not authorized for marketing in a given country but authorized elsewhere are not considered counterfeit. Substandard batches of, or quality defects or non-compliance with Good Manufacturing Practices/Good Distribution Practices (GMP/GDP) in legitimate medical products must not be confused with counterfeiting.
>
> Notes: (a) Counterfeiting is done fraudulently and deliberately. The criminal intent and/or careless behavior shall be considered during the legal procedures for the purposes of sanctions imposed.
>
> (b) This includes any misleading statement with respect to name, composition, strength, or other elements. (c) This includes any misleading statement with respect to manufacturer, country of manufacturing, country of origin, marketing authorization holder or steps of distribution. (d) This refers to all components of a medical product [13].

This definition stems from a similar version drafted at a workshop organized by the WHO and International Federation of Pharmaceutical Manufacturers & Association in 1992. Although revised in 2008 and generally accepted by many stakeholders, the definition was never formally adopted by member states and remains an area of great contention for many [9]. Some controversy originated from the initial use of "counterfeit" solely in conjunction with intellectual property or trademark violations. Only more recently has the scope of the definition been broadened to include falsified pharmaceuticals, where the identity or source of the medications have been misrepresented without necessarily violating intellectual property rights, as well as substandard medications where pre-specified quality standards are unmet [14]. The Institute of Medicine and the United Kingdom's Chatham House are continually refining their working definition of counterfeit medicines to emphasize the public health implications and not interfere with the trade in generics [14, 15].

More specifically, the concerns related to tougher legislation against counterfeits revolve around the role of WHO in the intellectual property debate. Some developing countries fear that the WHO's involvement in regulating counterfeit medications will negatively impact their ability to provide legitimate generic medications to their populations [16]. This fire was further fueled by the detention of 19 shipments of medications, which were under patent in Europe but came from or were sent to countries where the medications were considered generic [14]. Attempts to alleviate this concern resulted in the inclusion of the following phrases in the 2008 revised definition: "Violations or disputes concerning patents must not be confused with counterfeiting of medical products. Medical products (whether generic or branded) that are not authorized for marketing in a given country but authorized elsewhere are not considered counterfeit" [13].

Some countries, however, believe that the WHO should redirect their focus and address all substandard medications—in effect, those that threaten public health and safety—rather than focusing on counterfeits alone [14]. Some of these countries have thus adopted broader definitions that make no distinction between counterfeit and substandard medications, while others have clearly separated these out for fear of infringement on intellectual property considerations [15].

The debate over defining counterfeit medications is a subset of the larger issue regarding barriers to broad anti-counterfeiting policy adoption. Many of the policy measures suggested by advocacy and interest groups include mandatory reporting, greater transparency, cooperation between the private and public sector, and a multinational approach to tackling this issue. This approach is complicated by the hesitancy of some governments and pharmaceutical companies to publicize cases of counterfeits. Their concern is that such publicized awareness will harm the public's faith in medication, perhaps instigate a movement away from treatment all together, or damage the sales of the authentic pharmaceuticals targeted by counterfeiters [17]. Hence, disincentives exist to promoting awareness of this global counterfeit problem. Examples of the above actions are highlighted by SmithKline Beecham's decision not to act against counterfeiters when their meningitis vaccine was substituted for an inactive formulation by counterfeiters and distributed across Niger. The company was concerned that such publicity would damage their name brand [18]. Similarly, Schering took a whole month to distribute information that their oral contraceptive had been tampered with—by replacing the active pharmaceutical agent with wheat flower [18].

Regulation

The incidence of counterfeiting is greater in areas where regulation is weaker. With 30 % of countries lacking effective drug regulatory agencies, such nations become easy targets for counterfeiters [17]. Paradoxically, these are the same nations that exhibit the greatest burden of disease, least access to affordable medicines, and largest gap between the price of legitimate medicines and the price of counterfeits.

Therefore, it is essential that governments and international bodies regulate this issue. This was first addressed in 1985 when the issue of counterfeiting was raised at the WHO Conference of Experts on the Rational Use of Drugs in Nairobi, Kenya. It was suggested that the WHO facilitate global efforts to better understand the fight against counterfeit medicine through data collection, information sharing, and government alerts [14]. Three years later, a resolution was adopted against counterfeit and substandard medications at the 1988 World Health Assembly. They took an even stronger stance and asserted that the WHO should "initiate programs for the prevention and detection of export, import and smuggling of falsely labeled, spurious, counterfeited or substandard pharmaceutical preparations" [17].

This culminated in the creation of the International Medical Products Anti-Counterfeiting Taskforce (IMPACT) by the WHO in 2006. This partnership, charged with engaging stakeholders in a collaborative effort to protect individuals from counterfeit medications, has outlined critical areas for government intervention and legislative frameworks. Their multiple reports and guidelines are published and widely available.

International mobilization of this nature led to the Anti-Counterfeiting Trade Agreement (ACTA) in 2011. This multinational agreement aimed to create international legal framework and standardize enforcement guidelines to aid in detection and enforcement of counterfeit products. Although controversy centered on copyright infringement surrounding the agreement, it was ultimately adopted and remains an example of strong international collaboration.

In 2011, the European Union initiated efforts to both prevent and prosecute counterfeit activities, by drafting a convention on the counterfeiting of medical products and similar crimes involving threats to public health (MEDICRIME convention) [19]. The European Commission on Public Health further advanced this effort by publishing the Adoption and Publication of Commission Implementing Regulation on Pharmacovigilance Activities—a guide to help agencies apply new legislation targeted at combating counterfeits [20]. With an increasing amount of counterfeit medications sold online, the European Union also introduced the Directive on Falsified Medicines in 2011, increasing the regulation and safety of online pharmacies [21, 22]. Similarly, the National Association of Boards of Pharmacy (NABP), a North American-based organization, launched the Verified Internet Pharmacy Practice Sites (VIPPS) program in 1999. This program accredits sites with good compliance and licensure, thereby ensuring authenticity [23].

The American government has taken important steps to address the issue of counterfeits. With 40 % of pharmaceuticals sold in the United States and 80 % of all active ingredients made outside of American borders, the Food and Drug Administration (FDA) created a task force to identify high-yield recommendations aimed at government, industry, and the general public [24]. The agency's task force has completed border studies, developed an alert system, strengthened distribution systems, investigated new technologies, and engaged the public and private sector in this effort.

The FDA's work in this area is rooted in the Prescription Drug Marketing Act (PDMA) of 1987, which requires pharmaceutical wholesalers to track and trace drug distribution [25]. This act, modified in 1992 and with clear regulations for implementation published in 1999, laid the groundwork for the FDA's current mission of ensuring pharmaceuticals within the United States are protected by creating safeguards in the distribution system [26]. The FDA's first step in achieving this objective was the publication of the 2011 Pathway to Global Product Safety and Quality report that documented the agency's commitment to working seamlessly in the international environment [26]. The FDA has also worked with the United States Customs and Border Control to study pharmaceutical entry into the United States in an effort to delineate the problem and identify solutions [26]. Private trade organizations, including the International Federation of Pharmaceutical Manufacturers & Associations (IFPMA), have identified counterfeit medications as a public health concern and published position papers specifically targeting this issue. In 2010, the IFPMA circulated their Ten Principles on Counterfeit Medicines document, which aims to create a "policy environment that recognizes, prioritizes and effectively addresses the major threat to global health posed by counterfeit medicines" [27].

Detection is a critical step in the fight against counterfeit medications, and some legislative efforts have begun to focus on this specific aspect of anticounterfeiting. The FDA's system of reporting stems from an agreement made by US pharmaceutical companies in 2003, in which the FDA is notified within five business days of a suspected counterfeit; however, it remains a voluntary program that has no legal obligation for reporting. The WHO's Western Pacific Region also instituted a centralized database in 2005 that generates web-based "Rapid Alerts" to member countries following the detection of a counterfeit medication; these alerts aim to communicate real-time warnings across national borders [28]. Nonprofits organizations, such as the Partnership for Safe Medicines in the United States, have also started similar programs that publish weekly public alerts on suspected cases. However, all of these efforts depend on strong reporting, and the drug industry—often the first to know about counterfeits—is sometimes wary of the impact on their brand with public reporting. A private-industry collective, the PSI, has taken the lead on collecting data in this area: Their Counterfeiting Incident System (CIS) records the incidents of counterfeits, drug thefts, and diversions, drawing on direct reports from member pharmaceutical companies, nonmembers, the media, and the public sector. This database, which recorded 1,311 arrests for counterfeiting in FY2011 (a 14 % increase from FY2010), is confidential. Outside of the broad annual incident reports, its contents are neither shared with the WHO nor disseminated to the public [18].

Enforcement

In addition to the need for strong legislation to support safer practices in the manufacturing, distribution, and reporting of medicines, there also needs to be a strong legal system to prosecute perpetrators. Currently, the penalties for counterfeit medications are less onerous than those for counterfeiting a designer purse [29]. The FDA further reinforced this need by calling for higher penalties in its *Pathway to Global Product Safety and Quality* report [24]. In the United States, where the average jail sentence for a counterfeiting crime is 3 years, steps have been taken toward stricter penalties, most recently with the proposed Counterfeit Drug Penalty Enhancement Act of 2011. This act would increase the maximum prison sentence for counterfeiting medicines to 20 years for individual first-time offenders and increase the maximum fine that can be imposed on them to US$4 million [30, 31]. This legal disconnect is not unique to America. As of 2000, in India, which is the source of many counterfeit medications, the penalty for a convicted counterfeit drug manufacturing is imprisonment for at least 3 years and a fine of US$108 [32]. Although stricter penalties are needed, the challenge lies in the international nature of the crimes—often crossing many borders and with multiple minor infringements on manufacturing, shipping, importation, distribution, and documentation laws along the way.

Enforcement of the laws that do exist is a crucial step in better understanding the scope of the problem and effectively addressing proliferation of the counterfeit industry. Within the United States, the FDA created the Office of Criminal Investigations (OCI), which is tasked with taking the lead on investigations, working with local police to coordinate arrests, and working with local law enforcement to ensure these cases go to trial. Since its inception in 1992, the OCI has initiated 580 counterfeit drug investigations, resulting in 522 arrests and 414 convictions, with fines and restitutions totaling US$56,943,560 [33]. Most recently, in FY2011 the OCI initiated 59 counterfeit drug investigations—resulting in 30 arrests, 38 convictions, and US$1.3 million in fines [33]. Interpol has arguably played the largest role in this arena, mobilizing large international efforts around detection and enforcement. Its work over the last 15 years in many ways serves as a case study for effective, systematic partnership that acknowledges the transnational nature of the problem and works with multiple organizations and government agencies.

Interpol's multi-pronged approach hinges on collaboration between police officers, customs agents, health regulatory authorities, scientists, and the private sector while employing education, field support, and operational execution to support the work. Interpol uses training workshops to build international capacity for targeting transnational counterfeiting activities [34]. A seminar in Kenya in 2009 launched an effort to fight counterfeiting in Eastern and Southern Africa. A subsequent course in Senegal focused on Western and Northern Africa. Interpol's focus on skills and knowledge trains these representatives around the health risk of counterfeit medications and gives them tools to identify, investigate, and combat them. This education, taking place in the classroom and through online modules, lays the groundwork for field support. Through a series of interactive modules, Interpol has created a curriculum that fosters investigations, operations, and legal prosecutions. Lastly, Interpol's operations have proven that this type of multinational cooperation is not only possible, but, in fact, is also a highly-effective model.

Operation Storm was the first multi-country anti-counterfeiting operation led by Interpol, with the help of the WHO and World Customs Organization. This effort brought together customs, drug regulatory agencies, and policymakers of participating countries in an effort to disrupt the transnational criminal network of counterfeit trafficking in Southeast Asia. In keeping with Interpol's model, the operation began with planning meetings, helping to establish the political will and an international agreement to share intelligence. The scope of the operation was also clear; it had a particular emphasis on antimalarials, anti-TB drugs, anti-HIV drugs, and antibiotics.

Table 7.1 Operation Pangea successes [49, 66]

Results (no.)	Pangea II (2009)	Pangea III (2010)	Pangea IV (2011)
Countries involved	25	44	81
Websites identified as performing illegal activities	1,200	822	
Website shutdown	153	297	13,500
Packages inspected	21,200	278,000	45,500
Packages seized for with counterfeit medicines	2,356	11,349	8,000
Tablets seized		2,300,000	2,400,000
Suspects arrested or under investigation	59	87	55
Value of seized illegal or counterfeit medicines		US$6.77 million	US$6.3 million

Next, Interpol hosted training sessions for officials and personnel who would be participating in the operation. Collaboration extended beyond the public sector with buy-in from private facilities that could provide forensics analysis, such as the Health Science Authority Criminalistics Lab in Singapore. Pharmaceutical companies also offered additional intelligence and legitimate samples for comparison with counterfeits. This 5-month effort (April 15, 2008–September 15, 2008) was successful (Table 7.1) as an effective model for international cooperation. Operation Storm resulted in development of subsequent ongoing operations, targeting the disruption of transnational criminal networks of counterfeit trafficking in different parts of the world. Operation Mamba, in Eastern Africa, and Operation Cobra, in Western Africa, took similar systematic approaches to addressing this issue. Emerging from these successes was the creation of Operation Pangea, an annual week of action against the online sale of counterfeit pharmaceuticals. Small-scale alerts and large-scale programs, initiated by the private sector, have also been implemented to fight counterfeits. In 2002, Johnson & Johnson issued 200,000 letters to healthcare workers in the United States alerting them to the presence of fake ProCrit (medicine to treat anemia) on the market [18]. Larger efforts have come from companies, including Pfizer, Sanofi-Aventis, and Novartis, who have launched units dedicated to counterfeit detection and enforcement [35]. Working with investigators, police, the Secret Service, and customs, private companies have mobilized an effort to gather information through monitoring the Internet, distribution, and sales.

Communication/Public Awareness

Despite ongoing legislative efforts, drug counterfeiting continues to pose a serious public health threat, due to the public's profound lack of awareness of this critical problem. A 2003 survey in Benin demonstrated that 86 % of people interviewed thought medicines acquired from street vendors were of good quality [36]. A similar survey conducted in 2007 in a university setting in the United Arab Emirates and Tunisia revealed that approximately 50 % of students possessed some general knowledge about counterfeit medications. However, 93 % never considered the potential risk of purchasing counterfeits when filling prescriptions in the past [37]. Typically, when faced with a treatment failure, most consumers did not suspect counterfeit medication as the cause of the problem.

Thus, effective solutions for drug counterfeiting require risk communication, alerting the public to the potential dangers of counterfeit medications. Eliciting support from the media helps highlight this concern to the public. The target audience also requires education on how individuals can protect themselves from health risks associated with counterfeits. The ultimate goal is that these steps can change consumers' behaviors, so that procurement of medications is from a reliable source, such as an established pharmacy instead of an Internet vendor.

Several public awareness campaigns have been implemented to address this problem. In response to the 2003 Benin survey, a 9-month campaign was developed using primarily television and radio announcements to emphasize the dangers of the counterfeit drug market. In a follow-up survey, 90 % percent of respondents demonstrated understanding of this public health issue. In addition, investigators observed a subsequent decrease in purchase of medications from illicit vendors, as public health facilities and pharmacies became the dominant sources [38]. A poster-based campaign developed for school children in Northern Africa heightened awareness with 61 % of 3,182 school children having reported seeing the posters. More importantly, these children recounted having a conversation with their parents about illegal and counterfeit medicines [39].

Since 1998, the Global Anti-Counterfeiting Network has sponsored an annual World Anti-Counterfeiting Day as a way to simultaneously involve different stakeholders while attracting substantial media attention. In 2012, numerous countries, including Finland, France, and India, in collaboration with others, engaged in press releases, seminars, and open-forum discussions to curb drug counterfeiting [40]. In addition to promoting public awareness, these types of events elicit support from additional groups and may promote policies to achieve eradication of counterfeit pharmaceuticals. A global awards ceremony recognized organizations and individuals who had made exceptional contributions to the anticounterfeiting movement, further providing incentives to others to continue in their anticounterfeiting efforts.

With the rise of YouTube and widespread availability of the Internet, educational and promotional videos are a cost-effective means of spreading awareness about the problem of pharmaceutical counterfeiting. Numerous individuals and organizations have created documentaries on this topic, including the Global Fund to Fight AIDS video intended for Africans. In its production, the video beseeches Africans to "not be cheated and demand good medication" [41]. Other resources include IMPACT's videos, which give a case scenario of someone dying from a counterfeit medicine [42], and mPedigree, which produced a documentary filmed in Africa called "If Symptoms Persist," which suggests that consumers will consider counterfeit medications if their treatments are ineffective [43, 44]. A YouTube

Table 7.2 Online resources

SafeMeds Alert System	A free e-mail service that relays counterfeit drug alerts issued by the FDA
SAFEDRUG Checklist	An 8-step guide to boost medicine safety; tips on what to do if you suspect something
Safe Savings	A guide to government- and industry-sponsored programs offering high-quality, safe medicines at reduced prices
VIPPS Pharmacies	A direct link to legitimate online pharmacies recommended by the FDA
SafeMeds Blog	An expert-led discussion forum on safe medicines

Source: Pharmaceutical Security Institute (http://www.psi-inc.org/index.cfm) [46]

documentary entitled "Fake Medicines Mafia in Europe" also promoted awareness of the drug counterfeiting problem [45]. Similarly, Interpol launched an advertising campaign online on YouTube, called "Don't Be Your Own Killer" [42].

Several toolkits, both online and in downloadable forms, have been developed to provide patients and health professionals with action steps when counterfeiting activity is suspected. The PSI, in partnership with the Partnership for Safe Medicines (PSM), has created several online tools, all with the goals of protecting and empowering consumers and health professionals [46]. Their tools include e-mail alerts, tips for when one suspects counterfeiting, and links to legitimate online pharmacies and programs offering safe medications (Table 7.2). IMPACT has also created a BE AWARE Toolkit which provides basic education about drug counterfeiting, including when to suspect or report it [42]. It includes downloadable FAQ sheets, sample reporting forms, posters and brochures, checklists for patient waiting rooms, and helpful ways to broach topic with patients.

Promoting awareness should extend beyond just the end user or health professional and target those involved in policy decisions. In early 2012, PSM hosted a briefing on Capitol Hill entitled "The Continued Impact of Counterfeit Drugs in the United States." The event was part of a series designed to both raise awareness and develop policies to address the problem of counterfeit medicines [42]. This was partly prompted by counterfeit Avastin, a chemotherapy agent recently infiltrating the United States medical supply. PSM also hosts an annual Interchange Conference bringing together policymakers, pharmaceutical manufacturers, patient advocates, law enforcement, healthcare professionals, and anti-counterfeiting companies to discuss and solve this ever-growing issue [47]. PSM even has a Facebook page, publishing daily stories that highlight the global counter-feiting problem.

Information exchange on drug counterfeiting has been formalized in an attempt to streamline communication across national borders. In the Western Pacific Region, WHO created a Rapid Alert System, which is an electronic communication network involving representatives from numerous countries [48]. Alerts regarding suspected counterfeit activities are transmitted to the appropriate authorities. Once cases are confirmed, they are added to the WHO database for tracking and improved collaboration.

Ideally, this could develop into a resource that could be accessed by the entire global community—with a shared database of documented cases. IMPACT also created a "Model for a Network of Single Points of Contact" (SPOC), which also facilitates operational collaboration at national and international levels and enhances communication. This network has helped coordinate numerous large-scale operations, which were successful in stopping large groups of counterfeiting activities and making numerous arrests.

Taking advantage of these networks, Operation Pangea provides a great example of how international collaboration in conjunction with clear communication can successfully curtail counterfeiting. This multiphase international campaign has focused its efforts on the sale of online counterfeit medicines. Web-crawling software pinpointed suspicious websites worldwide, and as a result, the UK-based Medicines and Healthcare Products Regulatory Agency passed this information on to individual countries that researched the sites [49]. Designated SPOCs from each country reported daily activities, including closure of illegal websites, drug seizures, and arrests to Interpol, which posted that information on a secure exchange that was linked to other customs agencies. Information was also passed on to PSI, which kept track of ongoing investigations (so as to not duplicate efforts), thereby creating another communication loop.

Meanwhile, Interpol coordinated press releases on seizures and arrests at the end of week. All involved parties agreed on an identical opening message and simultaneous press release, generating a burst of international media attention. After the first phase in 2008, hundreds of newspaper and Internet articles picked up the story, and it was published in over 17 languages. Thus, the operation accrued a significant amount of media attention, transforming Operation Pangea into a powerful public health message. Operation Pangea was followed by an international debriefing session, allowing for feedback and ideas for future improvement.

Operation Pangea's results are impressive. The first phase, in 2008, was a 1-week event backed by the Permanent Forum on International Pharmaceutical Crime and Interpol and carried out in Australia, Canada, Ireland, Israel, Singapore, Switzerland, the United Kingdom, and the United States. The following year, Operation Pangea II expanded to 25 countries, with even broader involvement of police, customs agencies, and drug regulatory authorities simultaneously targeting Internet counterfeiting activities within their individual jurisdictions. Over 1,200 websites participating in counterfeiting or other illegal activities were closed [49]. Now an established annual event, Operation Pangea continues to expand (Table 7.1). Overall, great collaboration and communication among different agencies in different countries successfully fought against online counterfeiting and triggered a surge of media coverage. The international community was made aware of the public health hazards of counterfeit pharmaceuticals, with specific emphasis on hazards of purchasing medications from unreliable Internet sources.

Technology

Lastly, attention needs to be paid to technological innovations impacting anti-counterfeiting efforts. The technological savvy of individuals and corporations in the health field is growing exponentially. Ideally, as awareness of drug counterfeiting grows, the capacity for entrepreneurship, ingenuity, and technological innovation can be successfully applied to this problem. The global market for anti-counterfeiting packaging technologies has significantly increased, as more companies adopt sophisticated measures. Sales to food and drug industries amounted to US$59 billion in 2009, with a projected overall increase to US$74 billion in 2015 [50].

Technologic development should be conscious of both the cost and sustainability of project ideas in order to promote international compatibility. Ultimately, goals of anti-counterfeiting technologies include establishing the identity and authenticity of an item, thereby detecting counterfeits more easily and creating additional technological deterrents.

Anti-counterfeiting technologies can be broadly divided into authentication packaging technologies, both overt and covert, and track-and-trace technologies. As the name implies, overt technologies are easily visible by the naked eye. This includes marks as simple as the item's brand name as well as holograms, thermochromic inks, watermarks, or other security graphics [3]. These ideas have generated newer tamper-resistant technologies, such as HoloSeal™ or HoloCAP™, and apply the hologram idea to create security tapes and seals, thereby preventing the product from being adulterated or replaced. With any sort of tampering, a pill bottle cap may break a label and may convert to a void mark [51]. The visibility of these markings allows inspectors as well as end users to individually authenticate the item; however, this requires both awareness and education regarding the item's expected appearance. Otherwise, simple counterfeits can fool the average user.

Increased use of these technologies has unfortunately increased the incentive for counterfeiting. Since these packaging components are visible, they need to be complex and difficult to reproduce in order to deter imitations. This adds considerable cost to the development of overt technologies and does not eliminate the need for covert deterrents.

Unlike overt technologies, those that are covert require some form of equipment, for example, a special reader or chemical reaction, in order to establish a drug's authenticity. Invisible inks, digital watermarks, laser coding, and chemical tags all constitute forms of covert anti-counterfeiting measures. Covert technologies are typically of little benefit to consumers, since they will not even be aware of these markings, but rather are used at the manufacturing level. Once an outsider is aware of the covert technology, it loses its value, as these technologies are typically inexpensive and easy to copy [49]. Thus, strict secrecy is required. Initially proposed by one of the authors of this chapter (H.Z.) and presented at international meetings on counterfeits, the use of a cell phone to verify a code under a scratch-off label has been implemented by innovators in Africa [52]. Subsequently, in Ghana, a start-up

Fig. 7.4 A consumer scratches the panel on his medication to determine if it is genuine [43]

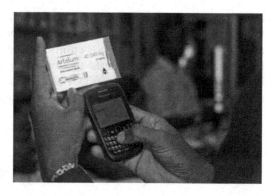

company called mPedigree worked with drug manufacturers and mobile phone companies to establish a mobile authentication system that empowered consumers to participate in the authentication process [43, 44]. Prior to distribution, manufacturers affix a scratch sticker to drug packaging (Fig. 7.4). When a consumer purchases that drug, he/she can simply scratch the panel to reveal a unique code. Texting this code, toll-free, to a designated data center prompts a quick response that proves or disproves the legitimacy of the product. The company has now grown considerably, receiving increased funding and expanding into Nigeria, with future plans for Kenya and possibly India [53]. This strategy, while not foolproof, is an example of an extremely accessible and consumer-friendly product that avoids the high costs of many other technologies.

Another authentication technology, ProteXXion®, uses the actual surface of the pill or drug packaging without any added markings to create a unique identifier. Lasers scan the item to create a biometric fingerprint; the item can then be re-scanned using a portable handheld scanner and the results compared. Non-identical images would indicate tampering with either the package or the drug itself [54, 55].

Forensic technologies require even more expertise and equipment. At the production level, microscopic or chemical tags can be added to a drug compound itself instead of using packaging markers. For example, radioisotopes, DNA tags, or photonic inks that emit unique wavelengths of light can be incorporated into the drug for identification purposes [49, 56]. More commonly, forensic technologies are applied to drug analysis in order to measure the potency of a drug's active ingredients and detect the presence of contaminants. For example, testing of antimalarial pharmaceuticals in Southeast Asia in 2001 demonstrated that 38 % lacked the active ingredient artesunate [57]. Similarly, a recent batch of Adderall (to treat attention-deficit disorder) sold over the Internet contained none of its intended active ingredients; these had instead been replaced with the painkiller tramadol [58].

Raman spectroscopy, one means of analysis, can noninvasively and nondestructively authenticate pharmaceutical products with high chemical specificity and accuracy [59]. The technology can penetrate pill capsules, bubble packaging, and plastic containers to establish a drug's chemical makeup. This technology has been applied to bottles of aspirin and antimalarials and is being developed as a handheld Raman analyzer [59]. Other handheld devices include portable ion mobility spectrometers that target drug analysis efforts. This technology is capable of screening large batches of pharmaceuticals and indicating which medications need further in-depth lab analysis. These methods have recently been applied to screening of dietary supplements, some of which have been found to contain excess amounts of sibutramine, an appetite suppressant, or sildenafil, an erectile dysfunction drug [60].

Limits of Anti-Counterfeiting Technology

While these high-tech strategies can establish a drug's authenticity with great chemical accuracy, they can be prohibitively expensive and require adequate laboratory infrastructure, including considerable human resources. Furthermore, many of the technologies are patented, which limits their availability globally. It can be very difficult for low-income countries to test their pharmaceuticals on a national scale. In response to the expense and technical capacity required to perform drug-quality monitoring, Global Pharma Health Fund (GPHF) developed inexpensive field test kits designated at GPHF-Minilabs, which could be used outside of a laboratory. More than 500 Minilabs have been supplied across 80 countries, with an emphasis on countries where tuberculosis, AIDS, and malaria are endemic [61].

Typically, product packaging authentication is combined with tracking and tracing technologies. 2D bar codes or serialization has been used primarily, which allows a batch of pharmaceuticals to be tracked through the supply chain. While not hidden, track-and-trace technologies identify the source of the pharmaceuticals, manufacturing data, product lot, and so forth, with the goal of preventing infiltration of the supply pathway. These simpler technologies have predominated, due to lower cost, complexity issues, and greater availability. Still, they require a central database which can be problematic in terms of ownership and management as the supply chain becomes increasingly global.

A newer but more costly technology, radio-frequency identification (RFID), uses a microchip imbedded in drug packaging to track pharmaceuticals wirelessly at the batch or item level [62]. RFID applications in the anti-counterfeiting realm are promising, because they allow for real-time, automatic e-documentation of pharmaceuticals. Tracking a product through the system using RFID would involve the following format: manufacturers include RFID tags into product and packaging materials; they release the tag number as a product identifier; various supply chain members and the retailer accept items only if they have a valid and plausible electronic pedigree; and the consumer uses an RFID-enabled mobile phone to ensure a drug is not counterfeit before purchasing it [63]. Databases have programs to spot duplicate sales or transactions, unreasonable transfers, or any other suspicious activity. Pressure from the FDA for an electronic tracking system has prompted many pharmaceutical companies to adopt RFID technology, but only in a piecemeal fashion for scheduled medications or a specific class of medication [64]. Unfortunately, attempts to standardize this in the United States have been unsuccessful, as legislation failed to pass [64].

Certainly, RFID technology offers easier identification, improved accuracy, and greater efficiency compared to bar codes [64]. Plus, the encryption of RFID tags makes counterfeiting difficult [62]. However, this sophistication comes at high cost, with estimates of US 20–50 cents per tag compared to US 2 cents for a 2D bar code [63]. Also, it is expensive to establish the necessary infrastructure, because all members of the supply chain would have to invest in compatible technology in order to successfully collect and share information about product movement [64]. Lastly, the RFID device could possibly be linked to personal information at the consumer or corporate level, prompting privacy concerns [64].

Conclusion

The issue of counterfeit medicines remains a major public health crisis in many regions across the globe, primarily in the developing world, but even in industrialized nations. Involving all types of pharmaceuticals—antibiotics, hormones, cancer therapies, vaccines, and antivirals, to name a few—the challenge for healthcare providers, public policy experts, manufacturers, and the consumer is to identify a workable collaborative strategy to combat this impending epidemic. As a multifaceted global problem, it requires the participation of all relevant stakeholders. To figure out the intricacies of such solutions, there must be frank exchanges, steadfast will, effective partnerships, and creative solutions. Efforts on the part of WHO and others to bring together key players has led to partnerships between the public and private sectors as well as increased visibility for an issue once perceived as more hype than fact.

Recently, ongoing debate has centered on the definitions of counterfeit, substandard, and falsified medicines. Despite efforts by leading organizations, including WHO and Institute of Medicine, to provide clarity on the terms, there remains the pragmatic issue of how the public health community tackles a growing scourge of bad medicines seeping their way into the pharmaceutical supply chain worldwide. Ultimately, these counterfeit or substandard medicines reach the hands and mouths of infirmed people on all continents. It has been the charge of public health specialists including those at FDA, European Medicines Agency, WHO, Interpol, World Customs Agency, PSI, Organization for Economic Co-operation and Development, International Federation of Pharmaceutical Manufacturers & Associations, and in Ministries of Health to develop the necessary fail-safe measures. Undertaking this task has also required the work of those within brand and generic companies, civil society, and foundations focused on global health.

Counterfeit drug trafficking is a $75 billion industry and tailors its products to the victim's needs. These statistics represent a 90 % increase in 5 years in worldwide sales. For example, in developing nations, counterfeiters focus on therapies for life-threatening conditions, such as malaria, tuberculosis, and HIV/AIDS. In industrialized nations, the attention is on the Internet sites providing lifestyle medications and steroids, which account for $14 billion in sales in Europe alone. WHO's International Medical Products Anti-Counterfeiting Taskforce (IMPACT) centered its efforts on five areas: legislation, regulation, enforcement, technology, and communication. Alliances between and among critical stakeholders have resulted in increased public awareness, effective regulatory strategies, harsher penalties, and creative technologies.

Overall, when considering new technologies to combat counterfeiting, these technologies should be developed and implemented in such a way as to be aligned with the various regulatory agencies, pharmaceutical groups, and other aspects of the industry to cohesively address this problem [65]. Key stakeholders should discuss ongoing issues, such as improving technological compatibility and legislation that addresses electronic tracking systems. Developed countries should continue to share their expertise and results with countries that lack sophisticated technologies. They must continue development and enhancement of low-cost technologies, as many lower-income countries are still dependent on those methods [65].

Urbanization has contributed to a rise in sales of counterfeit medications. With an estimated 50 % of people living in urban areas and an anticipated rise to 70 % by 2050, the health risks and new hazards from this population redistribution are notable. Chronic respiratory ailments, rapid spread of contagious infectious diseases, limited resources resulting in unsanitary conditions, physical inactivity contributing to obesity, and increased environmental pollutants will all result in an increased need for medical attention, with a shrinking pool of available health professionals. Inevitably, illnesses and injuries will require pharmaceutical products. With one in three urban dwellers living in slums (one billion people), limited access to quality health care, no financial resources for the purchase of effective medications, and inadequate supplies, it is conceivable that the urban environment is ripe for the sale of counterfeit medications.

An influx of people to the urban setting, coupled with increased birth rates, provides the foundation for overcrowding and an overburdened health system. Unable to receive adequate health care in this burgeoning populace, the poor will be subject to charlatans who sell their pharmaceutical wares promising treatment for ailments. Absent adequate and accurate health information about the counterfeit drug trade, a patient's condition will likely not improve and possibly deteriorate to the point of death. Combating drug counterfeiting must be comprehensive. As noted in this chapter, the problem of fake pharmaceuticals is of international concern. First, to achieve a strong hold on criminals involved in counterfeiting, stakeholders must reach consensus on definition of terms. Moreover, the public health community must come together on strategies for implementing changes regarding legislation, regulation, enforcement, technology, and communication, as they relate to counterfeit pharmaceutical products.

References

1. Poison pills. The Economist. September 2, 2012; print edition.
2. Putze E, Conway E, Reilly M, Madrid O. The deadly world of fake drugs. Washington, DC: AEI; 2012.
3. World Health Organization, IMPACT. Counterfeit drugs kill! 2008.
4. Board WHOE, editor. Counterfeit medical products: report by the secretariat. Geneva: World Health Assembly; 2008.
5. Bogdanich W, Hooker J. From China to Panama, a trail of poisoned medicine. New York Times. 2007.
6. Bogdanich W. F.D.A. tracked poisoned drugs, but trail went cold in China—New York Times. New York Times. 2007.
7. World Health Organization (WHO) | Counterfeit medicines. Fact sheet. WHO. 2006.
8. Mackey TK, Liang BA. The global counterfeit drug trade: patient safety and public health risks. J Pharm Sci. 2011;100:4571–9.
9. Clift C. Combating counterfeit, falsified and substandard medicines: defining the way forward? London: Chatham House; 2010.
10. International Narcotics Control Board, INCB. INCB warns of counterfeit medicines flooding markets. Press release, 2 Mar 2007.
11. Finlay BD. Counterfeit drugs and national security. Stimson Center, Washington D.C. Feb. 2011.
12. Pharmaceutical Security Institute. Incident Trends. 2012. http://www.psi-inc.org/incidentTrends.cfm. Accessed 24 Mar 2012.
13. IMPACT. Third IMPACT general meeting, 3-5 September 2008, Hammamet, Tunisia, Summary Report.
14. Clift C. Combating counterfeit, falsified and substandard medicines: defining the way forward? Center on Global Health Security, Chatham House. Chatham House Briefing Paper. November 2010.
15. World Health Organization. General information on counterfeit medicines. World Health Organization website. 2010.
16. Harper DE. EU customs blockade of India's generic medicines. The Student Appeal. 2011.
17. Newton PN, Green MD, Fernández FM, Day NP, White NJ. Counterfeit anti-infective drugs. Lancet Infect Dis. 2006;6:602–13.
18. Cockburn R, Newton PN, Agyarko EK, Akunyili D, White NJ. The global threat of counterfeit drugs: why industry and governments must communicate the dangers. PLoS Med. 2005;2:e100.
19. Council of Europe. Council of Europe Convention on the counterfeiting of medical products and similar crimes involving threats to public health. Council of Europe. 2012.
20. Health ECP, Editor. Pharmacovigilance—major developments. 2012. http://www.pharmacovigilance2012.nl/2012/06/21/adoption-and-publication-of-commission-implementing-regulation/.
21. Amending Directive 2001/83/EC on the community code relating to medicinal products for human use, as regards the prevention of the entry into the legal supply chain of falsified medicinal products. Directive of the European Parliament and of the Council. Official Journal of the European Union. July 1, 2011.
22. World Health Organization. Medicines: spurious/falsely-labelled/falsified/counterfeit (SFFC) medicines. Fact Sheet No. 75. May 2012. http://www.who.int/mediacentre/factsheets/fs275/en/index.html
23. Verified Internet Pharmacy Practice Sites (VIPPS). The National Association of Boards of Pharmacy (NABP). 2012. http://vipps.nabp.net
24. US Food and Drug Administration. Pathway to global product safety and quality. US Food and Drug Administration. July 7, 2011.
25. US Food and Drug Administration. Prescription drug marketing act of 1987. US Food and Drug Administration website. 2012.

26. Commissioner OOT. US Food and Drug Administration. Drug safety and availability—FDA initiative to combat counterfeit drugs. US Food and Drug Administration website. 2009.
27. International Federation of Pharmaceutical Manufacturers & Associations. Counterfeit: IFPMA. International Federation of Pharmaceutical Manufacturers & Associations. 2012. http://www.ifpma.org/global-health/counterfeits.html
28. World Health Organization Western Pacific Region (WPRO). Rapid Alert System for combating counterfeit medicine. WPRO. 2012.
29. Hellerman C. FDA commissioner talks counterfeit drugs. CNN. 2012.
30. H.R.3368. - Counterfeit drug penalty enhancement act of 2011. 112th Congress (2011–2012).
31. PhRMA. Counterfeit drug penalty enhancement act of 2011 can help crack down on counterfeiting crimes. PhRMA. Press release, November 17, 2011.
32. Green MD. Antimalarial drug resistance and the importance of drug quality monitoring. J Postgrad Med. 2006;52:288–90.
33. Hearing on H.R. 4223, the "Safe Doses Act"; H.R. 3668, the "Counterfeit Drug Penalty Enhancement Act of 2011"; and H.R 4216, the "Foreign Counterfeit Prevention Act". Subcommittee on Crime, Terrorism, and Homeland Security, Committee on the Judiciary. 2012.
34. Interpol. Training and operational workshops build capacity to fight counterfeit goods affecting consumer safety throughout Western and Northern Africa. Press Release, 21 May 2010.
35. Sanofi-Aventis. Press pack: Drug counterfeiting. Sanofi fights against counterfeit medicines. Sanofi-Aventis. 2012.
36. Abdoulaye I, Chastanier H, Azondekon A, Dansou A, Bruneton C. [Survey on the illicit drug market in Cotonou, Benin in March 2003]. Med Trop (Mars). 2006;66:573–6.
37. Fahelelbom KMS, Al-Zubiadi T, Abdulah A, Talal A. Drug counterfeiting problems (Survey study on public awareness of drug counterfeiting in UAE and Tunisia). In: 11th sci conference for Arab Pharm Colleges. Tripoli, Libya. 2007.
38. Abdoulaye I, Chastanier H, Azondekon A, Dansou A, Bruneton C. Evaluation of public awareness campaigns on counterfeit medicines in Cotonou, Benin. Med Trop (Mars). 2006;66: 615–8.
39. Cuchet-Chosseler M, Bocoum O, Camara M, Abad B, Yamani E, Ordre PM. Results of a survey to evaluate the efficacy of a regional awareness campaign on counterfeit street medicines in Bamako, Mali and Nouakchott, Mauritania. Med Trop (Mars). 2011;71:152–6.
40. World Anti Counterfeiting Day 2012. 2012. http://www.gacg.org/News/Read/53. Accessed 12 July 2012.
41. Inksure Technologies Inc. http://www.inksure.com/pharmaceutical-anti-counterfeiting. Inksure Technologies Inc. website. Accessed 12 July 2012.
42. The Partnership for Safe Medicines. Moving past the Avastatin incident: PSM counterfeit drug congressional briefing held on March 15. Partnership for Safe Medicines website. http://www.safemedicines.org/2012/03/psm-to-conduct-counterfeit-drug-congressional-briefing-on-march-8-.html. Accessed 9 July 2012.
43. Sharma Y. Fighting fake drugs with high-tech solutions. SciDevNet. 2011. http://www.scidev.net/en/features/fighting-fake-drugs-with-high-tech-solutions-1.html. Accessed 6 July 2012.
44. Dialing for development: how mobile phones are transforming the lives of millions. WIPO Magazine. 2010.
45. http://counterfeitdrugs.wordpress.com/videos/. Counterfeit Drugs Around the World website. Accessed 24 Sept 2013.
46. Pharmaceutical Security Institute. http://www.psi-inc.org/index.cfm. Pharmaceutical Security Institute website. Accessed 24 Sept 2013.
47. 2012 Partnership for Safe Medicines Interchange. http://www.safemedicines.org/counterfeit-drug-conference-2012.html. Accessed 9 July 2012.
48. World Health Organization. Rapid Alert System for combating counterfeit medicine. World Health Organization. 2005.
49. IMPACT. Facts|Activities|Documents developed by the Assembly and the Working Groups of IMPACT 2006–2010. Agenzia Italiana del Farmaco. 2011.

50. Research B. Anti counterfeiting packaging technologies in the US Pharmaceutical and Food Industries. 2011.
51. Shah RY, Prajapati PN, Agrawal Y. Anticounterfeit packaging technologies. J Adv Pharm Technol Res. 2010;1:368.
52. Keynote presentations by Howard Zucker at (1) WHO IMPACT Technology Working Group: Prague, Czech Republic, 13 Mar 2007. (2) Using cell phones to improve health, GSM International Conference, Barcelona, Spain, 13 Feb 2007 and (3) Combating counterfeit drugs: building effective collaboration, International conference on combating counterfeit medicine, WHO—AIFA Conference, Rome, Italy, 17–20 Feb 2006.
53. Sproxil. The fight against counterfeit drugs continues. 2011. http://tech.233.com.gh/posts/2011/unwired/sproxil-fight-against-counterfeit-drugs-continues/.
54. Eliminate counterfeit goods efficiently and effectively. http://www.protexxion.de/en/home.html. Accessed 9 July 2012.
55. Mehta R. Biometric fingerprints for anti-counterfeiting. The Packaging Professional. 2007.
56. Bastia S. Next generation technologies to combat counterfeiting of electronic components. IEEE Trans Compon Packag Technol. 2002;25:175–6.
57. Newton P, Proux S, Green M, et al. Fake artesunate in southeast Asia. Lancet. 2001;357:1948–50.
58. FDA warns consumers about counterfeit version of Teva's Adderall. 2012. http://www.fda.gov/NewsEvents/Newsroom/PressAnnouncements/ucm305932.htm. Accessed 9 July 2012.
59. Macleod NA, Matousek P. Emerging non-invasive Raman methods in process control and forensic applications. Pharm Res. 2008;25:2205–15.
60. Dunn JD, Gryniewicz-Ruzicka CM, Kauffman JF, Westenberger BJ, Buhse LF. Using a portable ion mobility spectrometer to screen dietary supplements for sibutramine. J Pharm Biomed Anal. 2011;54:469–74.
61. The GPHF-Minilab®—protection against counterfeit medicines. http://www.gphf.org/web/en/minilab/index.htm. Accessed 6 July 2012.
62. Kwok S, Ting JSL, Tsang AHC, Lee W, Cheung BCF. Design and development of a mobile EPC-RFID-based self-validation system (MESS) for product authentication. Comput Ind. 2010;61:624–35.
63. Choi S, Poon C. An RFID-based anti-counterfeiting system. IAENG Int J Comput Sci. 2008;35:80–91.
64. Coustasse A, Arvidson C, Rutsohn P. Pharmaceutical counterfeiting and the RFID technology intervention. J Hosp Mark Public Relations. 2010;20:100–15.
65. Guidance document on the use of detection technologies and overview of detection technologies for drug safety. APEC Life Science Innovation Forum Beijing, China. 2011.
66. Interpol. Global operation strikes at online supply of illegal and counterfeit medicines worldwide. Media release. September 29, 2011.

Chapter 8
Community Noise, Urbanization, and Global Health: Problems and Solutions

Charles M. Salter, Roy Ahn, Faiza Yasin, Rosemary Hines, Laurence Kornfield, Ethan C. Salter, and Thomas F. Burke

Introduction

Noise exposure is an environmental hazard that has been linked to a variety of health effects, including hearing loss, cardiovascular damage, learning deficits, and sleep disturbance. While occupational noise has been the focus of much literature, the adverse effects of community noise exposure are becoming more prevalent and should be emphasized as a growing public health concern [1–3]. According to the World Health Organization (WHO), noise is the presence of unwanted sound. The sources of community noise include all sources outside of the workplace, including road, rail, air traffic, and construction [4]. Noise pollution involves large-scale, cumulative health effects and is felt globally, both in developed and developing nations [5–7]. In the 1970s, the US Environmental Protection Agency (EPA) studied how noise levels increase with population (Fig. 8.1). This data suggests that urban noise problems will continue to grow with increasing population density [8].

To quantify noise pollution, intensity is measured on a logarithmic scale in decibel (dB) units. A 10 dB increase in noise is perceived as a doubling of noise [7, 8].

C.M. Salter, P.E. (✉) • E.C. Salter, P.E.
Charles M. Salter Associates, Inc., San Francisco, CA, USA
e-mail: charles.salter@cmsalter.com

R. Ahn, M.P.H., Sc.D. • T.F. Burke, M.D., F.A.C.E.P., F.R.S.M.
Division of Global Health and Human Rights, Department of Emergency Medicine,
Massachusetts General Hospital, Zero Emerson Place Suite 104, Boston, MA 02114, USA

Harvard Medical School, Boston, MA, USA

F. Yasin, M.P.H. • R. Hines, B.A.
Division of Global Health and Human Rights, Department of Emergency Medicine,
Massachusetts General Hospital, Boston, MA, USA

L. Kornfield
City and County of San Francisco, San Francisco, CA, USA

© Springer New York 2015
R. Ahn et al. (eds.), *Innovating for Healthy Urbanization*,
DOI 10.1007/978-1-4899-7597-3_8

Fig. 8.1 Day/night average sound level as a function of population density. Salter, Charles, et al. ACOUSTICS: Architecture, Engineering, the Environment. San Francisco, California: William Stout Publishers, 1998

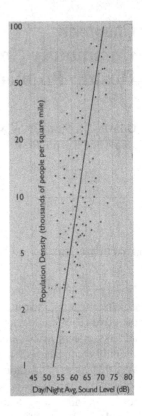

Environmental noise exposure assessments often use an A-weighted dB(A) scale, a filter weighted toward frequencies to which the human ear is most sensitive [4, 9]. As examples, the sound level of a whisper is 30 dB(A), while the sound of a gunshot can measure up to 140 dB(A) [7].

In order to protect people from the effects of noise exposure, WHO guidelines suggest that outdoor noise levels not exceed an average of 55 dB(A) in daytime or 45 dB(A) in nighttime [4]. Despite these guidelines, many people around the world experience much greater noise levels. One in three European Union residents, for example, are exposed to nighttime noise levels over 55 dB(A), a level sufficient to produce significant sleep disturbance and impaired physiological functions [4]. Average nighttime noise levels in residential neighborhoods in India range from 54 to 79 dB(A), and in Ilorin, Nigeria, from 44 to 66 dB(A) [10, 11]. Average noise levels in Karachi, Pakistan, exceed 66 dB(A) at all hours of the day with maximum measured levels reaching 100 dB(A) [12].

While noise pollution is prevalent in many areas of the world, the greatest environmental risk exposure is associated with low-income areas. Exposure to community noise is understood to be inversely correlated with socioeconomic status (SES) [8]. Data from the Urban Noise Survey of major US metropolitan areas showed an inverse correlation between income and 24-hour sound level exposure. The study indicated that those with income levels below US$10,000 experienced noise exposure levels approximately twice as loud as those with income levels above US$20,000 [13]. Lower SES is associated with diminished environmental quality that includes residential crowding, proximity to highways, and homes with less noise insulation. These factors increase an individual's exposure to noise pollution, which in turn increases the risk for associated adverse health effects [8, 14].

The differences in noise exposure and subsequent health consequences between the rich and poor highlight the need for targeted and contextual noise exposure studies and strategies. Promising interventions have been developed to mitigate community noise exposure, such as comprehensive noise assessments, alternative road pavement, noise barriers, and airport curfew systems [15–17]. These alleviation strategies, however, have been employed largely in developed countries, such as the UK, Australia, and the USA. With increasing crowding and urbanization in the developing world, exposure to community noise is on the rise, and the need for appropriate strategies is becoming ever more important.

This chapter will provide an overview of the sources of noise, followed by a description of the associated health effects. The chapter will then summarize the strategies and interventions that exist across the globe to reduce noise exposure, especially in urban areas. Interventions from the developed world can be utilized as a blueprint for cost-effective and successful interventions in low resource settings around the world.

Sources of Noise

Road Traffic

Road traffic noise is the most common source of community noise [4, 18]. It is produced primarily by running car engines, car horns, and the tires rolling on road surfaces. The level of noise depends on factors such as speed and road composition. At low speeds, most noise comes from the engine and exhaust, while at high speeds, most noise emanates from the wheels on the pavement. A doubling of traffic corresponds to a 3-dB(A) increase in noise [16]. Roads with a volume of more than 100,000 vehicles over a 24-hour period can cause sound levels that exceed 40 dB(A) in a 4-km-wide corridor [19].

Aircraft

Aircraft-related noise is another significant source of community noise. Most noise is produced during takeoff and landings. Larger and older aircrafts with turbojets produce the most noise. With the advent of new technologies, many modern aircrafts use quieter fans and engines to mitigate the severity of noise production [16].

Railroad

Railroad noise includes noise from the operation of train horns and bells, the mechanical sound of wheels rolling along the tracks, and the sound of the locomotive engine. Train noise increases with increasing speed, and speeds exceeding 250 km/h can sound as loud as an aircraft [4]. Rail activity also causes ground vibration, which causes a low-frequency rumbling noise [16]. Sound level, number of trains, and the vibration produced by rail traffic contribute to noise perception [20].

Construction

Construction noise is most prevalent in urban areas. Common sources are bulldozers, compressors, trucks, and pile drivers [21, 22]. Although the construction work may not last long, the disturbance often affects people who live or work in the vicinity of the construction site. A selection of commonly used construction tools and their associated noise levels are listed in Table 8.1.

Miscellaneous

Table 8.1 Noise levels of construction equipment [21, 22]

Equipment	Typical noise level (dB(A)) 50 ft from source
Air compressor	81
Impact pile driver	95
Concrete mixer	85
Crane, mobile	83
Jack hammer	88
Rock drill	98
Saw	76

Toys, air conditioners, vacuum cleaners, blenders, and other household appliances all contribute to daily noise exposure. A 2013 study from the USA assessed sounds emitted by a variety of popular children's toys and found that the toys produced an average sound level of 108 dB(A) when placed at the ear and 83 dB(A) at a distance of 25 cm [23]. This data suggests that many toys have noise levels that exceed guidelines and put children at risk for noise-related hearing loss.

Figure 8.2 shows the myriad noise sources in a residential building, including aircraft and road traffic, machinery noise, and noise intrusion from neighbors.

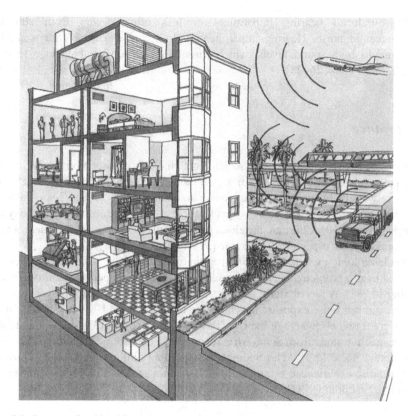

Fig. 8.2 Sources of residential noise exposure

Health Effects of Noise Pollution

Noise-Related Hearing Impairment and Loss

Hearing impairment and permanent hearing loss can result from noise exposure above recommended levels, with the probability of impairment increasing with exposure time and noise level. The World Health Organization (WHO) recommends that peak sound levels from impulse noise never exceed 140 dB(A) to avoid hearing problems [4]. The United States Environmental Protection Agency (US EPA) identifies a 24-hour average exposure level of 70 dB(A) as the threshold to prevent permanent hearing loss [24].

Despite these guidelines, individuals routinely experience much higher levels of noise, especially in urban areas [12]. Prolonged exposure to sound over 85 dB(A) is the leading cause of hearing loss after age-related loss and the most prevalent and preventable occupational hazard [4, 25–27]. A 2013 Italian study found a significant decline in the ability to hear mid-range frequencies common in regular speech and conversation among outdoor workers when compared to their indoor counterparts [27].

Noise-induced hearing impairment or loss often occurs from chronic environmental noise. Hearing impairment or loss can also arise after a single exposure to high sound levels, which cause direct mechanical damage to the cochlear hair cells [26–28].

Annoyance

Annoyance is an emotional state associated with feelings of discomfort, anger, anxiety, and helplessness [4]. It is the most common effect of noise exposure and most frequently studied metric in noise exposure assessments [18, 29, 91]. Many factors influence noise annoyance, such as age, stress level, noise sensitivity, and the type of noise source [30]. Children, the elderly, and people with preexisting illness, such as depression, are especially vulnerable [31].

Epidemiologic evidence suggests that annoyance may be a mediator of noise-induced health problems like cardiovascular disease and impaired cognitive functioning [4, 32]. A recent study demonstrated increased levels of annoyance with chronic aircraft noise exposure in school-age children in the UK, and similar findings were found elsewhere in the UK, Taiwan, and Germany [33–36]. A longitudinal prospective study from South Africa examined a cohort of 732 children exposed to different noise levels. The findings revealed that children exposed to chronic aircraft noise experienced significantly higher annoyance and subsequent impaired cognitive functioning [37].

Sleep Disturbance

Sleep disturbance is a significant burden of community noise and can lead to impaired physiological and mental functioning [38, 39]. Conservative estimates suggest a total of 903,000 disability-adjusted life years lost from noise-induced sleep disturbance in populations of the European Union living in towns of more than 250,000 inhabitants [40]. Similar to annoyance, evidence suggests that sleep disturbance is a connector between noise exposure and health problems, such as cardiovascular disease.

For restful sleep, some guidelines suggest that noise exposure levels should not exceed 45 dB(A) more than 10–15 times a night [41]. Lower nighttime noise levels, between 30 and 40 dB(A), may also cause sleep disturbances if they are experienced for prolonged periods of time [38]. The primary effects of sleep disturbance include problems falling asleep, alterations of sleep stages, and multiple awakenings during the night [38]. While asleep, physiological effects due to noise include increased blood pressure, heart rate, finger pulse amplitude, vasoconstriction, changes in respiration, cardiac arrhythmia, and increased body movements [31, 38, 42]. After a poor night's sleep, the secondary effects often involve fatigue, diminished mood or well-being, and decreased functionality, all of which can lead to more serious health problems, including mental illness and cardiovascular disease [38].

Cardiovascular Effects

The auditory system is directly linked to the autonomic nervous and endocrine systems. Noise exposure can generate a biological response with physiological changes such as increased blood pressure, increased heart rate, and vasoconstriction [18, 43, 44]. For example, data from a US study, showed an average increase of 3 beats per minute (bpm) for each 10 % increase in exposure time to peak noise [44]. A cross-sectional UK study confirmed adverse effects from aircraft noise on blood pressure in 9–10-year-olds [34].

In the long run, chronic noise can disrupt the homeostasis of an individual and cause an imbalance in the stress regulating mechanism, increasing an individual's risk for hypertension and ischemic heart disease [18, 45, 46]. WHO states that exposure to average nighttime noise levels above 55 dB(A) over the course of 1 year increases the risk for developing cardiovascular disease [38]. A supporting study from Germany comparing men exposed to traffic noise levels over 70 dB(A) to men exposed to levels less than or equal to 60 dB(A) found an association between exposure to high levels of noise and the risk of myocardial infarction (MI) [45].

A study from the Department of Environmental Health in Germany found that noise annoyance is positively associated with the risk of arterial hypertension [47]. Coordinated by the WHO in eight European cities, the Large Analysis and Review of European Housing and Health Status (LARES) study also confirmed the association between hypertension and other cardiovascular symptoms and chronic annoyance from traffic noise [48].

Effects on Cognition

Numerous studies have demonstrated the negative effects of noise on reading, attention, memorization, and problem solving [20, 46, 49–51]. Exposure to high levels of noise during the critical years of schooling could potentially disrupt longer-term development.

Studies from the USA and the UK have examined noise in schools and the resulting effects on children. For example, school children's ability to proofread and their level of persistence with challenging puzzles decreased with exposure to aircraft noise [50]. Impaired reading comprehension and recognition memory in school-age

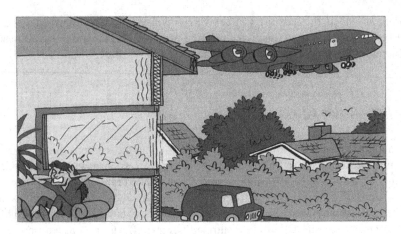

Fig. 8.3 Residential noise impact

children have also been associated with exposure to high levels of noise [49, 51]. Another study found that children in a classroom exposed to high levels of railway noise lagged 3–4 months behind in reading age compared to a classroom with lower noise levels [52].

Figure 8.3 is a cartoon indicting the significant impact that can occur on people living in poorly isolated homes near airports.

Strategies to Reduce Community Noise

In order to address the aforementioned health effects of noise exposure, strategies and tools are necessary and should include comprehensive noise assessment and mapping, creative design and engineering, and rules and regulations.

Management programs for noise control should be guided by these principles:

- Increased noise emissions may be permitted if there are no adverse effects or noise standards are not exceeded.
- Action should be taken to mitigate noise if adverse health effects are demonstrated or when noise levels exceed limits.
- The best available technology that does not involve excessive costs should be utilized.

This section will summarize several strategies that have been implemented in developed countries, including the USA, Germany, Sweden, and Hong Kong.

Various factors should be considered when evaluating the viability of noise abatement options. Given the resources of the region, the selected option must be technically and financially practical.

Noise Assessment

Evidence-based noise control recommendations and guidelines require data-driven noise risk assessments that evaluate hazards, population exposure, and appropriate exposure–response relations. Noise exposure mapping is a tool to help guide and optimize noise abatement policies [16]. Noise exposure maps show the total number of people living in areas exposed to noise from railways, airports, roads, and industry [53]. A good example is the noise exposure map launched by the European Environment Agency (EEA) in 2011, which underscores the extent to which European citizens are exposed to high levels of noise pollution [54].

Noise mapping can be expensive and require numerous resources. Alternatives to traditional noise mapping have found some success. For example, a 2013 study from Serbia on blood pressure and noise levels successfully used public transportation maps as proxy indicators of noise exposure [55]. By matching children's addresses with transport maps, the study avoided subjective measures of traffic levels, e.g., surveys, as well as the expense and resources required for more traditional noise assessments.

A variety of noise metrics are used in exposure assessments according to the type of noise and outcome assessed. Averaging the sound level over a specified period of time is the most common method to quantify noise pollution. The equivalent sound level (L_{eq}) is the descriptor for this average. European Union WHO guidelines suggest using L_{night} to assess sleep disturbance and L_{den} to assess annoyance [16]. L_{dn} is used to produce a combined average 24-hour day–night noise exposure level. For example, the L_{dn} levels vary from 67 to 89 dB(A) in Asansol City, India [56] (Table 8.2).

Table 8.2 Common noise exposure metrics [18, 20, 57]

Metric	Description
L_{den}	• Average day–evening–night long-term noise level • $L_{day}=0700$–1900, $L_{evening}=1900$–2300, $L_{night}=2300$–0700 • A 5-dB(A) penalty is applied to $L_{evening}$ and a 10-dB(A) penalty is applied to L_{night} to reflect greater noise sensitivity during these time periods
L_{night}	• Average A-weighted nighttime long-term noise level • $L_{night}=2300$–0700 • No added weighting
L_{dn}	• Average A-weighted day–night long-term noise level • $L_{day}=0700$–2300, $L_{night}=2300$–0700

San Francisco Noise Control Initiative: Innovations in Model Generation for Noise Planning Purposes

See Appendix for full case study.

Regulations were introduced into the California Building Code in 1974, requiring multifamily residential buildings to be constructed such that living spaces were acoustically protected if the site was exposed to noise levels greater than 60 dB. To identify noise-impacted areas, the San Francisco adopted a basic noise map. Over the years, an increasing number of noise complaints prompted a remapping project, the first step of a larger program to address urban noise in San Francisco.

Much of the modeling is founded on data developed through the San Francisco Chained Activity Modeling Process (CHAMP), an activity-based model used to predict future travel patterns for the city. Data was analyzed in a fine-grained 3D model of the city and included consideration of topography and urban development. An example of this noise mapping is shown below.

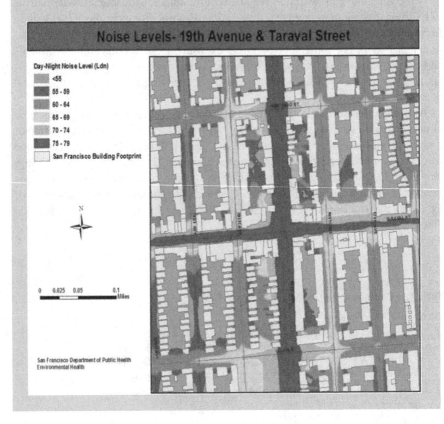

Source Interventions

Road Traffic

The most effective ways of lessening traffic noise are reducing the number of vehicles and making the vehicles quieter [15]. Promoting public transport can reduce traffic volumes. Better design of individual vehicles is imperative for maximum effectiveness in noise management [15].

In addition, the type of road surface can contribute significantly to traffic noise. Alternative road surfacing has been utilized to reduce road traffic noise at the source [15]. Porous asphalt is considered the quietest road surface and is an approved road surfacing in the UK [58]. Despite the acoustical benefits of porous asphalt, it is very expensive, and the risk for degradation and failure is higher than other surfaces. Stone mastic asphalt (SMA), another alternate road surface, reduces tire noise and is used in several European countries, including Germany and the Netherlands [58]. Like porous asphalt, however, studies indicate that it is significantly more expensive than the traditional asphalt concrete mixtures [59].

Rubberized asphalt pavement (ARFC), a mixture of recycled used tires and traditional asphalt, is a more promising approach in terms of cost and longevity in reducing road noise. Studies in Europe and Arizona have shown reductions in noise levels after resurfacing with ARFC by 3–5 dB(A) compared to traditional asphalt roads and by 6–12 dB(A) compared to concrete roads [60, 61].

Aircraft

With the advent of extensive commercial jet traffic, there has been an international effort to reduce aircraft noise emissions. The Federal Aviation Administration (FAA) adopted the Aviation Noise Abatement Policy (ANAP) in 1976, which spurred continual efforts over the past decades to reduce aircraft noise [60]. The federal noise abatement policy was a comprehensive effort to reduce aircraft noise and its effects [62]. It emphasized noise reduction at the source, requiring that older aircrafts with noisy four-engine jets be replaced by newer, quieter models [62]. Between 1976 and 2000, the FAA estimated that the number of Americans exposed to aircraft noise levels above 65 dB(A) (L_{dn}) dropped from 6–7 million to 500,000 [62].

While aircrafts are quieter, the number of flights has grown substantially. Airport curfews have been successful in reducing noise exposure in different cities. Heathrow Airport in the UK, for instance, utilizes a night flight plan set by the Department of Transport (DoT) with a Quota Count (QC) system. Each aircraft is categorized by noise level separately on takeoff and landing, with higher QC ratings corresponding to noisier aircrafts [17]. QC ratings are additive and count against the airports allotted maximum night noise quota. The night flight restrictions are reviewed every 5 years, and alterations are made based on new evidence, new technologies, and new data on noise management [17, 63].

In Sydney, Australia, airport curfew systems have been in place since 1995. The Sydney Airport Curfew Act established a curfew period from 11:00 pm to 6:00 am during which an aircraft cannot take off or land unless it is an international or freight aircraft or an aircraft that complies with noise standards [64].

Trains

In the US, the Department of Transportation Federal Railroad Administration's Quiet Zone program offers communities relief from railroad noise by designating quiet zones. A quiet zone is "a section of rail line at least one half mile in length that contains one or more consecutive public highway rail grade crossings at which locomotive horns are not routinely sounded" [65]. According to the US Department of Transportation, there are 549 quiet zones in the US. In Texas alone, there are 86 designated quiet zones in cities and towns throughout the state [65].

Modern high-speed trains (HSTs) are a promising alternative to conventional passenger and freight trains in terms of noise reduction. Although HSTs may produce some increased noise due to their increased speed, electrical power is quieter than diesel engines of conventional trains, and the noise impact is reduced because of the shortened duration of passby [66, 67].

Construction

Efforts to reduce construction noise include regulating work during nighttime hours and creating quieter machines. Using electrically-powered machinery instead of diesel engine-powered machinery makes construction noise quieter [22]. Alternatives to certain tools and operations can also provide some relief from construction noise. For example, vibration or hydraulic insertion methods may produce less noise than pile driving [22].

Noise-reducing additions to equipment, such as mufflers, sound aprons, noise absorptive mats, and sound enclosures for stationary machinery, are also options to reduce community noise exposure [22]. Muffler systems can reduce noise from the internal combustion engine of construction machinery, often the loudest part of the equipment [22]. Maintenance, replacement of old equipment, and lubrication of component parts are also important components of a construction noise reduction strategy [22].

Pathway Interventions

The following are examples of esthetically acceptable sound barriers around the world to control noise.

Barriers/Berms

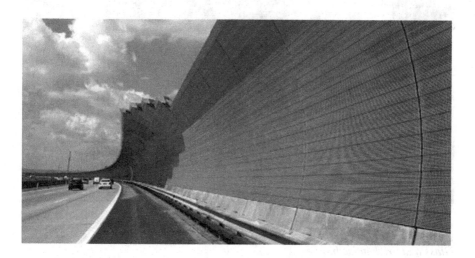

[67] *Vienna, Austria*
Steel highway noise barrier

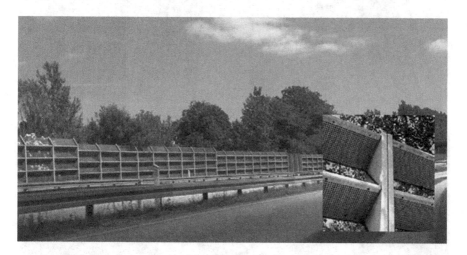

[67] *Copenhagen, Denmark*
Steel and glass barrier

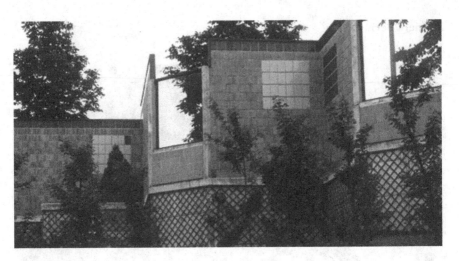

[67] *Paris, France*
Glass and brick noise barrier

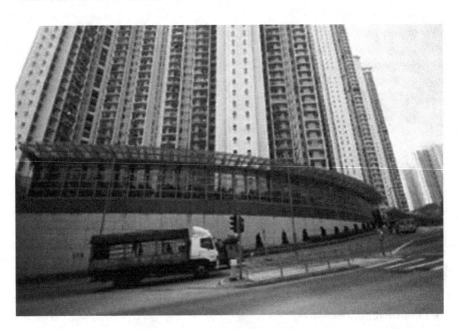

[68] *Hong Kong, China*
8-m-vertical transparent glass panels

Noise barriers can shield buildings, residences, and public spaces from excessive noise [16]. Steel, aluminum, concrete, glass fiber reinforced concrete, and landscaped earth berms are the most common materials used for barriers. The effectiveness of the barrier depends on shape, construction material, height, and distance from the noise source [16].

Barriers built between the source and receiver to reduce the impact of noise from existing roads and highways have been successful in multiple settings, reducing noise level by 10–15 dB(A) [16, 60, 69]. Noise annoyance among residents living within 150 meters of the road, as assessed by a survey questionnaire on a numerical scale, decreased from 64 % in 1976 to 34 % in 1988 after construction of noise barriers along four major highway routes in Germany [69]. A similar study in Sweden confirmed a reduction in reported annoyance from household residents within 100 meters from the road where a 2.25-meter high noise barrier was constructed [70]. In Ohio, noise barriers along an interstate highway reduced noise levels by up to 11 dB(A), and residents living next to the highway reported an improved quality of life [71].

Despite the acoustical benefits, noise barriers can be expensive to build and install. Material is the largest cost factor. Experience in Milwaukee, Wisconsin, has shown metal barriers to be the least expensive material for man-made barriers at $1.2 million per mile. Concrete has a unit cost nearly 65 % higher [72]. Washington State Department of Transportation estimates average construction costs at $53 per square foot [73]. Earth berms are made with available earth, and generally minimize capital costs but require more space than man-made barriers [73].

Land Use Planning

Land use planning helps reduce noise exposure by placing "noise-compatible" structures (such as parking garages and commercial shopping centers) closer to noise sources and noise-sensitive structures (such as residences) further away [68, 74]. Sufficient distances between residential areas and airports can minimize noise exposure. Additionally, ensuring availability of green space in urban areas may help alleviate noise-induced stress. Studies from Sweden have found that access to green space results in residents being significantly less annoyed in response to road traffic noise [75, 76].

Receiver Intervention

Façade Alteration

Façade insulation, such as noise-reducing windows and doors, can be used if the source or pathway interventions do not sufficiently reduce noise. Exterior windows, doors, and walls are the main surfaces that reduce sound intrusion. However,

ventilation openings can be a path for intruding noise and should be carefully evaluated to appropriately mitigate both intake and discharges. Double- or triple-pane
glass windows have noise reduction characteristics. Cheaper alternatives include
interior or exterior glass sashes and noise-reducing interior vinyl curtains [22]. In
Norway, a study found an average reduction of 7 dB inside dwellings with façade
insulation, and the percentage of residents annoyed by noise dropped from 42 to
16 % [77].

Internally lining ducts in ventilation systems, may reduce noise impact indoors
by acting as a sound-absorbing surface within air ducts. This process transforms
noise energy into heat [16, 78].

Figure 8.4 shows a noise reduction of 20 dB(A) with the addition of an acoustically rated window.

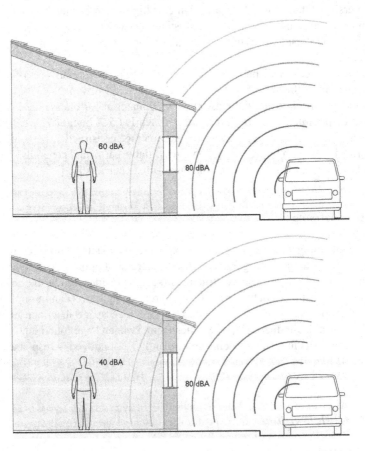

Fig. 8.4 Traffic noise exposure reduction with acoustically rated window

Design

Creative design strategies that place noise resistive portions of an office building or residence facing toward the source of significant noise should be considered to reduce noise exposure [74]. In Hong Kong, for example, some residential buildings are constructed with corridors, stairwells, and restrooms face the noise source. Noise-sensitive portions, such as bedrooms, face the opposite direction [68]. In one large residential building, Rhine Garden at Sham Tseng, creative design reduced noise by 5–10 dB(A) [68]. A similar study from Norway indicated that having access to a quiet side of a dwelling is associated with a comparatively lower noise annoyance [77]. The study estimated that having a bedroom facing a noise-shielded side of a dwelling corresponds to a 6 dB noise reduction [77].

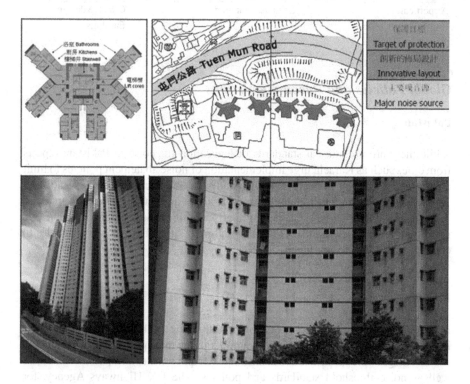

[68] *Environmental Protection Department. The Government of the Hong Kong Special Administrative Region*

Earplugs

Earplugs are another intervention that can reduce noise by up to 30 dB(A) if inserted correctly [79]. They are inexpensive noise-reducing devices made of plastic, rubber, or silicone. Earplugs can also be custom designed to fit the individual's ear canal perfectly and increase noise attenuation. Hospital-based studies found that the use of earplugs is a low-cost intervention to reduce noise exposure from the intensive care unit (ICU) while positively affecting sleep quality [80, 81]. Earmuffs with noise-canceling properties and selective amplification to permit the sound of speech have also been developed but costs are high, ranging from $150 to over $1,000 per set [82].

Table 8.3 summarizes the noise reduction interventions discussed herein.

Table 8.3 Noise reduction interventions, by type

Source interventions	Pathway interventions	Receiver interventions
Road resurfacing	Barriersfigberms	Façade alteration
Airport curfews	Land use planning	Creative design
Railway quiet zones		Earplugs

Global Policies and Recommendations

Pakistan

While there are no national standards or legislation for noise in Pakistan, reports from cities such as Karachi urge implementation of noise abatement policies to limit continued increase of noise levels. One study found maximum levels of noise at 110 dB(A) during the peak hours between 1:00 pm and 3:00 pm and 5:00 pm and 7:00 pm [83]. Other researchers have similarly identified the problem of high traffic noise with noise assessments in Pakistan, calling upon authorities to adopt rules to control and mitigate noise levels [83, 84].

Europe

Many European countries recognize noise pollution as a public health concern to be included in national standards and legislation. For the most part, European countries use an integrated approach that includes quieter pavements and noise barriers, as well as noise threshold standards and policies. The UK Highways Agency, for example, has adopted a policy that mandates use of lower noise surface materials when roads have to be replaced or resurfaced [57]. Denmark has a policy that prevents new houses from facing roadways. France uses thin, gap-graded, single-layer porous hot-mix asphalt pavements when possible, which can lower noise levels by 6 dB compared to dense-graded pavements [85].

Germany has implemented a product label that is awarded to eco-friendly products, such as low-noise machinery. The "Blue Angel" label has been successful in Germany, incentivizing the development of products that emit noise at significantly lower rates than EU guidelines suggest [86]. The label has pushed construction companies to develop quieter machinery [87].

Additionally, the Environmental Noise Directive (END) formed in 2002 mandated European Union states to create noise maps. These maps assess noise exposure near major roads, highways, airports, and railroads [88] and are currently available to the public. Each country has started to develop and publicize action plans to target the issues brought to light in the noise maps, with interventions such as quieter pavements [51, 88, 89]. EU member states must develop their own noise limits and mitigation strategies upon collection and analysis of their noise data [88].

Australia

Australia has regulations that limit the use of certain machines during specific periods of time and assign noise levels to different building types. The Environment Protection (Residential Noise) Regulations came into effect in October 2008 and utilized sections of an earlier noise policy implemented in Section 48A of the 1970 Environmental Protection Act [90]. Industrial and utility premises have higher assigned levels than noise-sensitive residences [90]. Furthermore, the regulations set standards for when certain products can be used. For example, the use of a lawn mower or electric power tool is not permitted Monday to Friday before 7:00 am or after 8:00 pm [90].

Future Directions and Recommendations for Action

Community noise is an accelerating global issue due to momentum from increased urbanization. This chapter has summarized the major sources of noise and associated health effects, and provided an overview for interventions to curb community noise.

We call for a participatory way to move forward in creating programs to alleviate urban noise impact. In the short term, a lack of resources may limit the implementation of these strategies. Nonetheless, by describing these interventions, we can better understand what is feasible in low resource settings in the longer term. By knowing what strategies exist, appropriate assessments and interventions can slowly be phased in.

As an example, the use of public transport maps in Serbia as proxy indicators of noise exposure is a low-cost solution that obviates more expensive noise mapping. Earth berms, which are less expensive than metal or concrete noise barriers, could be utilized as a noise reduction intervention. Focused efforts to acoustically separate new residential areas from existing noise sources can be considered. Similarly, new noise sources such as freeways and airports should not be added without assessing acoustic impacts on existing residences.

Noise level regulations, such as those in Australia, may be effective strategies because they do not require the capital costs of noise barrier construction or road resurfacing. Policy changes can produce positive changes, as seen in the slow phase-in of the European Environmental Noise Directive, which required each country to create their own noise map. Studies and assessments inform policy makers and residents about the increasing levels of noise and the associated health risks in their respective countries.

Beyond choosing an intervention, one universal point is that community noise reduction requires interdisciplinary collaboration. Effective policies, especially in the developing world, require that community residents, engineers, policy makers, and public health experts work together to create integrated and targeted approaches. Noise levels can be reduced by phasing in noise assessments and interventions in a participatory manner.

Given the link between noise exposure and health, strategies to reduce noise levels can improve the health and well-being of individuals throughout the world, especially in urban settings.

The push toward universal recognition of the problems that noise can produce in the environment will continue to be challenging. Progress and action on the governmental and commercial levels will be interspersed with periods of retraction and retrenchment.

Mitigation and interventions of the sources, pathways, and receivers will necessarily be balanced by the economic imperatives of stakeholders.

Governments may decide that short-term economic benefits from development (e.g., airport expansion, greater roadway networks, urban development) are balanced by the increased environmental noise levels. They may decide that "it's worth it" to become more modern. These decisions are not easy when the promises of urbanization and westernization bring with them louder urban areas. Noise pollution is recognized as an important environmental factor to control. To achieve meaningful reductions in urban noise exposure and a more comfortable environment, decisions charting a clear path forward are required by government, manufacturers, builders, engineers, designers, and citizens themselves.

Appendix A: San Francisco Community Noise Initiative

Lessons from San Francisco's Experiences in Urban Noise Mapping and Control

Laurence Kornfield
Chief Building Inspector for the city and county of San Francisco for 20 years

San Francisco has long strived to be on the cutting edge of urban regulations to assure a high standard for quality of life, health, and safety of its residents. Regulations include guidelines for building structural safety, fire prevention, air pollution control, and control of urban noise. This agenda is primarily the outcome of a vocal, public-oriented government that holds extensive public hearings and appeals on every issue. A majority of San Francisco residents are renters, a group that generally favor progressive, quality of life regulations.

Health concerns and environmental justice initiatives have also influenced governmental action in San Francisco. There have been decades of debate regarding the environmental health and justice implications of transportation planning decisions. A group called PODER (People Organizing to Demand Environmental and Economic Rights) along with the City of San Francisco Department of Public Health and the University of California School of Public Health researched the effects of transportation planning decisions, including the construction of an intra-urban freeway, on residents in a southeast San Francisco neighborhood (the Excelsior).[1] Their research states, "traffic related noise triggers community annoyance and sleep disturbance and is associated with hypertension and heart disease" (see footnote 1). Their research also revealed that air quality and noise modeling and monitoring provided evidence that traffic contributed significantly to environmental hazards in the Excelsior neighborhood. These results were alarming especially because the population was largely composed of families with children and people of color. The study found that the leading causes of death in this neighborhood were due to illnesses associated with exposure to traffic and traffic-related pollutants, including heart disease, lung cancer, and traffic collisions.

Despite many local regulations, noise complaints in San Francisco are common, particularly related to nighttime noise conflicts. These conflicts typically occur when residential development adjoins entertainment or commercial uses. Some of these noise conflicts would not exist if the newer buildings had been correctly built to meet applicable sound control standards, reducing noise intrusion to dwelling units. Some conflicts could be mitigated through regulation of noise sources or by other measures outside of the residential building.

Noise control requirements in San Francisco are found in state and local codes; there are currently no federal noise control mandates. Sound transmission requirements were introduced into the California Building Code in 1974, requiring new buildings to be constructed such that multifamily residential living spaces (including hotels and dormitories) are acoustically separated from outdoor areas when the city's General Plan indicates that a site may have noise levels potentially greater than 60 dB. To identify such noise-impacted areas, the city adopted a basic noise map in 1974. Over the following decades, that original noise map became less reflective of realistic patterns of city use, topography, and development. An increasing number of complaints of noise conflicts between various uses prompted a remapping project, the first step of a larger program to address urban noise in San Francisco.

The development of the new noise model for San Francisco was initiated and funded by the Department of Building Inspection as part of an effort to more

---

[1] For more information on this initiative, see Wier, Megan, M.P.H.; Sciammas, Charlie; Seto, Edmund, Ph.D.; Bhatia, Rajiv, M.D., M.P.H.; Rivard, Tom, M.S., R.E.H.S. "Health, traffic, and environmental justice: Collaborative Research and Community Action in San Francisco, California." Am J Public Health. 2009 November; 99(S3):S499–S504. doi:10.2105/AJPH.2008.148916 PMCID:PMC2774185. http://www.ncbi.nlm.nih.gov/pmc/articles/PMC2774185/.

diligently enforce the sound transmission requirements of the Building Code. The study was done by Senior Environmental Health Inspector Tom Rivard of the Department of Public Health with assistance from paid graduate students at the University of California at Berkeley, School of Public Health. Much of the modeling is founded on data developed through the San Francisco Chained Activity Modeling Process (CHAMP), an activity-based model used to predict future travel patterns for the city. Data was then analyzed in a fine-grained 3D model of the city, including considerations of topography and urban development. An example of this noise mapping is shown below.

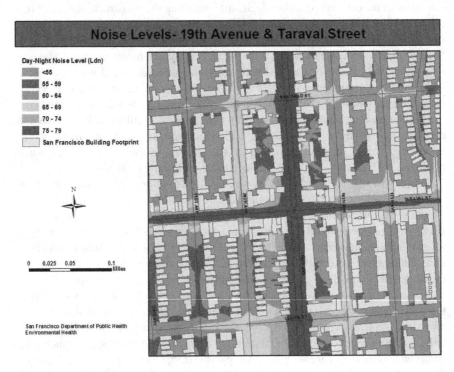

As urban noise is a complex interdepartmental problem, other city government agencies were involved in this modeling. The Planning Department reviewed and ultimately adopted the results of the model, and the County Transportation Agency provided critical data and analysis. The acoustical consulting firm of Charles M. Salter Associates generously provided expert advice. The remapping was a 5-year project of sampling data and building a robust noise model of San Francisco that reflected both current conditions and future development uses. The new noise map completed a public review process and was adopted into the Environmental Protection Element of the San Francisco General Plan in 2011. The noise-related issues in the Environmental Protection Element of the General Plan address vehicle and traffic noise; emergency sirens; building location, design, and construction; and planning for location of compatible uses.

Some of the challenges in updating San Francisco's noise model and the Environmental Protection Element included maintaining financial and other institutional support over the extended course of this work and finding staff with interest, expertise, and commitment to the subject (two of the principals retired at the end of the study). San Francisco may be unusual in that it benefits from being home to various expert acoustical engineering firms that could provide expert consulting services for the city study and the subsequent required analysis work.

Along with adoption of new planning maps and guidelines, San Francisco amended its Noise Ordinance to create a Noise Task Force, coordinated by Health Department staff, to bring together many government agencies to address enforcement issues, including such urban problems as motorcycle noise. The Task Force has had some successes but, like most city programs, significant improvements often require years of meeting, analysis, and regulatory adjustment. Another step forward in reducing urban noise has been the recent adoption of San Francisco's Eastern Neighborhoods Plan, which includes provisions to consider not just L_{dn} but to measure and mitigate likely "single event noise" within 500 ft of the site of a proposed project.

Compliance with Urban Noise Regulations

As a government official and former Chief Building Inspector for San Francisco, I believe that compliance with construction requirements regulating sound transmission can be most effectively implemented by regulatory mandate, not by encouragement or incentive.

The best practice is to incorporate such compliance mandates into the body of applicable building codes so that new building designs have sound transmission designs integrated into architectural, mechanical, structural, and other design works. Until the 1990s, the sound transmission requirements in the California Building Code were in a separate hard-to-find code section; they are now integrated into the general requirements of Chap. 12 for "Interior Environments," making the requirements much more accessible to building designers and city staff.

Under the California Building Code, a comprehensive acoustical analysis report and related sound control design elements must be submitted as part of a permit application for new multifamily residential projects. Adding these requirements to a permit submittal checklist would help assure that these elements are not neglected. This integration is in line with San Francisco's recent "Green Building" code requirements, in which the many building components of a LEED Gold or similarly highly sustainable building must be detailed on a standardized checklist as part of the permit submittal. In San Francisco, a permit application for a new residential building may not be accepted without both a "Green Building" checklist and an acoustical analysis report.

Most city plan reviewers focus on structural and life safety issues, often resulting in a lack of attention to acoustical requirements. Building Department staff training and oversight is critical to proper enforcement. Even a large city such as San Francisco has no acoustical engineers on staff, so the city relies primarily on the report prepared and signed by an experienced acoustical engineer. One continuing problem when relying on such outside experts is the lack of standardized licensure of professionals in the field of acoustics.

Cost is an issue in noise reduction compliance, with the additional construction elements typically paid for by the project owners. Owners may be reluctant to spend additional money to design, construct, and inspect noise mitigation elements that do not appear to add immediate value to a project. However, failure to comply at the time of construction can be expensive, as many sound transmission assemblies cannot be easily retrofitted and impacted residents are likely to complain and demand improvements.

Construction and inspection of sound control elements can be challenging. Most construction elements must be installed as designed or the systems will not perform properly. Something as simple as a screw in the wrong location or using the wrong caulking can "short circuit" a sound-rated assembly. Project sponsors, design professionals, and contractors often look for cost savings through "value engineering." This process can degrade the building design. Commonly, contractors substitute materials without understanding the possible negative effects on a carefully designed system. Building inspectors are unable to inspect the thousands of elements in the construction of a new building. Materials substitution or errors by contractor and a lack of detailed inspection have resulted in the construction of noncompliant buildings, leading to excessive urban noise intrusion. A solution to these construction and inspection problems lies in a process known as "Special Inspection," in which a licensed design professional assumes responsibility, overseeing field inspection of critical elements and submitting affidavits to the city attesting to proper installation. Another approach for compliance would be to require testing at the completion of construction to assure that sound transmission standards have been met; however, correction of defects at that time could be difficult.

After completion of construction, enforcement of noise regulations in San Francisco is primarily through the Municipal Code, which apportions enforcement authority to a variety of agencies, including Police for nuisance noise, Health Department for fixed-source equipment noise, Public Works for street and utility construction noise, etc. Additionally, San Francisco's Entertainment Commission regulates nighttime entertainment noise. This dispersion of noise enforcement results in uneven citywide enforcement, with some highly effective agencies and others failing to enforce even the basic requirements. Ideal enforcement would consolidate noise enforcement in a citywide Office of Noise Control. Failing that, inasmuch as possible, uniform training in noise control issues should be provided to the various city enforcement staff.

The experience in San Francisco is that properly designed, constructed, and maintained sound control systems in new buildings significantly reduce the intrusion of disturbing noise, helping ameliorate adverse health effects and supporting quality of urban life.

References

1. Ahmed HO, Dennis JH, Badran O, Ismail M, Ballal SG, Ashoor A, et al. Occupational noise exposure and hearing loss of workers in two plants in eastern Saudi Arabia. Ann Occup Hyg. 2001;45(5):371–80.
2. WHO. Occupational noise: assessing the burden of disease from work-related hearing impairment at national and local levels [Internet]. WHO. http://www.who.int/quantifying_ehimpacts/publications/9241591927/en/. Accessed 23 Sep 2013
3. Nelson DI, Nelson RY, Concha-Barrientos M, Fingerhut M. The global burden of occupational noise-induced hearing loss. Am J Ind Med. 2005;48(6):446–58.
4. Berglund B, Lindvall T, Schwela DH, Team WHOO and EH. Guidelines for community noise [Internet]. 1999. http://apps.who.int/iris/handle/10665/66217. Accessed 23 Sep 2013
5. Lang W. Global versus local issues in noise control policy. Noise Vib Worldw. 2003;34(2):17–22.
6. Sandberg U. Abatement of traffic, vehicle, and tire/road noise—the global perspective. 1999. http://trid.trb.org/view.aspx?id=651529. Accessed 23 Sep 2013
7. Begault DR. Fundamentals. Acoustics. San Francisco: William Stout Publishers; 1998. p. 27–36.
8. Evans GW, Kantrowitz E. Socioeconomic status and health: the potential role of environmental risk exposure. Annu Rev Public Health. 2002;23(1):303–31.
9. Begault DR. Measurements. Acoustics. San Francisco: William Stout; 1998. p. 45–50.
10. Banerjee D, Chakraborty S, Bhattacharyya S, Gangopadhyay A. Evaluation and analysis of road traffic noise in Asansol: an industrial town of eastern India. Int J Environ Res Public Health. 2008;5(3):165–71.
11. Oyedepo O, Saadu A. Evaluation and analysis of noise levels in Ilorin metropolis, Nigeria. Environ Monit Assess. 2010;160(1–4):563–77.
12. Mehdi M, Kim M, Seong J, Arsalan M. Spatio-temporal patterns of road traffic noise pollution in Karachi, Pakistan. Environ Int. 2011;37(1):97–104.
13. The Urban Noise Survey. Washington, D.C.: U.S. Environmental Protection Agency, Office of Noise Abatement and Control; 1977. Report no.: 550/9-77-100.
14. Kohlhuber M, Mielck A, Weiland S, Bolte G. Social inequality in perceived environmental exposures in relation to housing conditions in Germany. Environ Res. 2006;101(2):246–55.
15. Roads and Traffic Authority of New South Wales. Roads and traffic authority environmental noise management manual. 2001; RTA–Pub.01.142.
16. Rosen A. Environmental noise. In: Charles M. Salter Associates Inc., editor. Acoustics (Chapter 5). San Francisco: William Stout; 1998. p. 51–67.
17. Heathrow airport environmental noise directive noise action plan 2010-2015. London: Heathrow Airport; 2010.
18. Fritschi L, Brown A, Kim R, Schwela D, Kephalopoulos S, World Health Organization (WHO). Burden of disease from environmental noise: quantification of healthy life years lost in Europe; 2011.
19. Beckenbauer T. Road traffic noise. Handbook of engineering acoustics. Berlin: Springer; 2013. p. 367–92.
20. Gidlöf-Gunnarsson A, Ögren M, Jerson T, Öhrström E. Railway noise annoyance and the importance of number of trains, ground vibration, and building situational factors. Noise Health. 2012;14(59):190–201.
21. Office of Planning: Federal Transit Administration, US Department of Transportation. 12. Noise and vibration during construction. Transit noise and vibration impact assessment; 1995.
22. US Department of Transportation, Federal Highway Administration. 7.0 mitigation of construction noise. Construction noise handbook. NTIS no. PB2006-109102; 2006.
23. Weinreich H, Jabbour N, Levine S, Yueh B. Limiting hazardous noise exposure from noisy toys: simple, sticky solutions. Laryngoscope. 2013;123(9):2240–4.

24. Safety and Health Topics | Occupational Noise Exposure [Internet]. https://www.osha.gov/ SLTC/noisehearingconservation/. Accessed 23 Sep 2013.

25. Passchier-Vermeer W, Passchier W. Noise exposure and public health. Environ Health Perspect. 2000;108 Suppl 1:123–31.

26. Rabinowitz P. Noise-induced hearing loss. Am Fam Physician. 2000;1(61):2749–56.

27. Caciari T, Rosati M, Casale T, Loreti B, Sancini A, Riservato R, et al. Noise-induced hearing loss in workers exposed to urban stressors. Sci Total Environ. 2013;463–464:302–8.

28. Harrison R. The prevention of noise-induced hearing loss in children. Int J Pediatr. 2012;2012:473541.

29. Ising H, Kruppa B. Health effects caused by noise: evidence in the literature from the past 25 years. Noise Health. 2004;6(22):5–13.

30. Urban J, Máca V. Linking traffic noise, noise annoyance, and life satisfaction: a case study. Int J Environ Res Public Health. 2013;10(5):1895–915.

31. Stansfeld S, Matheson M. Noise pollution: non-auditory effects on health. Br Med Bull. 2003;68(1):243–57.

32. Niemann H, Maschke C. WHO LARES final report: noise effects and morbidity. Geneva: WHO; 2004.

33. Haines M, Stansfeld S, Brentnall S, Head J, Berry B, Jiggins M, et al. The West London Schools Study: the effects of chronic aircraft noise exposure on child health. Psychol Med. 2001;31(8):1385–96.

34. Clark C, Head J, Stansfeld S. Longitudinal effects of aircraft noise exposure on children's health and cognition: a six-year follow-up of the UK RANCH cohort. J Environ Psychol. 2013;35:1–9.

35. Wu TN, Lai JS, Shen CY, Yu TS, Chang PY. Aircraft noise, hearing ability, and annoyance. Arch Environ Health. 1995;50:452–6.

36. Babisch W, Schulz C, Seiwert M, Conrad A. Noise annoyance as reported by 8- to 14-year-old children. Environ Behav. 2012;1:68–86.

37. Seabi J. An epidemiological prospective study of children's health and annoyance reactions to aircraft noise exposure in South Africa. Int J Environ Res Public Health. 2013;10:2760–77.

38. World Health Organizations (WHO). Night noise guidelines for Europe; 2009.

39. Hobson J. Sleep. New York: Freeman; 1989.

40. Ristovska G, Lekaviciute J. Environmental noise and sleep disturbance: research in central, eastern, and south-eastern Europe and newly independent states. Noise Health. 2013;15(62):6.

41. Night aircraft noise index and sleep research results. In: Inter-noise 91—proceedings of the cost of noise; 1991.

42. Community Noise [Internet]. Stockholm: WHO; 1995. http://www.nonoise.org/library/who-noise/whonoise.htm

43. Sørensen M, Andersen Z, Nordsborg R, Jensen S, Lillelund K, Beelen R, et al. Road traffic noise and incident myocardial infarction: a prospective cohort study. PLoS One. 2012;7(6):e39283.

44. Lusk S, Gillespie B, Hagerty B, Ziemba R. Acute effects of noise on blood pressure and heart rate. Arch Environ Health. 2004;59(8):392–9.

45. Babisch W, Beule B, Schust M, Kersten N, Ising H. Traffic noise and risk of myocardial infarction. Epidemiology. 2005;16(1):33–40.

46. European Environment Agency. Good practice guide on noise exposure and potential health effects. EEA Technical report 11/2010.

47. Ndrepepa A, Twardella D. Relationship between noise annoyance from road traffic noise and cardiovascular disease: a meta-analysis. Noise Health. 2011;13(52):251–9.

48. Niemann H, Bonnefoy X, Braubach M, Hecht K, Maschke C, Rodrigues C, Robbel N. Noise-induced annoyance and morbidity results from the pan-European LARES study. Noise Health. 2006;8(31):63–79.

49. Stansfeld S, Berglund B, Clark C, Lopez-Barrio I, Fischer P, Ohrström E, et al. Aircraft and road traffic noise and children's cognition and health: a cross-national study. Lancet. 2005;365(9475):1942–9.

50. Cohen S, Evans G, Krantz D, Stokois D. Physiological, motivational, and cognitive effects of aircraft noise on children. Am Psychol. 1980;35:231–43.
51. Stansfeld S, Hygge S, Clark C, Alfred T. Night time aircraft noise exposure and children's cognitive performance. Noise Health. 2010;12(49):255–62.
52. Bronzaft A, McCarthy D. The effects of elevated train noise on reading ability. Environ Behav. 1975;7(4):517–28.
53. Murphy E, King E. Strategic environmental noise mapping: methodological issues concerning the implementation of the EU Environmental Noise Directive and their policy implications. Environ Int. 2010;36(3):290–8.
54. NOISE: Noise Observation and Information Service for Europe [Internet]. http://noise.eionet.europa.eu/. Accessed 23 Sep 2013.
55. Paunovic K, Belojevic G, Jakovljevic B. Blood pressure of urban school children in relation to road-traffic noise, traffic density, and presence of public transport. Noise Health. 2013;15(65):253–60.
56. Banerjee D, Chakraborty S. Monthly variation in night time noise levels at residential areas of Asansol city (India). J Environ Sci Eng. 2006;48(1):39–44.
57. Jones K, Cadoux R. Metrics for aircraft noise. Holborn: Civil Aviation Authority; 2009. Report no.: 0904.
58. Morgan P, Nelson P, Steven H. Integrated assessment of noise reduction measures in the road transport sector. 2003; PR SE/652/03.
59. Hassim S, Harahap R, Muniandy R, Kadir M, Mahmud A. Cost comparison between stone mastic asphalt and asphalt concrete wearing course. Am J Appl Sci. 2005;2(9):1350–5.
60. Manuel J. Clamoring for quiet: new ways to mitigate noise. Environ Health Perspect. 2005;113(1):A46–9.
61. Quiet Pavement Program [Internet]. http://www.azdot.gov/business/environmental-services-and-planning/programs/quiet-pavement-program/what_is_rubberized_asphalt.asp. Accessed 23 Sep 2013.
62. Federal Aviation Administration. Aviation noise abatement policy 2000, docket no.: 30109. Fed Reg. 2000;65(136):43802–24.
63. Government of the United Kingdom Department for Transport. Night flying restrictions at Heathrow, Gatwick and Stansted. Stage 1 consultation; 2012.
64. Van Renterghem T, Botteldooren D. Focused study on the quiet side effect in dwellings highly exposed to road traffic noise. Int J Environ Res Public Health. 2012;9(12):4292–310.
65. US Department of Transportation, Federal Railway Administration. Quiet zone locations. 2013. http://www.fra.dot.gov/eLib/details/L04490. Accessed 16 June 2013.
66. Wolf S, Riffey K, Barker J, Daniels A, van Ark R, California High Speed Rail Authority (CHSRA). High speed train sound fact sheet; 2010.
67. Bendtsen H. Noise barrier design: Danish and some European examples. 2010; UCPRC-RP-2010-04.
68. Environmental Protection Department. Housing design and mitigation measures to abate traffic noise in Hong Kong.
69. Kastka J, Buchta E, Ritterstaedt U, Paulsen R, Mau U. The long term effect of noise protection barriers on the annoyance response of residents. J Sound Vib. 1995;184(5):823–52.
70. Nilsson M, Berglund B. Noise annoyance and activity disturbance before and after the erection of a roadside noise barrier. J Acoust Soc Am. 2006;119(4):2178–88.
71. Mital A, Ramakrishnan A. Effectiveness of noise barriers on an interstate highway: a subjective and objective evaluation. J Hum Ergol. 1997;26(1):31–8.
72. Farnham J, Beimborn E. Noise barrier design guidelines. Final report, 1990. Center for Urban Transportation Studies, University of Wisconsin—Milwaukee.
73. British Columbia Ministry of Transportation and Highways. Noise control earth berms, guidelines for the use of earth berms to control highway noise. 1997. http://www.th.gov.bc.ca/publications/eng_publications/environment/references/Guidelines-Noise_Control_Earth_Berms.pdf

74. US Department of Transportation, Federal Highway Administration. The audible landscape: 4 physical techniques to reduce noise impacts; 2011.

75. Gidlöf-Gunnarsson A, Ohrström E. Attractive "quiet" courtyards: a potential modifier of urban residents' responses to road traffic noise? Int J Environ Res Public Health. 2010;7(9): 3359–75.

76. Gidlof-Gunnarsson A, Ohrstrom E. Noise and well-being in urban residential environments: the potential role of perceived availability to nearby green areas. Landsc Urban Plan. 2007;83:115–26.

77. Amundsen A, Klæboe R, Aasvang G. The Norwegian facade insulation study: efficacy of facade insulation in reducing noise annoyance due to road traffic. J Acoust Soc Am. 2011; 129(3):1381–9.

78. Ayers S, Fullerton J, Leed A, Miller S. Reducing HVAC noise with duct liner. HPAC Engineering. http://hpac.com/iaq-amp-ventilation/reducing-hvac-noise-duct-liner. Accessed 1 Jan 2012.

79. Verbeek J, Kateman E, Morata T, Dreschler W, Mischke C. Interventions to prevent occupational noise-induced hearing loss. Cochrane Database Syst Rev 2012;(10):CD006396.

80. Richardson A, Allsop M, Coghill E, Turnock C. Earplugs and eye masks: do they improve critical care patients' sleep? Nurs Crit Care. 2007;12(6):278–86.

81. Koo Y, Koh H. Effects of eye protective device and ear protective device application on sleep disorder with coronary disease patients in CCU. J Korean Acad Nurs. 2008;38(4):582–92.

82. Suter A. Construction noise: exposure, effects, and the potential for remediation; a review and analysis. Appl Sci Technol. 2002;63:768–89.

83. Zaidi SH. Noise level and sources of noise pollution in Karachi. J Pak Med Assoc. 1989;39:62–5.

84. Khan M, Memon M, Khan M, Khan M. Traffic noise pollution in Karachi, Pakistan. JLUMHS. 2010;9(3):114–20.

85. U.S. Department of Transportation Federal Highway Administration. Quiet pavements; lessons learned from Europe. FOCUS, accelerating infrastructure innovations. http://www.fhwa. dot.gov/publications/focus/05apr/04.cfm. Accessed April 2005.

86. Irmer V, Federal Environmental Agency. The Blue Angel Program in Germany to reduce noise levels from construction machines. 2000.

87. Federal Ministry for the Environment, Nature Conservation and Nuclear Safety. The Blue Angel. 2013. http://www.blauer-engel.de/en/. Accessed 19 July 2013.

88. European Commission. The environmental noise directive (2002/49/EC). 2012. http:// ec.europa.eu/environment/noise/directive.htm. Accessed 14 July 2013.

89. European Commission. Report from the commission to the European Parliament and the council on the implementation of the Environmental Noise Directive in accordance with Article 11 of Directive 2002/49/EC; 2011.

90. Environmental Protection Agency (EPA) Australia. Environment protection (residential noise) regulations 2008 (SR No 121 of 2008); 2008.

91. Sommerhoff J, Recuero M, Suarez E. Community responses to road traffic noise in Hanoi and Ho Chi Minh City. Appl Acoust. 2004;65(7):643–56.

Chapter 9
Modeling Vulnerable Urban Populations in the Global Context of a Changing Climate

Vijay Lulla, Austin Stanforth, Natasha Prudent, Daniel Johnson, and George Luber

Introduction

Climate change, an increase in overall average temperature and frequency of extreme weather events, will influence human populations and exert stress on the current and future built environment. Most contemporary climate models indicate that climate change will have heterogeneous impact globally, and its effects are expected to be more severe in urban centers. This is due to the increased density of human populations, materials used to construct the urban area, and land-use practices therein [44]. There are numerous health stressors present in urban locations, such as the urban heat island (UHI) effect and pollution, despite proximal access to health services. Understanding the effects of climate change on human health will become a central focus of the public health community in the twenty-first century. The anticipated consequences of climate change are not yet fully realized, but increased local risk disparities are apparent and will require a multidisciplinary paradigm of investigation to successfully identify vulnerable populations and mitigate environmental and social impacts. This chapter highlights several environmental and disease processes that are expected to be impacted by a changing climate. Following this introduction, a methodology of determining vulnerability using state-of-the-art data acquisition and computational techniques will be illustrated. Therefore, this chapter aims to be an introduction to climate effects on human health and to the vulnerability modeling of these effects.

V. Lulla, Ph.D. (✉) • A. Stanforth, M.S. (✉) • D. Johnson, Ph.D.
Indiana University Purdue University Indianapolis, Institute for Research on Social Issues, Indianapolis, IN, USA
e-mails: vlulla@iupui.edu; austin.stanforth@gmail.com

N. Prudent, M.P.H. • G. Luber, Ph.D.
Centers for Disease Control and Prevention, Atlanta, GA, USA

© Springer New York 2015
R. Ahn et al. (eds.), *Innovating for Healthy Urbanization*,
DOI 10.1007/978-1-4899-7597-3_9

Urbanization and Climate

As the world's population migrates from rural to more urban settings, understanding how urban forms (dense or spread out) alter local climate, and how climate change will uniquely impact urban environments, is critical. First, it is essential to understand the difference between weather and climate. Weather looks at short-term daily or monthly variations in precipitation, wind, and temperature within predefined geographical areas. Climate focuses on decadal trends of the above variables within those same or larger areas. Climate is influenced by energy added to and released from Earth's system over time, which influences weather patterns. The Sun provides energy to the system that is either radiated back into outer space or absorbed by oceans and land cover. Alterations in normal climate patterns can be attributed to disruptions in this energy balance. For example, increases in light-colored aerosols in the atmosphere serve to reflect solar radiance, decreasing the amount of energy that enters Earth's system; on the other hand, increasing amounts of greenhouse gases, concrete roads, and buildings serve to increase the amount of heat absorbed in Earth's system [51]. While large-scale energy fluxes influence global climate, urban centers can alter local energy budgets through UHIs and wind patterns to further impact local climate [45]. Increased commercial density, residential density, impervious surfaces (such as roads, parking lots, and other concrete features), and a reduction of green vegetation or large bodies of water all serve to modify temperature, precipitation, and wind, in comparison to rural areas [23]. Thus, climate investigations can be performed at either a global or urban scale.

The UHI effect is the phenomenon by which temperature in an urban setting is higher relative to the surrounding rural settings [1]. This steep gradient of temperature is driven by the man-made characteristics of urban areas. The composition of buildings and the decrease in cooling vegetation cause the retention of daytime heat. This heat is then radiated back out into the ambient air during the night, raising the local ambient temperature [68]. The steepness of the temperature gradient varies by climate zone, with temperate latitude cities seeing nighttime increases of 1–5 °C, while more tropical cities, during the dry season, exhibit gradients as high as 10 °C [37]. The size and density of the city also influence the intensity of the UHI effect [46]. Higher levels of light-colored aerosol-based pollutants, such as pure sulfates or salt particles, can have a cooling effect by blocking solar radiation. However, lower albedo or surface reflection levels within urban areas trap heat and offset any potential urban cooling experienced during altered radiation fluxes. In addition to lower albedo, larger street canyons typical of denser cities modify the intensity of urban temperatures through changes in wind speed and advection [23, 45].

Although the research is still developing, the UHI effect may also serve as one of the main drivers of changes in urban precipitation patterns [5, 6, 9, 40]. Warmer temperatures associated with the UHI effect increase thermal convection, leading to lower convergence [45, 63]. Cool, moist air is pulled toward the city for the formation of rain-bearing clouds downwind [9]. Intensification of precipitation has similarly been linked to urban canyons and the proximity of coastal bodies and rivers.

In addition, air pollution creates favorable conditions for water droplets to form and grow [4, 40]. Understanding precipitation dynamics over large cities is very complex, and studies show conflicting reports on the role urban form plays in changes to precipitation patterns. As human populations continue to expand the built environment through urban migration, understanding how urban forms influence local climate is necessary to assess climate change-associated negative health consequences within the context of urbanization.

Global Climate Change, Built Environment, and Health

Oppressive climates influence the health of human populations in various adverse ways. According to current climate change models, it is very likely that extreme heat events (EHEs) will become more severe and longer in duration. Future exposure to extreme heat has a significant impact on morbidity and mortality. One study estimates that by 2020—assuming current emission trends continue—44 large US cities will experience an increase of 2,260 excess summer deaths, and by 2050 those urban areas could experience total excess deaths of 3,190–4,478 [31]. In addition to the commonly experienced heat stroke, heat exhaustion, heat cramps, and dehydration cases, heat can also contribute to the formation of blood clots, aggravate chronic pulmonary conditions, cardiac conditions, kidney disorders, and psychiatric illnesses [67].

Climate change is also expected to exacerbate further poor air quality and pollution within urban centers. Ozone, particulate matter 2.5 µm in diameter (PM2.5), and aeroallergens are expected to be among the major air pollutants. Ozone formation increases with higher temperatures and increased sunlight [15]. Similarly, large particulate formation is partly dependent on temperature and humidity; thus, concentrations may increase with warmer temperatures [8]. Aeroallergens, like pollen, are airborne particles that elicit an allergic response in sensitive persons [34]. The warmer temperatures and increased carbon dioxide levels characteristic of urbanization and climate change contribute to earlier flower blooming and thus earlier and longer pollen seasons [58]. However, whether forecasted changes in the pollen season will result in an increase in allergic disease is yet to be definitively determined [34]. Health effects associated with poor urban air quality that climate change may exacerbate include decreased lung function, heart attack, arrhythmias, increased hospital admissions for respiratory illnesses (e.g., asthma, pneumonia, and rhinitis), and premature mortality [2, 8, 14, 15, 20, 24, 39, 41, 43, 49, 50, 55, 57].

Heavy rainfall events are expected to become more frequent and intense with climate change. This imposes an additional burden on already stressed urban infrastructure—particularly water and sanitation systems—and increases the potential for the spread of disease. Data on US waterborne disease outbreaks from 1948 to 1994 suggest a significant association with levels of extreme precipitation [10]. This relationship is not well understood, but is principally attributed to increased runoff transporting elevated levels of microorganisms (e.g., Giardia, Cryptosporidium) into surface water and groundwater [17]. The data also indicate that during heavy rainfall events, urban water sources are particularly susceptible to contamination due to overflows in pipes that transport both sewage and storm water (i.e., combined system overflows) [54].

Warmer temperatures and changing precipitation patterns characteristic of climate change may also alter the distribution of disease-carrying vectors and zoonoses. For example, rising temperatures may increase the rate of dengue virus replication in host mosquitoes [21]. Tick distribution is also highly correlated with temperature and humidity. It is suspected that change in climate may affect incidence of tick-borne diseases, such as Lyme disease and Rocky Mountain spotted fever [21]. West Nile virus and Saint Louis encephalitis virus are associated with drought-like conditions and high temperatures [21]. However, despite known correlations between temperature, precipitation, and distribution of vectors and zoonoses, increases in transmission rates are affected by a host of other ecological factors [13, 18, 38, 42, 47, 52, 59, 66]. The public health impact of changes to the distribution of disease-carrying vectors and zoonoses depends on non-climatic factors as well, such as access to prevention methods (e.g., air conditioning and sealed structures) [51]. Better holistic urban climate change models need to be developed before we can truly identify the best methods for dealing with the negative effects of climate change [18].

The emerging threats of climate change within the context of urban health provide an engaging framework for addressing anticipated health stressors [16]. The field of public health includes a continually evolving evidence-based body of tools, such as vulnerability assessments, that identify segments of the population facing the greatest risk of direct exposure. These tools can serve to promote resilience and form sustainable policies in communities disproportionately burdened with negative health consequences associated with climate change and urban development.

Vulnerability and Urban Population Health

New Spatial Vulnerability Assessment Approaches

Population vulnerability results from the inability of a population to cope with a hazard due to increased sensitivity, susceptibility, or lack of adaptive capacity [22, 23]. Within the public health literature, an understanding of vulnerability lies within the environmental justice thesis, which suggests that risks incurred from environmental hazards are greater among marginalized populations [22]. The study of population vulnerability, then, seeks to identify conditions that render certain populations more prone to exposures and measure the adaptive capacity of the population within a socioeconomic context [11].

Traditionally, population vulnerability is the cumulative negative pressure exerted by biophysical and social ramifications. Social vulnerability is composed of variables derived from the social or economic environment, encompassing age, education, income, gender, ethnic/racial composition, and population density of individuals in the population. Biophysical vulnerability includes risk to direct environmental exposures, such as extreme heat and flooding. It also includes built environment factors, such as the UHI effect, and other land-use patterns that exacerbate biological risks. Social vulnerability is well-researched, while assessments of biophysical vulnerability are a more recent endeavor [65]. Integrating social and biophysical risk factors into an assessment of population vulnerability allows for a more cohesive and useful understanding of how climate change will influence populations in expanding urban environments.

It is at the finer scale within cities that intra-urban vulnerability becomes most pronounced, i.e., social and biophysical risks are disproportionally distributed across an urban area [61]. For example, a vulnerability study in Phoenix, Arizona, demonstrated that pockets of communities within the study area faced greater exposure to heat stress, due to higher social and biophysical vulnerabilities (e.g., age and less vegetation), than the surrounding communities [22]. Spatial distribution of vulnerable populations overlapping with climate hazard segments within a city has yet to be fully explored [28]. Less utilized city-specific analyses may provide more information on social and biophysical vulnerability than larger, less spatially resolute studies at the regional and national levels [53]. Thus, vulnerability metrics should be aggregated at the city level, where decisions are more likely to reflect information on vulnerability within intra-urban populations and can therefore be the most informed methods of response [33]. Implementing vulnerability mapping techniques that incorporate social and biophysical vulnerabilities into a place-based, or location-specific, assessment allows for improved integration of historically disparate information. This can lead to improved implementation and monitoring of risk reduction policies within rapidly growing urban communities at the local level [11, 28, 33].

Satellite-Based Remote Sensing as a Surveillance Tool

Remote sensing is the process of acquiring data about an area of interest without direct contact, be it one or 100 m way. Common examples of remote sensing include X-rays, photography, and even human vision. These are all examples of practices that gather information from a distance, whether it is through a handheld device or incorporated into an orbiting satellite. For environmental research, the process is most similar to photography, where a sensor will "take a picture" of an area while recording data from within and outside the visual spectrum. Visual light is created by the Sun, which also emits other wavelengths of electromagnetic radiation (EMR), such as X-rays, infrared, thermal, and radio waves. Unlike the human eye, remote sensing devices can be calibrated to collect data across many diverse and distant wavelengths [25]. Analysts can use these multispectral, diverse wavelength images to interpret data not available to the human eye. A common application of nonvisual spectrum data is the use of thermal or infrared vision goggles.

Remote sensing allows for the analysis of environmental features through imagery and quantitative calculations through pixel values. Thermal imagery, for example, can be used to distinguish areas of the city that have increased thermal characteristics through calculation of land surface temperature (LST) [27]. This technique is used to identify the UHI or the hot spots within a city that are disproportionally warmer than the surrounding features. Johnson et al. [26] summarizes various possibilities by including remotely sensed data to examine vulnerability (e.g., understanding the variability of heat between intra-urban neighborhoods). The application of remote sensing can also be useful for identifying other additional stress factors, such as a lack of vegetation. Plants can be responsible for reducing LST and filtering pollutants out of the atmosphere.

Photosynthetic vegetation utilizes blue, red, and thermal wavelengths of EMR during photosynthesis while reflecting green and near-infrared wavelengths. This process gives plants their green color. Since this process occurs in healthy, photosynthetic vegetation, the health and quantity of local vegetation can be calculated by creating an index from reflection measurements of red and near-infrared light [19, 25]. This process is commonly utilized in remotely sensed projects and is known as the Normalized Difference Vegetation Index (NDVI). The higher NDVI value recorded, the more protection vegetation should provide, both through decreased thermal impact to the area and by filtering pollutants out of the air during respiration [11]. A similar scale, the Normalized Difference Built-up Index (NDBI), utilizes the reflection properties of cement and other constructed materials to identify areas of impervious surfaces. Higher NDBI values are normally associated with increased urban construction, which is linked to increased temperature, air pollutants, and precipitation runoff. Incorporating LST, NDVI, and NDBI allows for the consideration of environmental impacts on vulnerability—previous studies have not integrated environmental properties and socioeconomic vulnerability in this way [62]. These indices can be used to represent the influence—either positive or negative—of environmental variables on the vulnerability of local populations [28].

An Example Methodology: Modeling Vulnerability to an Extreme Heat Event

Vulnerability to EHEs is normally considered only from a statistical perspective. That is, an area is considered to be under extreme weather conditions when the weather station, commonly located outside the city limits, has observed adverse conditions (high temperature, high relative humidity, or a combination of these two) similar to historical events that had a statistical increase in mortality/morbidity. While this approach can be applicable to a broad understanding of a vulnerability event over a large area, such as a county or city boundary, it is insufficient for city planners and emergency management personnel to identify specific areas of high risk. Mitigation strategists and planners need a more detailed view of vulnerability. Hence, there is a trend in the research community to include environmental factors (provided by remotely sensed data) in combination with socioeconomic factors to understand vulnerability at a much finer scale [29, 53, 64]. Gauging vulnerability to EHEs is particularly challenging, because EHEs occur without clear warning signs. Other natural hazards, such as tornadoes or blizzards, approach as clouded weather fronts and are typically associated with drastic changes in wind and temperature. The public must rely on advisories, warnings, and watches issued by weather agencies to become aware of an EHE. As previously mentioned, these warnings are often based on data collected from a weather station located outside of the urban core, where temperatures are not as extreme. While the reported maximum temperature and heat index describe predicted temperatures across large urban areas, they do not represent the true exposure of various intra-urban areas to EHEs, because vulnerability to heat is not uniform across the entire urban space. For example, densely populated areas with old and dilapidated buildings, commonly found within inner city cores, may experience temperatures 3–5° higher than what is indicated by the issued advisory recorded by the weather station [27].

Our research aims to (a) understand the spatial distribution of vulnerability for EHEs within an entire urban setting and (b) develop maps identifying areas of increased risk. In our method, socioeconomic data collected and disseminated by the US Census Bureau is combined with environmental factors (LST, NDVI, and NDBI) to generate an index representing the vulnerability of an enumeration unit (census block/block group/tract) during an EHE. Therefore, an accurate understanding of the spatial distribution of vulnerability is a useful tool for risk management and mitigation strategists. This index can be generated using either principal component analysis (PCA) or an artificial neural network (ANN) (Fig. 9.1).

Vulnerability Indices Using Principal Component Analysis

A method of data reduction is needed to better understand how the vulnerability input variables interact to create the severity of an area's risk. PCA can be used to identify the underlying constructs of the variables, identify trends, and designate which features are most important [12]. This method can be used to see which input variables are similar in order to create a simpler set of factors to represent the variables that most heavily affect vulnerability. Data reduction reduces the number of input variables in order to streamline calculations including many factors [30]. The PCA's data reduction method simplifies a multivariable dataset, by identifying the input variables' correlation among themselves. It then creates new factors by restructuring the data into new combined components that individually express a larger portion of the variance found in the original variables. PCA results can be compared between studies by the number of components they produce. The fewer components needed to demonstrate the variance, the more correlated/similar the original data is—and the stronger the model that is produced.

These components can be utilized in mapping EHE mitigation. If the components are plotted against a heat mortality-dependent value, the primary components will contain an identification of mortality risk. The components can then be mapped

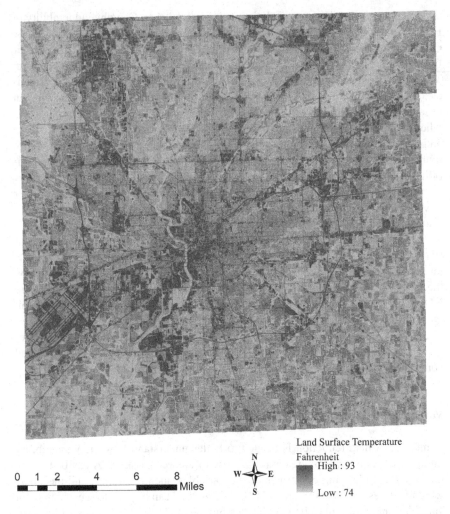

Land Surface Temperature

Fahrenheit
High : 93

Low : 74

0   1   2   4   6   8
Miles

N
W ← → E
S

Fig. 9.1 LST image of Indianapolis, IN, acquired by the Landsat 5 TM satellite platform acquired on July 1, 2011

to identify areas that feature a majority of the characteristics related to heat mortality during an EHE.

The socioeconomic variables included in this model, extracted from decadal census data, include population counts by race, age, educational attainment, household income, and elderly living alone. These factors are combined with environmental factors (LST, NDVI, and NDBI) known to contribute to vulnerability. This analysis can be carried out at both the census tract and census block group enumeration levels, which are political boundaries based on population density. The output from this analysis yields an index of vulnerability. Organizing enumeration units into

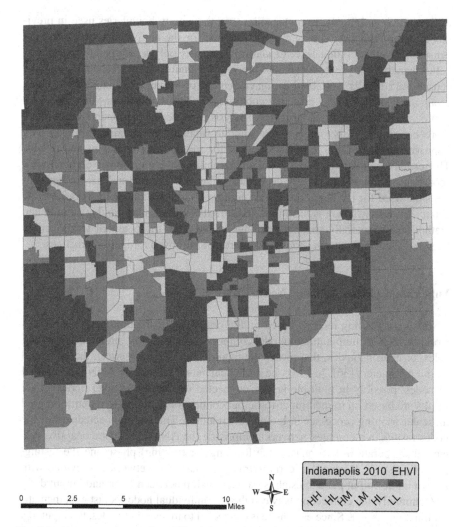

Fig. 9.2 An extreme heat vulnerability index analysis map of Indianapolis, IN, utilizing 2010 census socioeconomic data and environmental data collected by the Landsat 5 TM satellite on July 15, 2011

classes based on this vulnerability score provides a clear picture of vulnerability levels across specific micropopulations. The analysis of the 1995 Chicago, IL, heat wave by Stanforth [62] is an example of how PCA can be used to determine vulnerability utilizing these input variables (see Fig. 9.2).

The study by Stanforth [62] also aimed to evaluate the significance of spatial resolution, and utilization of residential vs. commercial land use, for this type of analysis. The results supported the hypothesis that vulnerability to EHE mortality and morbidity can be appropriately measured and predicted within boundaries (census track and block groups) smaller than the county boundaries used in previous systems. The best explanation of variance for the study occurred during the census tract enumeration level of analysis, but was only a few percentage points better than the analysis using smaller block group enumeration levels. Although the census tract results contained a higher percent of variance explained, the block group analysis had fewer principal components. This demonstrates that the block group, smaller spatial boundary, PCA analysis resulted in components which were more correlated. This suggests that similar smaller-scale models could greatly improve spatial resolution, or accuracy, of the incorporated variables and results. The results demonstrated that, overall, vulnerability is very specific to certain socio-economic variables and is very dependent on spatial resolution. This further suggests the need for increased spatial resolution of variables and analysis beyond the county boundary, which is used in most current NWS warnings and is an outdated method. New, spatially-specific warnings would have the potential to save more lives and reduce disaster response costs through improved mitigation practices.

Vulnerability Using Artificial Neural Networks

ANNs is a modeling method based on the principles of the biological neural network. ANN is a computational model comprised of a series of interconnected variables, or neurons/nodes, that model the relationship of data between the input and output parameters [36]. Just like the biological neural system, an ANN is composed of nodes, possibly in multiple layers, connected to a series of other nodes. ANN results are based on trained input-to-output connections, similar to repetition-based muscular training processes in biological creatures. The interconnectedness of the nodes results in a complex network comprising the ANN. ANNs are adaptive systems that operate in two phases: the learning (or training) phase and the testing/predicting stage. During the learning/training phase, the network is provided with known input-output pairs to establish a relationship between input and output data.

Commonly, the connection between the two individual nodes is just a mathematical function $f:X \rightarrow Y$. Since each node is connected to many other nodes, the input to a node is the summation of all the incoming connections, and the output is the function f applied to this summation [36]. The interconnectedness of the nodes provides an opportunity for modeling many different kinds of relationships, by changing the mathematical function used for the connections or by adjusting the weights to different inputs to precisely control the input of all the different inputs (Kohonen 1990). The connections between the nodes are adjusted so that the network converges toward, or learns, a model that is actually represented by the data. The number of nodes, number of layers, learning function, rate of learning, number of iterations required to converge on a solution, and least acceptable error are all parameters that can be modified, by trial and error, to develop a model to fit the study's requirements.

There has been a recent increase in ANN use, because they have some very useful characteristics. ANNs do not pose any restriction on the distribution characteristics of the collected data [32, 48]. Linear regression, on the other hand, requires data used for modeling to be normally distributed. ANNs also allow the incorporation of many different types of variables (categorical, nominal, and/or ordinal data) to be included in the analysis [3, 7]. Finally, ANNs are not affected by variable outliers in the data as much as PCA. ANNs do, however, have some drawbacks. They are complicated and often require extensive setup to initiate. The final drawback is the issue of model over-fitting. Model over-fitting occurs when ANN trains noise to result's nodes along with the signal, when the number of input variables is larger than the number of training cases, and/or the input variables are highly correlated with each other [56, 60].

We describe below how we used ANN for some preliminary analysis. As described earlier, the input variables are comprised of socioeconomic and environmental factors. Mortality data was obtained from the respective cities, and only deaths related to the EHE were selected and geocoded, located spatially based on a postal address. The predicted number of aggregate deaths within each census enumeration unit (census tract or block group) was used as the output for the ANN. Once the model was created, after training and testing, it predicted the number of deaths per census boundary and compared them to recorded deaths from a historical EHE. The figures below show the neural network predicted mortalities compared to the actually observed mortality.

The difference in the scatter plots is due to the different number of enumeration units and different number of deaths for the cities of Dayton (a) and Phoenix (b) (Fig. 9.3). As can be seen from the images, the predicted mortality appears to follow the trend of observed mortality. This suggests a strong positive predictive ability of the ANN and suggests a possibility of improving the neural network model, either by tweaking the parameters used during training or refining the data by incorporating only residential areas, as demonstrated by Stanforth [62].

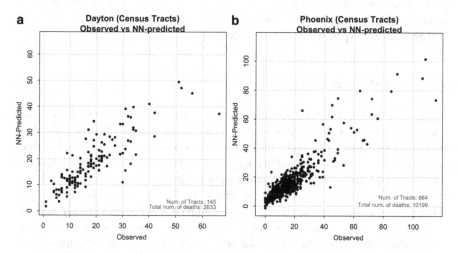

Fig. 9.3 Scatter plot of NN predicted vs. observed mortality for (**a**) Dayton and (**b**) Phoenix. Analysis was carried out at census tract enumeration level

Future Directions for Research and Improvement

Hyperspectral Remote Sensing

As discussed earlier, satellite-based remotely sensed data is now commonly used in modeling vulnerability, but there are limitations to the use of such data. First, temporal resolution, or frequency at which the data is collected, does not allow for continuous measurement, as the sensor is only in position a couple days per month. For example, the temporal resolution for Landsat data is 16 days; in other words, an image is taken at the same location once every 16 days and will sometimes miss the heat wave window or be blocked by cloud cover. There are some satellites that have a temporal resolution of one day, but their spatial resolution is too coarse to be of much use for the study of intra-urban areas. Aircraft-based hyperspectral remote sensors can alleviate both the issues of spatial and temporal resolution. Hyperspectral remote sensors are very analogous to their multispectral counterparts, but differ in that they measure the electromagnetic reflectance in very narrow, contiguous bands. This provides a much more representative sample of the reflectance curve of the underlying feature. The spatial resolution of aircraft-collected data can also be much better than the satellite-based multispectral data, depending on the altitude at which the aircraft passes over the area of interest. This availability of higher spectral and spatial resolution provides more fine-grained data, which can improve the performance of models using this data. The methods and techniques used for hyperspectral analysis are slightly different than those for multispectral data. Increased spectral bands require higher computer processing power, and the preprocessing methods are also different. Since hyperspectral data are aircraft collected, they contain errors attributable to the movement of the aircraft (roll, yaw, and pitch). These errors need to be removed by preprocessing the data. This is not a complicated problem, as most of these sensors come with utilities and tools with customizable settings for each flight, allowing for correction of errors later on. Still, hyperspectral sensors are very expensive; therefore, they not practical for widespread use.

Web-Based Modeling Tools

While most vulnerability-related modeling is carried out in university labs and research centers, there is a possibility of creating a Web-based tool/framework. This tool could be specifically designed to allow local planners to input data for their localities and generate vulnerability maps for planning and mitigation purposes. This Web interface could allow a municipality to identify areas at an increased risk to weather disasters and to efficiently distribute the data and test/implement mitigation plans. In a digital format, the application could allow the vulnerability maps to be distributed to hospitals or nonprofit groups so that medical assistance could be positioned in high-risk areas before the adverse conditions occur. The application could also allow city planners to test how a new mitigation practice would impact risk, such as planting trees in areas of high UHI. The Web application could also allow for the quick update of data during oppressive seasons. If a wild fire or tornado destroyed a large portion of the urban canopy, as during the 2011 Alabama disasters, new mitigation maps could be produced "on the fly" to assist with the cleanup and preparation for the next disaster. Work is currently being conducted on creating such a Web framework used for generating EHE vulnerability maps specific to a city or county.

Concluding Remarks

With increased awareness about climate change and its impact on the environment and society, there is an ongoing trend to move toward collaboration among different areas of the research community. While vulnerability has traditionally been studied primarily by sociologists, it now involves researchers from diverse fields who aim to collect, analyze, and model data in new and meaningful ways. These collaborations present a unique opportunity to better understand and model vulnerability through more comprehensive studies. While only EHE has been discussed in this chapter, these same principles can be applied to model vulnerability to other natural and anthropogenic hazards throughout the developed and developing world. The procedures previously described for heat mitigation could be adapted easily to cold weather disasters as well or be utilized to create location-specific mitigation plans for flash flooding and identification of Lyme disease-infested tick populations. Understanding the improved benefits of incorporating environmental and societal risk elements has provided a new holistic view of vulnerability. This view will hopefully lead us to a safer and more prepared future.

References

1. Arnfield AJ. Two decades of urban climate research: a review of turbulence, exchanges of energy and water, and the urban heat island. Int J Climatol. 2003;23:1–26.
2. Bell ML, Dominici F, Samet JM. A meta-analysis of time-series studies of ozone and mortality with comparison to the national morbidity, mortality, and air pollution study. Epidemiology. 2005;16:436.
3. Benediktsson JA, Swain PH, Ersoy OK. Neural network approaches versus statistical methods in classification of multisource remote sensing data. IEEE Trans Geosci Remote Sens. 1990;28:540–52.
4. Braham R. Cloud physics of urban weather modification—a preliminary report. Bull Am Meteorol Soc. 1974;55:100–6.
5. Braham RR, Semonin R, Auer AH, Changnon SA, Hales JM. Summary of urban effects on clouds and rain. In: Changnon SA, editor. METROMEX: a review and summary. Boston: American Meteorological Society; 1981. p. 141–52.
6. Burian SJ, Shepherd JM. Effect of urbanization on the diurnal rainfall pattern in Houston. Hydrol Process. 2005;19:1089–103.
7. Carpenter GA, Gopal S, Macomber S, Martens S, Woodcock CE, Franklin J. A neural network method for efficient vegetation mapping. Remote Sens Environ. 1999;70:326–38.

8. Confalonieri U, Menne B, Akhtar R, Ebi KL, Hauengue M, Kovats RS, et al. Human health. In: Parry ML, Canziani OF, Palutikof JP, Van der Linden PJ, Hanson CE, editors. Climate change 2007: impacts, adaptation and vulnerability. Contribution of working group II to the fourth assessment report of the intergovernmental panel on climate change. Cambridge: Cambridge University Press; 2007. p. 391–431.

9. Cotton WR, Pielke RA. Human impacts on weather and climate. New York: Cambridge University Press; 1995.

10. Curriero FC, Patz JA, Rose JB, Lele S. The association between extreme precipitation and waterborne disease outbreaks in the United States, 1948–1994. Am J Public Health. 2001;91:1194–9.

11. Cutter SL, Boruff BJ, Shirley WL. Social vulnerability to environmental hazards*. Soc Sci Q. 2003;84:242–61.

12. DeCoster J. Data analysis in SPSS. 2004. http://www.stat-help.com/notes.html. Accessed 31 May 2011.

13. Degaetano AT. Meteorological effects on adult mosquito (Culex) populations in metropolitan New Jersey. Int J Biometeorol. 2005;49:345–53.

14. Dominici F, Peng RD, Bell ML, Pham L, Mcdermott A, Zeger SL, Samet JM. Fine particulate air pollution and hospital admission for cardiovascular and respiratory diseases. JAMA. 2006;295:1127–34.

15. Ebi K, Balbus J, Kinney P, Lipp E, Mills D, O'Neill M, et al. Synthesis and assessment product 4.6: chapter 2, effects of global change on human health (final review draft). CCSP; 2008.

16. Frumkin H, Hess J, Luber G, Malilay J, Mcgeehin M. Climate change: the public health response. Am J Public Health. 2008;98:435.

17. Gaffield SJ, Goo RL, Richards LA, Jackson RJ. Public health effects of inadequately managed stormwater runoff. Am J Public Health. 2003;93:1527.

18. Gage KL, Burkot T, Eisen RJ, Hayes EB. Climate change and vector-borne diseases. Am J Prev Med. 2008;35:436–50.

19. Glenn EP, et al. Relationship between remotely-sensed vegetation indices, canopy attributes and plant physiological processes: what vegetation indices can and cannot tell us about the landscape. Sensors 8.4. 2008: 2136–2160.

20. Gryparis A, Forsberg B, Katsouyanni K, Analitis A, Touloumi G, Schwartz J, Samoli E, Medina S, Anderson HR, Niciu EM. Acute effects of ozone on mortality from the "air pollution and health: a European approach" project. Am J Respir Crit Care Med. 2004;170: 1080–7.

21. Haines A, Patz JA. Health effects of climate change. JAMA. 2004;291:99–103.

22. Harlan SL, Brazel AJ, Prashad L, Stefanov WL, Larsen L. Neighborhood microclimates and vulnerability to heat stress. Soc Sci Med. 2006;63:2847–63.

23. Hughes K. The impact of urban areas on climate in the UK: a spatial and temporal analysis, with an emphasis on temperature and precipitation effects. Earth Environ. 2006;2:54–83.

24. Ito K, De Leon SF, Lippmann M. Associations between ozone and daily mortality: analysis and meta-analysis. Epidemiology. 2005;16:446.

25. Jensen JR. Remote sensing of the environment: an earth resource perspective. Upper Saddle River: Pearson Prentice Hall; 2007.

26. Johnson DP, Lulla V, Stanforth AC, Webber J. Remote sensing of heat-related risks: the trend towards coupling socioeconomic and remotely sensed data. Geogr Compass. 2011;5(10): 767–80. doi: 10.1111/j.1749-8198.201.00442.x.

27. Johnson DP, Stanforth AC, Lulla V, Luber G. Developing an applied extreme heat vulnerability index utilizing socioeconomic and environmental data. Appl Geogr. 2012;35(1–2):23–31. ISSN 0143-6228, 10.1016/j.apgeog.2012.04.006.

28. Johnson DP, Wilson JS. The socio-spatial dynamics of extreme urban heat events: the case of heat-related deaths in Philadelphia. Appl Geogr. 2009;29:419–34.

29. Johnson D, Wilson J, Luber G. Socioeconomic indicators of heat-related health risk supplemented with remotely sensed data. Int J Health Geogr. 2009;8:57.

30. Jolliffe I. Principal component analysis. New York: Wiley; 2002.
31. Kalkstein LS, Greene JS. An evaluation of climate/mortality relationships in large US cities and the possible impacts of a climate change. Environ Health Perspect. 1997;105:84.
32. Kanellopoulos I, Wilkinson GG. Strategies and best practice for neural network image classi-fication. Int J Remote Sens. 1997;18:711–25.
33. Kienberger S, Lang S, Zeil P. Spatial vulnerability units? Expert-based spatial modelling of socio-economic vulnerability in the Salzach catchment, Austria. Nat Hazards Earth Syst Sci. 2009;9:767–78.
34. Kinney PL. Climate change, air quality, and human health. Am J Prev Med. 2008;35:459–67.
35. Kohonen T. Self-organized formation of topologically correct feature maps. Biol Cybern. 1982;43:59–69.
36. Kohonen T. Self-organization and associative memory. Berlin: Springer; 1989.
37. Kovats S, Akhtar R. Climate, climate change and human health in Asian cities. Environ Urban. 2008;20:165–75.
38. Kunkel KE, Novak RJ, Lampman RL, Gu W. Modeling the impact of variable climatic factors on the crossover of Culex restauns and Culex pipiens (Diptera: Culicidae), vectors of West Nile virus in Illinois. Am J Trop Med Hyg. 2006;74:168–73.
39. Laden F, Schwartz J, Speizer FE, Dockery DW. Reduction in fine particulate air pollution and mortality. Am J Respir Crit Care Med. 2006;173:667–72.
40. Landsberg HE. The urban climate. New York: Academic; 1981.
41. Levy JI, Chemerynski SM, Sarnat JA. Ozone exposure and mortality: an empiric Bayes metaregression analysis. Epidemiology. 2005;16:458.
42. Mccabe GJ, Bunnell JE. Precipitation and the occurrence of Lyme disease in the northeastern United States. Vector Borne Zoonotic Dis. 2004;4:143–8.
43. Mudway I, Kelly F. Ozone and the lung: a sensitive issue. Mol Aspects Med. 2000;21:1–48.
44. O'Neill M, Jackman D, Wyman D, Manarolla X, Gronlund C, Brown D, Brines S, Schwartz J, Diez-Roux A. US local action on heat and health: are weprepared for climate change? Int J Public Health. 2010;55:105–12.
45. Oke TR. Boundary layer climates. New York: Psychology Press; 1988.
46. Oke TR, editor. Urban climates and global environmental change. London: Routledge; 1997.
47. Ostfeld RS, Canham CD, Oggenfuss K, Winchcombe RJ, Keesing F. Climate, deer, rodents, and acorns as determinants of variation in Lyme-disease risk. PLoS Biol. 2006;4:e145.
48. Paola JD, Schowengerdt RA. A review and analysis of backpropagation neural networks for classification of remotely-sensed multi-spectral imagery. Int J Remote Sens. 1995;16: 3033–58.
49. Pope III CA, Burnett RT, Thun MJ, Calle EE, Krewski D, Ito K, Thurston GD. Lung cancer, cardiopulmonary mortality, and long-term exposure to fine particulate air pollution. JAMA. 2002;287:1132–41.
50. Pope III CA, Burnett RT, Thurston GD, Thun MJ, Calle EE, Krewski D, Godleski JJ. Cardiovascular mortality and long-term exposure to particulate air pollution epidemiological evidence of general pathophysiological pathways of disease. Circulation. 2004;109:71–7.
51. Prospero JM, Lamb PJ. African droughts and dust transport to the Caribbean: climate change implications. Science. 2003;302:1024–7.
52. Purse BV, Mellor PS, Rogers DJ, Samuel AR, Mertens PPC, Baylis M. Climate change and the recent emergence of bluetongue in Europe. Nat Rev Microbiol. 2005;3:171–81.
53. Reid CE, O'Neill MS, Gronlund CJ, Brines SJ, Brown DG, Diez-Roux AV, Schwartz J. Mapping community determinants of heat vulnerability. Environ Health Perspect. 2009;117: 1730.
54. Rose JB, Epstein PR, Lipp EK, Sherman BH, Bernard SM, Patz JA. Climate variability and change in the United States: potential impacts on water-and foodborne diseases caused by microbiologic agents. Environ Health Perspect. 2001;109:211.
55. Samet JM, Dominici F, Curriero FC, Coursac I, Zeger SL. Fine particulate air pollution and mortality in 20 US cities, 1987–1994. N Engl J Med. 2000;343:1742–9.

56. Sarle WS. Stopped training and other remedies for overfitting. In: Proceedings of the 27th symposium on the interface of computing science and statistics. 1995.
57. Schwartz J. Short term fluctuations in air pollution and hospital admissions of the elderly for respiratory disease. Thorax. 1995;50:531–8.
58. Shea KM, Truckner RT, Weber RW, Peden DB. Climate change and allergic disease. J Allergy Clin Immunol. 2008;122:443–53.
59. Shone SM, Curriero FC, Lesser CR, Glass GE. Characterizing population dynamics of Aedes sollicitans (Diptera: Culicidae) using meteorological data. J Med Entomol. 2006;43:393–402.
60. Smith M. Neural networks for statistical modeling. Boston: International Thomson Computer Press; 1996.
61. Smoyer KE. Putting risk in its place: methodological considerations for investigating extreme event health risk. Soc Sci Med. 1998;47:1809–24.
62. Stanforth A. Identifying variations of socio-spatial vulnerability to heat-related mortality during the 1995 extreme heat event in Chicago, IL, USA. M.S. Thesis. IUPUI: USA. 2011. http://hdl.handle.net/1805/2643.
63. Thielen J, Wobrock W, Gadian A, Mestayer P, Creutin JD. The possible influence of urban surfaces on rainfall development: a sensitivity study in 2D in the meso-[gamma]-scale. Atmos Res. 2000;54:15–39.
64. Uejio CK, Wilhelmi OV, Golden JS, Mills DM, Gulino SP, Samenow JP. Intra-urban societal vulnerability to extreme heat: the role of heat exposure and the built environment, socioeconomics, and neighborhood stability. Health Place. 2011;17:498–507.
65. Vescovi L, Rebetez M, Rong F. Assessing public health risk due to extremely high temperature events: climate and social parameters. Climate Res. 2005;30:71.
66. Wegbreit J, Reisen WK. Relationships among weather, mosquito abundance, and encephalitis virus activity in California: Kern County 1990–98. J Am Mosq Control Assoc. 2000;16:22–7.
67. WHO. Preventing harmful health effects of heat-waves. Copenhagen: World Health Organization; 2006.
68. WMO. Climate and urban development. WMO no. 844. 1996.

Chapter 10
Urbanization and Unintentional Injury in Low- and Middle-Income Countries

John D. Kraemer

Introduction

Urbanization has a complex relationship with injury. The movement of people from rural to urban areas, and their accumulation in cities, changes the risk of injury and its causes. Particularly in developing countries, urbanization exposes people to a host of dangers they often do not encounter in rural areas. It does this through two primary means. In a general sense, urbanization in low- and middle-income countries (LMICs) is often unplanned and rapid, overwhelming urban infrastructure and its margin of safety. Urbanization outpacing its infrastructure is a major determinant of urban road crashes, for example. Additionally, rapid urbanization often results in great social inequality, with many people living in informal settlements or other substandard housing and working in conditions that are not conducive to safety [33, 38, 124]. Combined with the weak safety enforcement and limited resources for prevention and treatment of injuries, residents of urban LMIC areas often face unacceptably high injury risks.

At the same time, urbanization reduces certain injury risks and often increases the likelihood that an injured person will receive adequate treatment. As with most causes of morbidity, injury risk is correlated with socioeconomic status. In cities, people are more socially mobile and are more likely to acquire higher standards of living, thus lessening their risk of many types of injuries (such as childhood burns). Similarly, access to trauma services—such as emergency surgery and blood transfusions—is much improved in urban areas in most low- and middle-income settings, enhancing the chance that an injured person will survive without long-term

J.D. Kraemer, J.D., M.P.H. (✉)
Department of Health Systems Administration, Georgetown University School of Nursing & Health Studies and O'Neill Institute for National & Global Health Law, Georgetown University Law Center, Washington, DC, USA
e-mail: jdk32@georgetown.edu

© Springer New York 2015
R. Ahn et al. (eds.), *Innovating for Healthy Urbanization*,
DOI 10.1007/978-1-4899-7597-3_10

complications. The opportunity for social organization and governmental action that can exist in urbanized areas also allows for risk mitigation [150].

Throughout history, urbanization has been recognized as a double-edged sword. In antiquity, Rome faced a constant, serious fire risk and repeatedly burned. However, its highly organized state authority also allowed it to regulate fire risks and respond to fires as previously had not been possible. In Industrial Revolution era Europe and America, the shift of laborers from agricultural to manufacturing enterprises created a multitude of new dangers but also allowed for regulation of workplace safety, which, over time, drastically reduced workplace injuries and deaths. During the Gold Rush in California, the population of San Francisco exploded, and hastily assembled hovels became fire traps. Soaring death rates in these districts, however, caused housing codes to be better enforced—something that had been difficult in previously rural areas set beyond the efficient reach of regulators [168]. As shown, the lesson of history is that urbanization can at times increase the risk of injury but also can create opportunities for individuals and governments to prevent injury by enabling resources to be pooled and organized.

This chapter explores the relationship between urbanization and injury, with particular focus on the three major causes of unintentional injury that are prevalent in LMIC cities: road crashes, burns, and falls. Two common causes of unintentional injury—drowning and poisoning—are not addressed in detail, because they comprise a substantially lower percentage of the burden of injury in most LMIC urban areas, urbanization decreases their risk (at least for drowning), and the evidence base for interventions in LMICs is very limited. Similarly, this chapter does not address intentional injuries, whether inflicted by oneself or others, even though in many urban areas, intentional injury is a major cause of morbidity and mortality. Intentional injury—especially criminal violence—often springs from causes distinct from those that lead to unintentional injury, and its prevention involves a range of different strategies and actors that are less relevant to the public health approach to unintentional injury.

The main focus of this chapter is on innovations to reduce the injury risks of urbanization and decrease the extent of the burden of injury in urban areas. It focuses separately on the prevention of road crashes, burns, and falls, and it discusses strategies for improving treatment of injuries of all causes. For the most part, the innovations this chapter will present are not high-tech; while high-tech approaches to safety have a role to play, most durable solutions to the risk of injury require improved systems of managing risks in the physical and social environment, supporting safer behavior by individuals, and delivering emergency care. By and large, the tools for doing so are known; the challenge is in implementation.

Epidemiology of Injury in Urban LMIC Areas

Injuries are a neglected tropical disease. Though unintentional injuries comprise a substantial proportion of the burden of ill health, especially in LMICs, very little data exist to describe their distribution, especially, for LMICs. Even less research has sought to understand the coverage of safety interventions and barriers particular to developing settings.

Nonetheless, certain aspects of global injury epidemiology are clear. Injuries result in approximately one-tenth of the global burden of years of life lost, reflecting, in part, the disproportionate risk of injury borne by adolescents and young adults. As a proportion of all causes of death, injury has the largest impact in middle- and high-income settings, where injuries cost between 10 and 15 % of all years of lost life. However, this reflects the lower overall burden of disease and death in emerging and developed economies, not a greater risk of injury. In fact, adjusting for age, the risk of death from injury is three times higher in low-income countries (LICs) than in high-income countries (HICs) (124 vs. 41 deaths per 100,000 people), with middle-income countries having intermediate risk [164]. Of the approximately four million people who lose their lives to unintentional injuries annually, more than 90 % live in LMICs, reflecting both the greater risk of injury and the greater number of people who live in less well-developed regions [24].

The primary causes of unintentional injury are constant across countries' income levels and regions, but their distribution varies substantially. Globally, one-third of all injury deaths result from road crashes. There is substantial variation across regions and country income levels (see Table 10.1), though comparisons are limited by a substantial amount of incomplete reporting and attribution of injury deaths in LMICs. However, road traffic accidents appear to cause a disproportionately high percentage of unintentional injury deaths in sub-Saharan Africa (45 %) and the World Health Organization's (WHO's) Western Pacific region (40 %), compared to Southeast Asia (23 %). On the other hand, burns, which represent a very small percentage of the burden of unintentional injury death in sub-Saharan Africa and the Western Pacific (approximately 2 %), cause one-seventh of all unintentional injury deaths in Southeast Asia [24, 54].

Major data gaps prevent a complete understanding of how the causes and distribution of injury differ in rural and urban areas and how the process of urbanization alters the risk of injury. Whether the risk and severity of injury increases in urban areas varies by location, though comparative data are limited, and higher quality

Table 10.1 Percentage of all injury deaths by cause and WHO region/national income level

Region	Road crashes (%)	Falls (%)	Burns (%)	Poisoning (%)	Drowning (%)	Other (%)
Africa	45	12	2	7	7	27
Americas	41	4	10	8	13	24
E. Med.	23	14	4	19	6	34
European	45	8	9	5	9	24
SE Asia	23	9	14	7	8	39
W. Pac.	40	16	2	7	16	19
LMICs	33	10	8	9	10	30
HICs	34	22	3	9	5	27

data exist for injury mortality than morbidity. In general, though, it appears that urbanization often decreases the risk of injury and subsequent death, particularly when urbanization is associated with increased wealth (as opposed to entrenched poverty) and in countries where emergency services tend to be more available in cities.

In Asia, the injury risk for adults in Pakistani cities—particularly in poorer communities—is higher than in rural areas, and injured urban residents are more likely to have lasting disability (though this may reflect a better emergency services resulting in a lower likelihood of dying) [38]; however, there is no significant difference in the risk for children [39]. In India, the mortality rate from injury is about 20 % higher in rural areas, with rural children about twice as likely to die before their fifth birthday [67]. Similarly, data from Hubei Province, China, found mortality rates from injury in rural areas to be more than twice those in urban areas. Though the most pronounced gaps were from deaths due to suicide, unintentional injury deaths were also higher [94]. In Africa, a different pattern emerges. A study in Ghana showed the risk of injury is higher in rural areas, but that there are more injury-related deaths in urban areas [103]. This is broadly consistent with research from Uganda, which found the risk of all injuries to be higher in urban areas, with the greatest relative increase for fatal and disabling injuries [83]. In Tanzania, the risk of injury was found to be higher in rural areas, but major injuries were equally common in rural and urban settings [110]. While researchers have highlighted urbanization as an issue for injury prevention in Latin America, data on urban and rural injury rates are scarce [124]. Understanding better what drives this regional and country-to-country variation would enable better targeted injury prevention programs.

While more detailed cause-specific epidemiology will be discussed in this chapter, a few key points about the causes of injury in urbanized areas are worth noting. The most important is the increase in the relative impact of road crashes in most LMIC urban areas. In many countries, there is an increase in absolute risk of road crash injuries in urban settings—particularly among adults—and a reduced risk of other types of injuries (such as lacerations from farm work), which make road crash injuries relatively more important [103]. This is particularly true in African settings, where road crashes comprise a much higher percentage of injuries in urban than rural areas and lacerations and drowning a much lower percentage. For example, a review of injuries treated at an urban tertiary hospital in Cameroon found that road traffic injuries comprised 60 % of all injuries and three-quarters of unintentional injuries over a 1-year period. Excluding intentional injuries, falls, burns, and bites represented 11, 4, and 4 % of recorded injuries [71]. For urban children, however, falls tend to be the leading cause of injury. One study, which assessed childhood (under 12 years of age) injuries treated at urban emergency departments—which likely serve primarily urban and periurban populations—in 4 cities in Asia, Latin America, and North Africa, found that falls were the most common cause of injury (56 %) [64]. Similarly, a study of injuries among urban children in a poor part of Lima, Peru, found that falls caused half of the serious injuries documented, with road crashes (22 %) and burns (15 %) trailing [33].

Epidemiology of Urban Road Safety

Unlike in HICs, where most road deaths occur among drivers and occupants of four-wheeled vehicles, deaths in LICs and MICs are concentrated among vulnerable road users, particularly pedestrians (especially in LICs) and motorcyclists (disproportionately in MICs) [112]. While data are limited (a common refrain when assessing injury outside of HICs), the risk of road deaths appears to be highest as countries reach lower- and middle-income status, with a peak risk of death per motor vehicle when gross national income is approximately US$2,000 per capita and a peak overall risk of road traffic death in the population occurring around US$3,000 per capita. Most of this relationship appears to be mediated by the increase in interaction between pedestrians and motorized vehicles that occurs as countries develop, as well as increased use of motorcycles [121]. Though the existing data are not detailed enough to infer causality, this phase of economic development often coincides with increased urbanization, and potentially harmful interactions between pedestrians, motorcyclists, and automobiles will usually be most intense in urban areas [52]. For example, in Kenya, rates of road injury and deaths—as recorded in police statistics—are about 50 % higher in Nairobi than in any other area of the country, but this may partially reflect stronger data systems in the capital [12] (Fig. 10.1).

Population-based surveys produce mixed results about the relative risk of road crash injury in rural and urban areas. In Ghana, one study found approximately comparable rates of injury in rural and urban areas [104], while another found a higher rate of minor injuries in rural areas and major injuries in urban areas [103]. Similar results were found in Tanzania [110]. In China, road crash deaths were

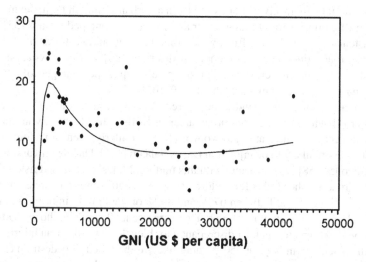

Fig. 10.1 Road traffic deaths per 100,000 people by per capita gross national income. Reprinted from Paulozzi et al. [121]

found to be substantially lower in rural than urban areas [94], and the risk of road crash injury was found to be equal in rural and urban areas in Pakistan [38]. Regardless of the absolute risk of road crash injury and death, across LMIC urban areas, road crashes consistently comprise a higher proportion of injuries in urban areas than in rural ones—a finding that is consistent across regions [67, 83, 127].

The class of road users most injured in crashes varies between urban and rural areas in LMICs. In Africa, pedestrian injuries and deaths comprise a higher percentage of all road crash casualties in urban areas than in rural areas. Depending on the location, they tend to be the most commonly-injured urban road users or make up about the same percentage as motor vehicle occupants [6, 104]. Bicyclists tend to comprise a lower percentage of injured road users in Africa [110], though different studies produce radically different levels of bicycle-related injury [6]. In Asia, fatalities are concentrated much more among motorcyclists, though some studies find nearly half of nonfatal injuries (46 % in Guangzhou, China) occurring among bicyclists. In Southeast Asia, about half of road crash fatalities are among motorized two wheelers; in the western Pacific, they comprise about 20 % of fatalities. Similar results have been found in Latin America, though road crash fatalities tend to be distributed more evenly among motorcyclists, four-wheeled motor vehicles, and pedestrians in Latin America than in Africa, South Asia, and Southeast Asia [25, 112]. Much of the variation across regions reflects the distribution of road users; for example, in places where motorbikes are a substitute for cars (and where a substantial proportion of the population is wealthy enough to purchase them), crash deaths will be concentrated among motorcyclists.

In urban areas, the risk of road crash injury generally increases with age, both in Africa [103, 110] and Asia [94], though data are very limited. A very high percentage of children who are injured or killed, though, in urban areas, are pedestrians [64]. This is particularly true as children become old enough to go to school and walk to school by themselves. For example, in an urban setting in Peru, the majority of road traffic injuries for children under age 15 were among pedestrians [33]. This is consistent with data from Africa, which found that about two-thirds of child and adolescent road injuries occurred among pedestrians [63]. In South Asia, pedestrians and bus occupants comprise approximately equal percentages of children injured in road crashes, with each about 30 % [64].

Across all settings, men tend to be injured in road crashes at a higher rate than women [154]. This is true across urban areas in LMICs. In Aleppo, Syria, men are injured at a 50 % higher rate than women [101]. Similarly, men were found to be about 70 % more likely to be injured in Dar es Salaam [110]. Data from Turkey [127] and Mexico [56, 58] are consistent with this finding. Males' heightened risk of being injured in road crashes holds for children as well as adults in urban areas. In South Asia, it is estimated that between 67 % and 80 % of youth road injuries are among boys [172]. In urban Peru, boys were found to represent 60 % of childhood road crash injuries, with the greatest gender discrepancy for bicycle and pedestrian injuries [33]. In South Africa, urban boys are 50 % more likely to be killed in pedestrian crashes, though the gap is much smaller for fatalities as motor vehicle passengers (which comprise a much smaller number of childhood fatalities in South Africa) [23].

Epidemiology of Urban Burn Injuries

Burns from fires kill approximately 300,000 people annually, with an uncertain additional number of people killed by non-fire burns (such as scalds and chemical burns). Almost all burn deaths—over 95 % by WHO estimates—occur in LMICs [163]. Data on the distribution of burn injuries in LMICs are limited, but, in most settings, burn injuries disproportionately affect children and adult women. For adults, the risk of burns largely tracks occupations risks, with women facing higher risks in settings with traditional gender roles (i.e., very high risk in Southeast Asia), though men face heightened occupational risks in some settings [24, 44]. For pre-adolescent children, boys generally have a greater risk than girls [122].

Data comparing burn risks in rural and urban areas are very limited. A study in Uganda found somewhat higher risk of burn-related injury in urban areas [83], similar to evidence from South Africa that burn deaths were common in cities [21], though the latter may have been influenced by incomplete mortuary registry of rural deaths. Research from China [95] and Bangladesh [100] found the opposite pattern, however, with children from rural families being overrepresented among burn victims. However, the Chinese study classified children of migrant workers from rural areas who move to cities as rural, so it may have undercounted burns that resulted from factors in the urban living environment. Similarly, a survey of households in India found a substantially lower risk of death from burns among urban dwellers [67]. Finally, research from Ghana found a lower risk of minor burns in rural areas, but no difference in major burns [103].

In urban areas in LMICs, almost all burns occur within the home. For example, a study in Abidjan, Cote d'Ivoire, found that 95 % of burns requiring hospitalization occurred at home [149]. This is consistent with research from other African settings [9], China [95], Iran [8, 88], and elsewhere [119]. Studies from several urban settings, including in Peru [33] and Bangladesh [30], have identified particular aspects of the home environment as contributing to burn injuries [119]. In particular, overcrowding, poverty, residence in low-income and informal settlements, and physical spaces where cooking implements could not be easily placed out of reach of children played a role in the occurrence of burns.

In most LMIC urban settings, scalds predominate as the cause of burns and are usually due to incidents in the kitchen [64, 119]. For example, about two-thirds of burns in a study in Abidjan were due to scalds [149], as were more than half of pediatric burns in a study in Tehran [8]. However, burns from fires also comprise a substantial portion of burns. For example, a study of pediatric burns in Mombasa found that the majority of burn injuries resulted from flames [9]. In many urban settings, the proportion of burns from fires increases among older children and adults, as do electrical burns (which tend to comprise a small proportion in LMICs) [8, 95]. Additionally, severe and fatal burns are often due to fires instead of scalds, including fires in occupational settings, such as factories [149].

Epidemiology of Urban Fall Injuries

Globally, falls kill more than 400,000 people each year (second only to road crashes as a cause of death from unintentional injuries), with four-fifths of those deaths occurring in LMICs. In both HICs and LMICs, the greatest risk of death from falls is among those over the age of 60, who are often most likely to fall and often suffer the greatest complications [161]. Because of an older age structure, the highest cause-specific mortality rates for falls are in Western Europe [173]. However, within particular age groups, the risk tends to be greatest in LMICs. Though data are uncertain, it appears that the burden of fall injuries is higher in Asia than in Africa, with too little data to make sound comparisons with Latin America [62]. In LMICs, almost all data on falls focus on children, making a detailed understanding of adult falls difficult.

There is very little research on the epidemiology of falls in LMICs, so it comes as no surprise that comparisons of risk in urban and rural areas are limited. One study of childhood injury in Pakistan determined that falls comprise a higher proportion of all injuries in urban areas than rural areas, though this may be in part due to relatively fewer burns in urban Pakistan [39]. Research from Tanzania came to the opposite conclusion, with falls being about 60 % more common in rural areas than in urban areas [110]. Similarly, in India, falls comprised a slightly higher percentage of all injury deaths in urban areas than in rural areas, but the overall risk of dying from a fall was lower in urban areas (as was true for most other causes of injury) [67]. In Hubei Province, China, the mortality rate from falls was found to be indistinguishable between rural and urban areas [94].

In any event, falls remain a substantial cause of injury in LMIC cities. For example, 40 % of childhood injuries in Cape Town were found to be due to falls. Though the prognosis for children in Cape Town whose injuries were due to falls was better than for most other causes of injury, the sheer frequency of fall injuries resulted in falls being the second only to road crashes as a cause of severe injury [55]. A study in a low-income part of Lima, Peru, found that falls caused 56 % of serious pediatric injuries [33]. Similarly, a study in Ilorin, Nigeria, found that falls were responsible for one-third of childhood head injuries requiring hospitalization [118]. In Aleppo, Syria, nonfatal falls were more likely than road crashes or poisonings to result in temporary or long-term disability [101].

Falls most commonly occur in the home, with this being particularly the case in cities [62]. For example, in Tanzania, almost two-thirds of urban fall injuries occurred in or around the home, with a quarter of injuries occurring within dwellings. In rural areas, at-home falls tended to occur outside, and occupational falls (while farming) comprised a much higher percentage of the total in rural areas than in urban ones [110]. The predominance of falls in homes is consistent with data from Cape Town [55] and Sao Paulo [45] as well as national data from India [67] and Pakistan [39]. In some settings, falls in urban areas are more likely to be from greater heights [103].

In general, men tend to have a higher risk of fall injuries and deaths than women, both as adults and children. Research from Dar es Salaam found that men were more likely to be injured in falls than women [110]. There is, however, some data that older women are more likely to fall than men, albeit with less severe injuries [161]. In general, boys appear more likely to be injured in falls than girls in LMICs, though data specific to urban areas is limited [62]. For example, among children in Lima, boys were significantly more likely to be injured in falls than girls were [33].

Falls cause a high proportion of occupational injuries and deaths in LMIC cities. For example, a study in Shanghai, China, found that falls comprised one-third of all occupational deaths, including almost half of construction deaths—with the greatest risk during the period of fastest urban expansion [170]. Urbanization has been associated with increased occupational injury in other settings, such as research in an urbanizing commune in Vietnam that found the risk of occupational injury to be about 20 % higher among those doing nonagricultural work [99]. Research in Brazil found that, while only 14 % of falls were occupational, these falls were more likely to be from greater heights and result in worse injuries [98]. This is consistent with data from China that found urban falls were more likely to be from greater heights when work-related and less likely to be on-level falls [125]. Finally, most research has found that occupational injuries, including falls, are more likely among men than women [27, 98]. However, research from Managua, Nicaragua, suggests that—at least in some settings—this results from under-inclusion of the informal sector and home-based work by women. In Managua, when work conducted in any location was included, falls were approximately equally common among men and women, and falls were by far the most common cause of occupational injury for women [116].

Public Health Approach to Interventions for Injury Prevention

A public health approach to preventing injuries and resultant deaths requires a consideration of many levels of risk factors and potential opportunities for intervention. For example, preventing deaths from structure fires might focus on housing codes, educating occupants about safe kerosene use, providing smoke detectors, equipping emergency responders to safely enter burning buildings, improving burn care, or reducing social stigma for people with serious burns. Each of these interventions focuses on a different target—from at-risk individuals to components of the built environment and public policy arena—and moment in the continuum of events that lead to injury, from primary prevention to emergency treatment and rehabilitation.

The Haddon Matrix

		FACTORS		
PHASE		HUMAN	VEHICLES AND EQUIPMENT	ENVIRONMENT
Pre-crash	Crash prevention	Information Attitudes Impairment Police enforcement	Roadworthiness Lighting Braking Handling Speed management	Road design and road layout Speed limits Pedestrian facilities
Crash	Injury prevention during the crash	Use of restraints Impairment	Occupant restraints Other safety devices Crash-protective design	Crash-protective roadside objects
Post-crash	Life sustaining	First-aid skill Access to medics	Ease of access Fire risk	Rescue facilities Congestion

Fig. 10.2 The Haddon Matrix, applied to road safety. Reprinted from WHO's *World Report on Road Traffic Injury Prevention* [154]

Though there are many ways to conceptualize the interactions between these dimensions, the injury prevention community has been well served by primarily adopting a single approach: the Haddon Matrix. Proposed by William Haddon in 1970, the matrix organizes factors that contribute to injury along axes of time and ecologic proximity to the injured individual. Events with the potential to cause injury are temporally divided into pre-event (event prevention), event (injury prevention for those involved in the event), and post-event (rescue and emergency services) phases. For each phase, risk factors are organized into various categories: human, agent/vehicle, and environmental—both social and physical—factors [50, 136]. (See Fig. 10.2 for an example of the Haddon Matrix applied to road safety.)

Interventions to Reduce Urban Injuries

The remainder of this chapter will examine particular classes of injury, with a focus on risk factors and interventions particular to urbanized areas. Especially in areas of rapid urbanization and informal settlement—where people are often at the greatest risk of injury—individuals may be constrained in their agency to prevent injury. That is, even with information about workplace risks, a resident of Nairobi's enormous Kibera slum may be compelled by economic considerations to continue working a dangerous job with minimal protective equipment. For this reason, priority will often be given to interventions that address distal factors through changes to the risk environment, enforceable policy, or sustainable changes to systems. Because post-event interventions are, to a large extent, common across types of injuries, they will be discussed once at the end of the chapter and not divided between injury types (Table 10.2).

Table 10.2 Summary of preventive interventions by hazard and target

Hazard	Target		
	Injury environment	Person	Vehicle, agent, or equipment
Road crashes	Road network planning	Motorcycle helmet promotion, including laws and enforcement	Periodic motor vehicle safety and inspection standards
	Pedestrian facilities and separation	Bicycle helmet promotion	Safety standards for sale or registration of vehicles
	Traffic calming, including speed bumps	Restraint availability and use	
		Improved licensure standards and enforcement	
		Improved traffic enforcement	
		Behavior change communications	
		Enhanced social pressure	
Burns	Improved used of fire detection and warning equipment, both by law and behavior change communications	Improved cook stove design	Textile flammability standards
	Fire code enforcement and inspection	Shatter-resistant or non-kerosene lanterns	Burn safety education
	Improvement of water temperature regulation		
Falls	Housing and building safety codes	Education and support to elderly persons at risk of falls	
	Improved occupational safety standards and enforcement	Fall risk assessment by health care workers	

Road Crashes

Urbanization and road safety have a complex relationship. When urbanization occurs rapidly, extreme stress is often placed on traffic infrastructures. The sheer number of motor vehicles, pedestrians, and pedal cyclists that occupy overlapping space overwhelms efforts to plan and control their interactions, creating particular dangers for vulnerable road users—those who are not protected by enclosed vehicles. Though data are limited, rapid urbanization likely spills over into rural areas, as the increased amount of traffic moving between urban areas may substantially alter the road crash risks for people in rural areas. At the same time, the relatively privileged economic status of many urban areas may allow governments to better implement interventions to improve the traffic environment and enforce safety regulations. Paradoxically, there is some evidence that heavy traffic congestion found in many urban areas in LICs and MICs sufficiently reduces traffic speeds, making severe injury less likely in the event of a road crash [154].

Road Safety Interventions for Urban Areas

To the extent that there are limited data about the epidemiology of urban road injuries in LMICs, this is doubly true for interventions. Very few studies have been conducted to assess the implementation of road safety interventions outside of high-income settings. However, limited data do exist, as well as experience from other settings, which can be applied to urban LMIC contexts. As noted above, interventions will be divided into environmental, vehicle, and human levels and subdivided by precrash and at-the-moment-of-crash interventions. Postcrash interventions—primarily emergency services—will be addressed later in the chapter, because they tend to be applicable to a wide range of injury causes.

Interventions Targeting the Traffic Environment

Interventions aimed at the traffic environment have a major advantage over other types of road safety interventions: they work at a systems level, acting without the need for conscious compliance or judgment by individuals. Insofar as environmental interventions are durable, they can often be highly cost-effective, because they may be less likely to require ongoing expenditures than other interventions, such as improved traffic law enforcement. While environmental interventions exist that operate at the moment of crash or after, the most practical environmental interventions operate before crashes to mitigate risk.

In sub-Saharan African cities, a particular focus on pedestrian safety is warranted by the high proportion of road deaths that occur among pedestrians, though pedestrian safety is a major concern in all settings. In terms of the traffic environment, there are two classes of interventions that can improve pedestrian safety. The first are interventions to keep cars and pedestrians from occupying the same road space, thereby reducing the risk of collision. The second are interventions to reduce the severity of injury should collisions occur, usually by reducing the speed with which motorized vehicles travel in areas also occupied by pedestrians.

Ideally, such interventions are conducted as urban areas are being planned. For example, freeways, which are designed to facilitate high-speed travel with few interruptions, will often be closed to certain vehicles and pedestrians. Arterial roads will shunt high volumes of traffic within urban areas, while residential roads will have lower speeds and be intended for widespread use by vulnerable road users. Appropriate design of road networks can substantially reduce the risk and severity of crashes [154]. However, retrofitting a planned road network onto the existing and overstretched infrastructure that is characteristic of many LMIC cities—or planning adequately in rapidly urbanizing areas—often proves to be difficult and cost prohibitive.

In busy urban environments, pedestrians often interact with vehicles in unsafe ways [174]. Physical separation of pedestrian walkways from roadways is highly effective at reducing collisions involving pedestrians. While it is probably better to have sidewalks adjacent to streets and at the same level as the roadway than to have no sidewalks at all, the best option is to design pedestrian walkways that are physically separated from the roadway or have a raised curb to prevent motorized vehicles from using them. Many studies in high-income settings have demonstrated the benefit of raised or separated sidewalks [52, 154]. Very little evaluation data exist from LICs, but a modeling study of the traffic environment in Addis Ababa suggests that constructing sidewalks with a raised curb can reduce the risk of crashes involving pedestrians by almost half. While its effect was less, widening and paving sidewalks were also found to reduce pedestrian crashes, probably because both made their use more hospitable and encouraged pedestrians not to walk in the street [18]. The latter interpretation is consistent with data from urban Peru and Mexico, which found that children were more likely to be struck by cars in areas with a high density of street vendors, because they impede sidewalk use and may block visibility [34, 57].

The haphazard growth of many cities makes large-scale reengineering of the pedestrian environment difficult in low-income settings. In such settings, while sidewalks with paved surfaces would be ideal, planners may have to seek other ways to protect pedestrians. In parts of Nairobi, for example, pedestrian walkways are not separated from the roadway, but small poles—separated by a few feet—are inserted into the walkway. In other places, small asphalt bumps are added to the walkway. Both are designed to prevent automobiles or motorbikes from easily using the sidewalk. While these approaches have not been evaluated, both operate by the same mechanism as raised curbs—by providing physical barriers to motorized vehicles using pedestrian spaces—and are likely to be beneficial. Significantly, these improvements can be added to existing walkways without significant construction.

Similarly, pedestrians' risk of crashes can be lessened by physically removing them from the space used by automobiles. In some instances, this takes the form of physical barriers between the walkway and roadway that are difficult for either cars or pedestrians to cross. Pedestrian overpasses are also becoming more common, especially in situations where pedestrians would otherwise be tempted to cross multiple lanes of quickly moving traffic. However, just as studies of neighborhood walkability in HICs suggest a need for improvements to the environment to be coupled with behavior change information [113], an evaluation of a pedestrian overpass in Uganda found low rates of use and no reduction in pedestrian crashes. This underscores the need for changes to the built environment to be based on sound pre-intervention assessments and appropriate communications to the intervention's target population [111], as well as enforcement, when possible. There is some data to support the effectiveness of pedestrian education campaigns to improve children's

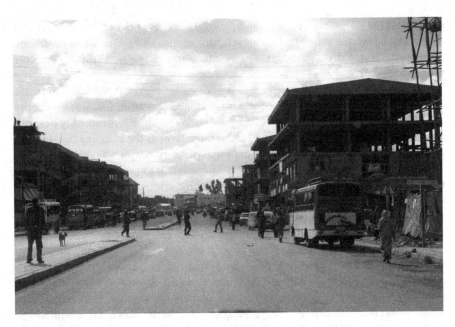

Fig. 10.3 Pedestrians in a suburb of Addis Ababa walking in the street instead of on a raised sidewalk. Environmental interventions often must be coupled with behavior change communications

safety in urban settings in HICs [35], but none in LMICs. Similarly, while formal evaluations do not exist, the greater frequency with which pedestrians in Kigali (than in many other sub-Saharan African cities) use sidewalks when they are present likely reflects more rigorous enforcement (Fig. 10.3).

Speed also plays a critical role in both the likelihood a pedestrian will be involved in a crash and the probability that the crash will be survived. WHO counsels that most pedestrians will survive being hit at 20 miles per hour, but most will die if hit at 30 miles per hour [158], though newer data suggests a higher likelihood of surviving higher-speed crashes [134]. In addition to pedestrian safety, reducing the speed of motor vehicles protects bicyclists, motorcyclists, and vehicle occupants, so it has substantial benefits in urban settings where pedestrians comprise a smaller portion of road crash victims, such as urban areas in Asia and Latin America. Intersection collisions above 30 miles per hour pose a much greater risk of serious injury for vehicle occupants, with tolerable speeds being even lower for vehicles of marginal safety often found in cities in LMICs [158].

Speed bumps are the primary environmental intervention to reduce the speed of traffic. Increasingly common in LMICs, evidence strongly supports their efficacy, especially when drivers along higher-speed routes are nearing congested pedestrian areas or intersections. Research in Ghana has found that speed bumps and rumble strips substantially reduces vehicle speed and sharply reduces the risk of crashes, including a reduction in pedestrian injuries by more than half [4, 5]. Because a relatively small percentage of intersections are involved in a fairly high percentage of collision deaths, it is likely that targeted placement of speed bumps would be highly effective at both protecting pedestrians and drivers. Similarly, placing speed bumps on the margins of urban areas, where high-speed traffic meets lower-speed city traffic, has been shown to substantially reduce crashes [4]. Furthermore, because speed bumps are inexpensive and durable, targeting the sites with greatest risk is cost-effective, with estimates of less than $100 per life saved in sub-Saharan Africa, South Asia, and Latin America and less than $150 in other LMICs [19].

Other approaches to area-wide traffic calming, such as the utilization of one-way streets, using roundabouts in place of intersections, and other changes to the road environment, have also been found to be beneficial in cities in HICs. While data suggest little or no impact of many traffic calming interventions on the number of crashes, there is convincing evidence that they can reduce injuries by reducing the speed at which crashes occur [22]. Research is lacking from LMICs, but it is reasonable to believe that the effect in LMICs would be similar to in HICs. Additionally, some approaches, such as the installation of roundabouts, which can be placed at high-risk intersections, could be feasibly retrofitted into existing urban road networks. Roundabouts have shown to reduce injury-causing crashes by up to 75 % [130].

Interventions Targeting Person-Level Factors

Many interventions oriented toward drivers, motor vehicle passengers, motorcyclists, bicyclists, and pedestrians can greatly reduce the risk and severity of road crashes in urban settings. Though person-level interventions often lack the durability of many environmental interventions, they frequently benefit from being relatively low-cost and, in particular, not requiring the up-front capital of many construction projects. Further, to the extent that many person-level interventions provide individuals with knowledge or commodities they would not otherwise have, these interventions give people more control over their own safety. Providing individuals with greater agency over their own health and safety is both productive and ethically important [85].

Moment of Crash Interventions

Many person-level interventions to improve urban road safety operate at the moment of crash to reduce the severity of injury and augment prevention efforts designed to prevent crashes. For motorcyclists—who are ubiquitous in cities across LMICs, particularly in many Asian cities—correct use of a high-quality helmet is the most important intervention. In a crash, motorcycle helmets reduce the risk of death by more than 40 % and the risk of head injury by about two-thirds [93].

Achieving high rates of motorcycle helmet usage is possible. For example, 95 % of motorcyclists in urban parts of Guangdong Province, China, were observed to correctly wear helmets [169]. However, usage rates tend to be quite low in most urban settings in LMICs. For example, studies in urban settings in Ghana found that only 34 % of drivers and 2 % of pillion passengers were helmeted [1]. Studies in other urban settings have found similar results: 56 % use in Karachi, Pakistan [82]; 65 %–82 % in Phnom Penh, Cambodia, depending on the time of day [13]; 30 % in urban and periurban Hai Duong province, Vietnam [61]; 40 % in Mar del Plata, Argentina [89]; and 55 % correct usage (though 89 % total usage) in Yogyakarta, Indonesia [28]. Studies of hospitalized crash victims in urban India [43] and Nigeria [117] found very low rates of helmet use, though it is likely that hospitalized riders wear helmets less often than the general public—with helmet-preventable injuries being one reason they end up in the hospital. Even in places where helmets are common, frequent use of substandard helmets has been recorded, such as the 55 % of helmeted delivery drivers in urban areas of Malaysia observed wearing substandard helmets [87]. Research from high-income settings has found that motorcyclists using nonstandard helmets are more likely to suffer head injury in a crash than those wearing standard helmets and also at rates higher than those of motorcyclists wearing no helmets (though the latter conclusion must be interpreted with caution)[123].

Laws mandating motorcycle helmet use are highly effective and strongly supported by the WHO. Evidence suggests that helmet laws should form the basis of helmet promotion programs and be reinforced by other behavior change modalities [155]. Data are limited from sub-Saharan Africa, but studies in Asia have found substantial benefits from helmet laws. For example, Vietnam's law was associated with 16 % less head injuries and 18 % less road crash deaths in a hospital-based study [120]. Other studies found similar results, including a 14 % reduction in deaths among motorcycle riders in Taiwan [145]. In Vietnam, helmet use was found to be much more common on streets where it was compulsory than on streets where it was not [61], and in urban Indonesia, motorcyclists frequently reported being more likely to wear helmets when they thought enforcement of the law was likely [28]—both of which support a causal link between helmet laws and reduced motorcyclist deaths; this causal association is well-established in high-income settings [59].

Motorcycle helmet laws are not self-implementing. While laws may occasionally impact usage purely through their own normative force, increasing urban helmet use rates in LMICs requires that laws be clear and comprehensive in scope, enforced well, and coupled with behavior change communications. In general, helmet laws are less effective when they exempt certain locations, such as particular roads in Vietnam [61], or classes of riders, such as the ambiguity over whether children had to wear helmets (also in Vietnam) [126]. They should also be specific about exactly what types of helmet meet the regulatory standard and that the helmet must be worn—not merely carried—to avoid enforcement [28]. Similarly, nonenforcement leads to suboptimal impact, as has been seen in urban settings in Nigeria [140]. Modeling studies suggest that only a small number of motorcyclists need to be cited in order to drive higher rates of helmet use, because people violating the law have a low probability of evading detection—but riders do have to perceive a chance of being cited [19]. Finally, helmet laws will work best when they are coupled with information about the law and its requirements as well as the benefits of helmet use; and when helmet promotion is tied to local data about barriers and facilitators of use [13, 155].

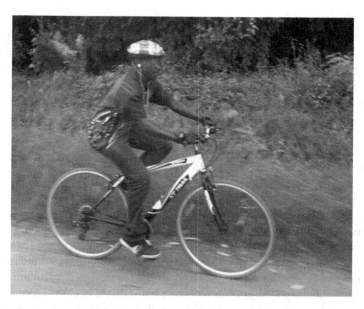

Fig. 10.4 A man wearing a bicycle helmet in a suburb of Nairobi. Bicycle helmet use is highly effective against head injuries but exceedingly rare in most LMIC cities

As with motorcyclists, the most important intervention for protecting bicyclists in crashes is helmet use. Bicycle helmets are highly effective at preventing deaths and head injuries—even when cyclists are hit by cars [143], which is a major cause of urban cyclist death—and helmet laws are effective at increasing usage, at least in the high-income settings where legislative approaches have been evaluated [96]. The few existing studies on bicycle helmet use rates in urban LMIC settings suggest almost complete nonuse, including in cities in China [91, 172], Singapore [53], Malawi [86], and Mexico [105] (Fig. 10.4).

In high-income settings, legal mandates are highly effective at increasing helmet usage [74, 96]. No data exist on bicycle helmet laws in LMICs, but they are likely to be as effective as motorcycle helmet laws in these settings, because they operate through the same likely mechanisms (penalties to deter nonuse, generating a norm of use, and providing an opening for education and behavior change). Further, as with motorcycle helmet laws, identifying violators is relatively easy and cheap, making enforcement likely [19]. Cost-effectiveness modeling suggests that bicycle helmet legislation is the single most cost-effective intervention to prevent road deaths in sub-Saharan Africa, even under a wide range of assumptions about its effectiveness. Also, it has been found to be cost-effective, as part of combination approaches in Asia [26].

In the same vein as interventions to increase helmet use, interventions to increase the use of seat belts and other restraints would provide substantially improved protection at the point of crash—assuming that vehicles have seat belts in the first place, which is a frequent problem in many LMICs (though data suggest that installation of seat belts in cars that lack them would be cost-effective) [153]. Seat belt and child restraint laws have been effective at reducing injuries and fatalities in HICs [132]. Limited data suggest similar effects in cities in LMICs [17, 114], but that motorists must perceive a likelihood of enforcement in order for benefits to be obtained [2]. Car seat used by small children—and legislation to require it—is also highly effective in HICs. In LMICs, it is often limited by the availability of low-cost car seats, but WHO recently announced that a prototype optimized for use in LMICs is close to entering the market [162].

Precrash Interventions

A number of other person-level interventions could reduce the frequency or severity of crashes in urban areas and focus on the precrash period. Most of these aim to improve the knowledge, skill, or behavior of road users. While data tend to be very scarce from LMICs, all are routine and well-validated in high-income settings.

Safe use of roadways begins with an understanding about likely hazards and how to prevent and respond to them. Such knowledge (as well as a minimum level of skill) is generally assessed prior to receiving one's driver license. Though assessment of licensure standards is very difficult, their efficacy is logical and widely incorporated in both HICs and LMICs. For example, China requires passage of a rather detailed (and often somewhat amusing—at least for non-test takers) computerized test, much of which focuses on the mix of vehicles and pedestrians common to rapidly urbanizing areas [131].

In many HICs, school-based driver education is a rite of passage; however, data suggest that it does not reduce the frequency of crashes and, by facilitating younger licensure, may increase risks [65, 148]. Similarly, data do not support the efficacy of post-licensure or remedial education [81]. Rather, the weight of the evidence suggests that licensure regimes should maximize driving experience under controlled circumstances, not merely education [166]. This is the theory underlying graduated driver license programs in high-income settings, which restrict new drivers from driving at night, with passengers, and/or without supervision, and which consistently have been found to reduce crashes and fatalities among youth [40, 137].

Given the extremely hectic driving environment in many urban areas in LMICs, as countries strengthen driving regulations, strengthening licensure requirements with a preference for graduated or other experience-based requirements would likely be beneficial. In one study in urban Nigeria, for example, a high proportion of motorcycle drivers lacked a license, and the majority of licensed drivers had not passed a road test [66]. This approach, which has been adopted in countries such as Zambia—which requires 3 months of supervised driving prior to passing a driving test—turns on the ability to enforce the graduated license's conditions. This, however, requires officials to be able to identify drivers who are not meeting the conditions of their licenses and to possess adequate resources and will to engage in enforcement. The Zambian approach of clearly marking vehicles driven by a supervised driver with special plates is likely to partially achieve the first initiative, by at least making it clear that drivers are violating their conditions when driving alone [129].

Road users' behavior can also be influenced by the vigor with which officials enforce enacted safety regulations. Almost all jurisdictions regulate drivers' speed and alcohol consumption, as well as recklessness of all classes of road users. Traditionally, however, most LMICs have had substantial enforcement gaps, leading to low compliance with speed limits, traffic controls, and intoxicated driving laws. Additionally, many jurisdictions' laws are insufficient for urban safety. For example, several Middle Eastern countries have urban speed limits in excess of 60 miles per hour, which is double what WHO recommends [160]. To optimally deter unsafe driving, the law must prohibit unsafe conduct, motorists must believe they are likely to be penalized if they violate the law, and penalties must be sufficiently large to change behavior [156].

In high-income settings, speed and red-light cameras have become commonplace, and both have been found to be effective at reducing crashes [3, 167]. Data from LMICs are limited, but one study in Johannesburg found that speed enforcement cameras reduced crashes and average driving speed [70]. While there are concerns about the cost of automated enforcement, cost-effectiveness modeling suggests that using cameras to enforce speed limits (at least when targeted to high-risk locations) is highly cost-effective in Africa and Asia whether used alone or in combination with other interventions [26], based on WHO cost-effectiveness thresholds [165]. Additionally, in settings where citizens are wary of interactions with police, enforcement cameras may have greater legitimacy, due to their ability to objectively verify infractions.

Alternatively (or, even when cameras are deployed, in addition), enforcement can be conducted by traditional police patrol. While either cameras or physical police presence can be very effective at reducing infractions at defined, high-risk locations, traditional enforcement can convince road users they may be cited at any location, which may have effects throughout cities [158]. Optimally, then, police will be trained to routinely cite drivers observed to violate traffic laws and to have screening checkpoints for both alcohol and speed. Both routine and checkpoint-based enforcement increase the likelihood of detecting violators, and the latter may serve to underscore that traffic safety laws are vigorously enforced, which facilitates behavior change [156]. In one study in Uganda, increased police presence reduced crash deaths by about one-sixth and was highly cost-effective [20].

Enforcement improves road safety by increasing the costs of safety violations. Of course, there are inherent costs to unsafe road use in the form of injuries, and many behavior change approaches focus on awareness of, and reductions in, risks the road user can influence. There is a robust literature on health promotion strategies for road safety behavior change, including a number of approaches that capitalize on the availability of signage or other media in the urban driving environment [7, 36, 90, 108, 142]. In general, as is usually the case, the most successful approaches are layered and incorporate behavior change communications along programs that make compliance easier (such as subsidized helmet programs for helmet use) and noncompliance more costly (such as enforcement) [152].

Most efforts to change the safety behavior of road users focus directly on motor vehicle operators or pedestrians themselves. Emerging research, however, suggests that in settings where passengers comprise a high proportion of crash victims, prompting passengers to encourage drivers' safe practices may be fruitful. For example, in Kenya, where a high percentage of traffic deaths are among passengers in matatus (minibuses), posting simple signs in the matatu encouraging passengers to speak up if conditions are unsafe can reduce the risk of crashes by half. Simple and cost-effective, such approaches bear serious consideration, both for urban minibuses and for long-haul minibuses, which are commonly used by people traveling between cities or cities and rural areas [49].

Interventions Targeting Vehicle-Level Factors

The last set of interventions to prevent road crash injuries in urban areas deal with vehicles themselves. In most LMICs, a high percentage of motor vehicles are relatively old, poorly maintained, and lack safety features common in many higher-income areas. These factors contribute to the likelihood of crashes and exacerbate injuries when crashes happen. For example, a study of vehicles in Pretoria, South Africa, found that almost three-quarters had been driven more than 100,000 km, and 40 % had at least one significant defect that posed a safety hazard. The rate of defects was even higher for minibus taxis, the majority of which were found to have unsafe tires. Assessments of crashes in LMICs have found between 2 % and 16 % of road crashes to be attributable to mechanical defects [147].

Beyond defective vehicles, the older fleets of vehicles often found in LMICs also tend to be inherently less safe: less likely to have adequate protective space or crumple zones to protect occupants, less likely to be designed with faces that are protective of pedestrians, and less likely to have working seat belts and airbags. In many cities in LMICs, taxi services are frequently provided by locally manufactured scooter taxis, which provide minimal protection in the event of a crash [109, 154].

In HICs, there are three major strategies to ensure the roadworthiness of vehicles: manufacturing standards for vehicles sold in the country, safety inspections when vehicles are registered, and routine traffic citations for unsafe vehicles. While data are limited about the effect of inspections on crash risk [154], their benefits are plausible, based on the assumption that they remove some high-risk vehicles from the streets and encourage maintenance and repair of other vehicles. In particular, targeting inspections and citations to commercial vehicles may be useful, because research suggests that mechanical defects are common [147] and also because operators (or their insurers) may have greater ability and more incentives to ensure safety.

Creating and enforcing standards for what vehicles can be sold has been clearly shown to work in high-income settings. For example, airbag standards in the United States have substantially reduced deaths from crashes [42, 72]. The same is true for requiring vehicles to include seat belts [48]. Most countries have vehicle safety inspection standards, such as Kenya's standards for pre-export inspection of vehicles to be sold in Kenya [69] and inspections prior to registration [80]. There is a broad range of options for safety standards, ranging from minimal (the vehicle must have minimum safety features and be in working order) to requiring advanced features (such as side airbags and pedestrian-protecting designs) that are increasingly common in HICs [154]. No data exist on the effectiveness of vehicle safety standards in LMICs, but it is likely that their effectiveness is a function of two factors: the contents of the standards and their likelihood of enforcement. Both involve political and economic tradeoffs for authorities, which can complicate stringent safety regulation.

Burns

The relationship between urbanization and burns is complex and, even more than is the case for road crashes, high-quality data on this relationship is scarce. Greater wealth in urban areas often allows people to shift away from using open fires and charcoal stoves and the significant risk that comes from them. On the other hand, the poor housing conditions and overcrowded circumstances common for the urban poor may make burns—especially scalds—more common. In all settings, indoor fires become much more common when poverty requires fuel oils or flames to be used for heating and light—as is often the case for both the rural and urban poor [9, 119].

Interventions to Combat Urban Burns

The fact that burn injuries have become far less common in HICs gives reason for optimism in LMICs. Unfortunately, as the WHO noted in its recent burn prevention and care plan, few of the interventions that have been successful in HICs have been adopted in LMICs, and many face substantial barriers to implementation. Of these approaches, some may be effective in MICs, but few are available to the urban poor in LICs [159]. To a great extent, burns are injuries of poverty—even more so than road crashes, which tend to increase as economic development increases the availability of motor vehicles before safety regulation can catch up [121]. As such, the greatest success against burns will likely come as LMICs accelerate economic and human development, enabling people to inhabit safer and less crowded homes, cook and heat with safer appliances, and be protected by rigorous and well-enforced building codes. In the meantime, though, a number of strategies exist to reduce urban burn injuries in LMICs, albeit with generally weak evidence bases.

Interventions Targeting the Injury Environment

As with road crashes, to the extent possible, environmental interventions are often favored, because they can serve to reduce the risk of injury without the active participation of people at risk. It is no surprise, therefore, that most of the mainstays of burn prevention in HICs focus on environmental factors: the presence of smoke detectors and alarms and sprinklers; building codes; escape routes that are clearly marked, navigable, and accessible to persons with disabilities; and temperature regulators on hot water heaters. Some of these are applicable in LMICs—particularly MICs—but some are unlikely to bring down the rate of burn injuries substantially among those at greatest risk. For example, temperature regulators on hot water heaters presuppose that one's water is warmed by a hot water heater in the first place—an uncommon occurrence in most of sub-Saharan Africa.

Though fires do not cause the majority of burn injuries in low- and middle-income cities, they often cause severe injury or death. In the United States and other HICs, smoke detectors and alarms play a key role in fire prevention—allowing fires to be detected early and residents to escape safely from a burning building. In HICs, they are both highly effective as an injury prevention tool and produce a net savings of costs [163]. In LMICs, however, their use is rare outside of commercial buildings or other settings where inspection and enforcement are likely—especially among those who are not relatively affluent. For example, two studies in Monterrey, Mexico, assessed smoke detector use. Even among the most affluent households, smoke detector use was rare; in households of lower socioeconomic status, it was essentially nonexistent [105]. Rates of usage did not increase after an educational intervention, likely because of the scarce availability and perceived cost of smoke detectors in the community [107].

These findings are consistent with data from HICs that often find that multiple barriers to using alarms sometimes prevent generally favorable perceptions about their efficacy from being translated into long-term, consistent usage. Successful interventions overcome barriers of knowledge, availability, affordability, and motivation to maintain detectors in working order, and interventions targeted only to a single barrier (such as community giveaway programs) often do not have lasting effect [31, 133, 135]. At the same time, when the right conditions are in place, health promotion campaigns to promote smoke detector use can be effective [75]. Especially in middle-income settings, smoke detector programs should be promoted more aggressively and incorporate a comprehensive approach that focuses on education and behavior change, provision of smoke detectors, and ongoing use and maintenance (such as replacement batteries). Because the evidence base on successful programs is nonexistent for LMIC cities, implementation research is badly needed to guide successful programs [163]. In commercial settings, including apartment complexes, use of smoke detectors should be mandated by law and supported by inspections and fines.

A number of other changes to the environment would reduce the risk of burns from fires. For example, public spaces in HICs are universally required to have and mark exit routes, keep them clear of obstructions, and comply with building codes and other regulations to reduce the risk of fire or slow its spread to enable escape. Fire safety regulations have been a mainstay of public health law for several hundred years, and there is no debate over their value. Most LMICs have adopted similar standards, either as guidance [77] or binding regulations [78], but enforcement is variable. To date, no research assesses strategies for improving fire safety compliance in LMICs. However, as with other safety regulation, increasing the chance of detecting violators (as through routine fire safety inspections) and levying penalties to incentivize compliance are likely to succeed.

To prevent scalds, the primary approach used in HICs is limiting the maximum temperature that can be produced by hot water heaters. This approach has been highly successful in HICs, and it would be likely to be similarly effective in LMICs—at least where the primary source of hot water is a hot water heater. Though education programs have been successful in HICs, an educational intervention to encourage parents to check their home water temperature was not successful in Monterrey, Mexico; rates were very low both before and after the intervention [105, 107]. Data from HICs suggest that in many settings, educational programs alone are insufficient and will be most effective when coupled with laws that regulate the maximum water temperature. There is also some evidence that education about the extra energy costs incurred by overheating water may be effective [163].

Unfortunately, while these environmental approaches may bear dividends in cities in MICs and among more affluent residents in LICs—which would certainly be something to celebrate—they will not, in the short term, address the primary causes of injuries and deaths from burns in urban areas in LICs. Burn deaths in LICs often result from low-quality housing, overcrowding, and minimal separation between areas used for cooking and other areas of the home [163]. There is some evidence that basic modifications to cooking spaces and other aspects of the home environment, such as raising cooking surfaces and guarding fires, may be beneficial [119], but very little research either to confirm the efficacy of particular intervention approaches or implementation research to maximize the effectiveness of interventions.

Interventions Targeting Agents of Burn Injuries

The most interesting innovations to reduce the risk of burns in LMICs involve attempts to make the generation of household light and heat safer. As noted previously, a high percentage of scalds in urban areas—particularly in impoverished neighborhoods or informal settlements—results from liquids being heated at ground level on traditional stoves and tipped over. Similarly, many serious fires result from unstable or breakable kerosene lanterns and stoves being upset, and many serious flame burns result from open fires being used to cook or heat dwellings. Designing safer means of cooking food, heating homes, and generating light that are affordable for the urban poor would produce substantial safety benefits.

In recent years, a number of safer heat sources have been developed. Though data are limited, research suggests that substituting a simple wood stove for an open fire for home cooking will reduce the risk of serious childhood burns (as well as improve pulmonary health). One study in Guatemala did not find that the stoves were associated with a reduction in the total number of childhood burns, but it did find that the most serious—those that resulted from falling into fires—declined. Of importance, though, the researchers found that improvements from merely changing stove designs were suboptimal because households continued to use open fires for other purposes, suggesting, as always, that innovative technologies need to be coupled with education and behavior change initiatives [163].

Similarly, simple design modifications to kerosene lanterns can make them much safer. The most dangerous lanterns are homemade, unstable, and fragile—as when households repurpose burned-out light bulbs as lanterns. In some settings, local production of simple and cheap lanterns that are made of thick, shatter-resistant glass and with spill-preventing lids is being implemented. While these lanterns have not been formally evaluated, their design should be much safer than those currently used in many settings. Their simple production makes them amenable to micro-finance or other initiatives to stimulate decentralized production and increase availability [163].

Both safer cooking implements and safer lights are usually promoted as innovations for rural areas. However, in many LMICs, they would also find frequent use in urban areas, particularly in informal settlements or other very poor settings where electricity and safer, in-home cooking gas are unavailable or too expensive to be used regularly. Additionally, in some cities, the supply of electricity and cooking gas is irregular or subject to large price fluctuations [15], resulting in households using less safe methods as a backup—which puts urban households at unnecessary risk.

Interventions Targeted at Person-Level Factors

In some LMICs, individuals' burn risk is increased by the clothes that they wear. In particular, long, flowing clothes made from flammable materials pose a significant danger when they come into contact with open heat sources. Burns that result from clothing fires pose a very high risk of death or serious injury [73]—more so than burns from other causes because they tend to be more severe and cover a greater portion of the body. In some settings, serious childhood burns due to clothes constructed of man-made fibers melting are also a problem [30]. Similarly, flammable bedding can create a high risk of serious injury, particularly in settings where people are crowded closely to heat sources when they sleep, as is often the case in informal urban settlements [119].

In high-income settings, much of this risk has been removed by legal requirements governing the flammability of clothes, mattresses, and other materials. In LMICs, some countries have imposed similar standards, but no data exist yet about their effectiveness. The WHO endorses both regulatory and social marketing approaches to improving the safety of clothing and household materials [163]. The effectiveness of this approach will likely depend on the extent to which materials are produced in the formal sector (vs. at home) and, thus, amenable to regulation, the availability of safer alternatives, and the extent to which consumers can be persuaded to purchase safer materials.

Additionally, all burn interventions should be accompanied by health promotion approaches to increase knowledge and safer practices among those at risk. For example, experts have recommended targeting burn safety education to urban mothers, who often bear primary responsibility for managing children and the kitchens in which many burns occur [30]. Several studies have identified low maternal education as a key risk factor for childhood burns [33, 44], underscoring both the importance mothers play in household injury prevention and the complex social etiology of burns and other injuries. Though no data exist from LMICs, research in HICs has found parental education programs to be effective at reducing burn injuries [76].

Falls

Falls are a leading cause of injury, particularly for the very young and the elderly. Nonetheless, in LMICs, very little data exist about the frequency of falls, risk factors, or approaches to prevent them. Nonetheless, aspects of urbanization can make falls more likely, or more likely to have severe consequences if they occur. Because urban dwellers are more likely to live in vertical spaces—multistory dwellings and apartment buildings—they may be more likely to encounter falls from greater heights. Similarly, many jobs that are common in rapidly growing urban areas, such as construction, pose a heightened risk of falls. These risks, as is all too common in both HICs and LMICs, are likely to land heaviest on people who live in poverty.

Interventions to Combat Urban Falls

Good data on interventions to reduce the frequency and severity of fall injuries in urban LMIC settings are very limited. Nonetheless, interventions will target three major classes of falls: falls at home, particularly for children; falls at work; and falls among the elderly. More than for other causes of injury, however, interventions are tentative and based only on the general experience of other settings.

Interventions Targeting the Injury Environment

In HICs, falls in the home are reduced by common household features, such as slip-resistant flooring materials, steps with surfaces and grades that are designed to reduce fall risk, and handrails and railings where falls are likely. Similar approaches in LMIC homes would be likely to be effective and currently are often absent—particularly in lower-income housing [33]. The physical environment can be made more safe through behavior change interventions that work to get residents or outside inspectors to inspect and improve their premises in many cases, though this may not be feasible when environmental risks (such as unsafe stairs) are used by multiple housing units [157]. In HICs, this approach has been demonstrated to work [47].

Alternatively, regulatory approaches are used in many countries to improve the safety of the physical environment in both residences and workplaces. In most HICs, owners of apartment buildings have a legal duty to ensure the safety of the premises, including by ensuring safe stairwells, balconies, windows, and other fall risks. Similarly, employers generally have the legal responsibility to ensure safe workplaces, and workplace safety laws are generally credited with substantially reducing occupational injures [139]. Data evaluating these approaches in LMICs do not exist, but countries are increasingly enacting comprehensive safety regulation—including protection against falls. Kenya, for example, recently passed a detailed Occupational Safety and Health Act that, if rigorously enforced, will substantially reduce the risk of injuries and deaths from falls [79]. Similarly, Singapore has enhanced workplace standards and penalties for unsafe conditions for maids after several—most of whom were immigrants from less developed countries—died in falls while washing windows [10].

Interventions Targeted at Person-Level Factors

Most evidence-based approaches to fall reduction that target person-level factors are aimed at elderly persons or the parents of children, and data are absent from LMICs. Nonetheless, research from HICs has consistently found that such approaches can be effective. For example, educational interventions for parents—alone or paired with home visits and support—have been found to reduce the risk of childhood injuries, including fall risks [76]. Data are less supportive of educational interventions alone to reduce injuries among elderly persons [102].

However, a number of other approaches have been shown to substantially reduce the risk of falls among the elderly. In HICs, multifactorial assessment of fall risk accompanied by home-based support is likely to reduce injuries [47, 102]. In HICs, such assessments are often conducted by a combination of clinical providers and home nurses or home health aides; in LMICs, it is possible that community health workers could play a similar role, but such an approach has not been evaluated. Strength training and other exercise interventions have also been shown to be effective in HICs, and at least some studies suggest that vitamin D supplementation and assessment (and withdrawal if necessary) of medications posing fall risks may be beneficial, though data are particularly mixed for the last intervention [47, 102]. None of these interventions, however, have been evaluated in LMICs.

Minimizing the Effect of Injuries After They Happen: Emergency Services

Up to this point, the interventions discussed to address urban injuries have focused on prevention, which, in LMICs, is often a primary focus because of its relative cheapness. However, any effort to reduce the burden of injuries must also involve systems of care to urgently treat injuries. When it comes to treatment, urban residents are often better off than rural residents, because in LMICs most health facilities that can treat significant trauma are located in cities. Nonetheless, major gaps continue to exist in many settings, including an insufficient number of trained health professionals, very limited prehospital care and transport, issues of quality, and difficulty summoning emergency services (especially for the most impoverished). Fortunately, innovations from other areas of global health—especially maternal mortality initiatives—provide templates for improving emergency services.

Prehospital Care and Issues

In many LMICs, emergency services are rarely used. For example, data from Ghana found that 40 % of people injured in urban areas did not receive medical care. While this was substantially better than people injured in rural areas (three-quarters of whom did not receive treatment), it is a rate that is far too high and predisposes people to preventable, long-term disabilities and prolonged recoveries. Similarly, for road crash victims in Kenya, fewer than 10 % were transported by emergency responders [154].

There are, of course, many reasons for low utilization of emergency services, and these issues are not specific to injuries. For example, research on causes of maternal death suggests that many factors—including limited transportation options, difficulty summoning care, cost barriers to services or transportation, poor perceptions of care, and a low availability of services [16]—all impede use of emergency services.

In the immediate aftermath of an incident causing serious injury, two things are critical: the provision of immediate first aid and procuring transport to a facility that can provide more in-depth emergency care. In HICs, the latter is generally provided by the injured person or a bystander phoning for an ambulance, generally on a universal phone number (such as 911 in the United States or 112 in the European Union). WHO strongly recommends adopting a national emergency phone number. However, many countries—particularly LMICs—have not adopted this guidance or have different numbers for different regions of the country, which can impede dialing the correct number [160]. This is a particularly important missed opportunity in urban areas because, even in countries where phone ownership is relatively low, use of mobile phones by urban populations tends to be very high. For example, 91 % of urban households in Angola possess a mobile phone [29]; in Liberia and Malawi, urban mobile phone ownership rates are 78 % and 73 %, respectively [92, 97].

Of course, phoning for paramedics only works in settings where a formal first responder system exists. Prehospital care tends to be better in urban areas than in rural areas [115]. However, in many low (and sometimes also middle-income) countries, ambulance services are limited and, when they exist, are often for transport only and do not have personnel trained to provide emergency care [84]. In such settings, people are often transported to medical facilities by other types of vehicles. For example, research in Ghana found that more than half of injured persons in an urban area were transported by taxi, and more than two-thirds by some sort of commercial vehicle. To take advantage of this, researchers trained commercial drivers on basic first aid. Though data were not collected on injury outcomes, participants, more than half of whom subsequently provided emergency first aid, retained skills and were more likely to provide emergency care after being trained [106]. In particular, trained drivers were able to maintain an open airway and control bleeding better than untrained drivers [144]. Similarly, research in Kampala, Uganda, found that providing training and a first aid kit to police, taxi drivers, and community leaders resulted in significantly more provision of emergency services, and participants retained knowledge and skills for at least 6 months. Importantly, the Kampala program was found to be cost-effective for low-income settings, with the estimated cost per life-year saved being $27 [68].

Though it has not been broadly adapted to other emergencies, commercial drivers have also been used to reduce maternal mortality. Several countries either reimburse commercial drivers for costs incurred by transporting women to medical facilities [37, 138] during obstetric emergencies or incentivize drivers to do so [46]. While these interventions have primarily been used in rural areas, they may have applicability in urban areas also, particularly among residents of informal settlements or others in poverty for whom cost may be a barrier to promptly seeking care. While data are limited, the evidence that does exist suggests that such programs are both effective and relatively inexpensive [138].

Hospital and Rehabilitative Care

Hospital-based emergency care tends to be much better in urban settings than in rural settings, as there is usually a greater availability of higher-level hospitals with more advanced clinicians and better facilities. For example, blood transfusions are often much more readily available in urban settings [128]. However, major gaps continue to exist, particularly for burns, with many secondary hospitals that can address other injuries having relatively limited capacities to treat burns. For example, specialized burn surgeons are extremely rare in LMICs [11].

While substantial barriers exist to increasing the quantity of emergency care, recent innovations in other areas of emergency services may be applicable for injury treatment. Checklists have emerged as a key tool for improving the quality of care, with the highly publicized success of WHO's Surgical Safety Checklist [51] and preliminary results from its Safe Childbirth Checklist [141] catalyzing their use for other purposes. WHO is currently developing a trauma care checklist which, when available, is likely to produce similar benefits for emergency services.

Rehabilitative services are highly neglected in LMICs, where the focus of medical care is frequently triaged in favor of lifesaving care. Unfortunately, this results in many people with addressable disabilities not receiving services. However, a number of interesting technologies have recently been developed to mitigate this problem. For example, the Jaipur Foot, a prosthetic designed for use in LMICs, has seen rapid increases in use and has returned mobility to many people with disabilities, though access to prosthetics remains limited in many settings [60]. Similar advances have been made in low-cost wheelchair availability for use in sub-Saharan Africa and other LMIC settings [151], though the accessibility of public spaces in many urban settings in LMICs remains limited [14, 146].

Conclusion

Urbanization impacts unintentional injury in complicated ways—sometimes increasing, sometimes decreasing, and sometimes merely changing risks. HICs have been very successful at mitigating these risks, especially in cities, where access to emergency services often limits the effect of injuries and prevent deaths and lasting disabilities. In LMICs, progress has been much slower. However, as this chapter details, there are ample opportunities for cities and their residents and health systems to innovate to prevent and ameliorate injury. These innovations, while occasionally high-tech, will generally focus on improvements to the physical, social, and policy environment using approaches that are well established in HICs but require adaptation to LMICs. In doing so, cities can create space for urban dwellers to live safer lives, i.e., less at risk of premature death or avoidable disability.

References

1. Ackaah W, Afukaar FK. Prevalence of helmet use among motorcycle users in Tamale Metropolis, Ghana: an observational study. Traffic Inj Prev. 2011;11:522–5.
2. Aekplakorn W, et al. Compliance with the law on car seat-belt use in four cities of Thailand. J Med Assoc Thai. 2000;83:333–41.
3. Aeron-Thomas AS, Hess S. Red-light cameras for the prevention of road traffic crashes. Cochrane Database Syst Rev 2005;(2):CD003862.
4. Afukaar FK. Speed control in developing countries: issues, challenges, and opportunities in reducing road traffic injuries. Inj Control Saf Promot. 2003;10:77–81.
5. Afukaar FK, Damesere-Derry J. Evaluation of speed humps on pedestrian injuries in Ghana. Inj Prev. 2009;16:A205–6.

6. Afukaar FK, Antwi P, Ofosu-Amaah S. Pattern of road traffic injuries in Ghana: implications for control. Inj Control Saf Promot. 2003;10:69–76.
7. Aigle J, Rossiter JR. Fear patterns: a new approach to designing road safety advertisements. J Prev Interv Community. 2010;38:264–79.
8. Alaghehbandan R, Rossignol AM, Lari AR. Pediatric burn injuries in Tehran Iran. Burns. 2001;27:115–8.
9. Albertyn R, Bickler SW, Rode H. Paediatric burn injuries in sub Saharan Africa—an overview. Burns. 2006;32:605–12.
10. Alpert E. Singapore restricts window washing after maids plunge to deaths. *Los Angeles Times*. 2012.
11. Atiyeh B, Masellis A, Conte C. Optimizing burn treatment in developing low- and middle-income countries with limited health care resources. Ann Burns Fire Disasters. 2009;22:121–5.
12. Bachani AM, et al. Road traffic injuries in Kenya: the health burden and risk factors in two districts. Traffic Inj Prev. 2012;12:24–30.
13. Bachani AM, et al. Helmet use among motorcyclists in Cambodia: a survey of use, knowledge, attitudes, and procedures. Traffic Inj Prev. 2012;13:1–6.
14. Banda-Chalwe M, Nitz JC, de Jonge D. Participation-based environment accessibility tool (P-BEAAT) in the Zambian context. Disabil Rehabil. 2012;34:1232–43.
15. Barasa L, Konuche J. Kenya: acute gas crisis hits towns. Daily Nation (Nairobi). 2007
16. Barnes-Josiah D, Myntti C, Augustin A. The three delays model as a framework for examining maternal mortality in Haiti. Soc Sci Med. 1998;46:981–93.
17. Benjamin AL. The use of seatbelts in Port Moresby 12 years after the seatbelt legislation in Papua New Guinea. P N G Med J. 2007;50:152–6.
18. Berhanu G. Models relating traffic safety with road environment and traffic flows on arterial roads in Addis Ababa. Accid Anal Prev. 2004;36:697–704.
19. Bishai DM, Hyder AA. Modeling the cost effectiveness of injury interventions in lower and middle income countries: opportunities and challenges. Cost Eff Resour Alloc. 2006;4:2.
20. Bishai D, et al. Cost-effectiveness of traffic enforcement: a case study from Uganda. Inj Prev. 2008;14:223–7.
21. Blom L, van Niekerk A, Laflamme L. Epidemiology of fatal burns in rural South Africa: a mortuary register-based study from Mpumalanga Province. Burns. 2011;37:1394–402.
22. Bunn F, et al. Traffic calming for the prevention of road traffic injuries: systematic review and meta-analysis. Inj Prev. 2003;9:200–4.
23. Burrows S, van Niekerk A, Laflamme L. Fatal injuries among urban children in South Africa: risk distribution and potential for reduction. Bull World Health Organ. 2010;88:267–72.
24. Chandran A, et al. The global burden of unintentional injuries and an agenda for progress. Epidemiol Rev. 2010;32:110–20.
25. Chandran A, et al. Road traffic deaths in Brazil: rising trends in pedestrian and motorcycle occupant deaths. Traffic Inj Prev. 2012;13:11–6.
26. Chisholm D, et al. Cost effectiveness of strategies to combat road traffic injuries in sub-Saharan Africa and South East Asia: mathematical modelling study. Br Med J. 2012;344:e612.
27. Concha-Barrientos M, et al. The global burden due to occupational injury. Am J Ind Med. 2005;48:470–81.
28. Conrad P, et al. Helmets, injuries and cultural definitions: motorcycle injury in urban Indonesia. Accid Anal Prev. 1996;28:193–200.
29. Cosep Consultoria, Consaúde, and ICF International. Angola Malaria Indicator Survey 2011. Calverton: Cosep Consultoria, Consaúde, and ICF International; 2011.
30. Daisy S, et al. Socioeconomic and cultural influence in the causation of burns in the urban children of Bangladesh. J Burn Care Rehabil. 2001;22:269–73.
31. DiGuiseppi C, Goss CW, Higgins JPT. Interventions for promoting smoke alarm ownership and function. Cochrane Database Syst Rev 2001;CD002246.
32. Donroe J, et al. Falls, poisonings, burns, and road traffic injuries in urban Peruvian children and adolescents: a community based study. Inj Prev. 2009;15:390–6.

33. Donroe J, et al. Pedestrian road traffic injuries in urban Peruvian children and adolescents: case control analyses of personal and environmental risk factors. PLoS One. 2008;3:e3166.
34. Duperrex O, Roberts I, Bunn F. Safety education of pedestrians for injury prevention. Cochrane Database Syst Rev 2002;(2):CD001531.
35. Elliott MA, Armitage CJ. Promoting drivers' compliance with speed limits: testing an intervention based on the theory of planned behavior. Br J Psychol. 2009;100:111–32.
36. Essien E, et al. Community loan funds and transport services for obstetric emergencies in northern Nigeria. Int J Gynaecol Obstet. 1997;59:237–44.
37. Fatmi Z, et al. Incidence, patterns and severity of reported unintentional injuries in Pakistan for persons five years and older. BMC Public Health. 2007;7:152.
38. Fatmi Z, et al. Incidence and pattern of unintentional injuries and resulting disability among children under 5 years of age: results of the National Health Survey of Pakistan. Paediatr Perinat Epidemiol. 2009;23:229–38.
39. Fell JC, et al. An evaluation of graduated driver licensing effects on fatal crash involvements of young drivers in the United States. Traffic Inj Prev. 2011;12(5):423–31.
40. Ferguson SA, Schneider LW. An overview of frontal air bag performance with changes in frontal crash-test requirements: findings of the blue ribbon panel for the evaluation of advanced technology air bags. Traffic Inj Prev. 2008;9:421–31.
41. Fitzharris M, et al. Crash characteristics and patterns of injury among hospitalized motorized two-wheeled vehicle users in urban India. BMC Public Health. 2009;9:11.
42. Forjouh SN. Burns in low- and middle-income countries: a review of available literature on descriptive epidemiology, risk factors, treatment, and prevention. Burns. 2006;32:529–37.
43. Gawryszweski VP, et al. Treatment of injuries in emergency departments: characteristics of victims and place of injury, Sao Paulo State, Brazil, 2005. Cad Saude Publica. 2008;24: 1121–9.
44. Ghana News Agency. Central region drivers curb maternal deaths. Ghana News Agency. http://www.ghananewsagency.org/details/Health/Central-Region-drivers-curb-maternal-deaths/?ci=1&ai=23802. Accessed 24 Dec 2010.
45. Gillespie LD, et al. Interventions for preventing falls in elderly people. Cochrane Database Syst Rev 2003;CD000340.
46. Glassbrenner D. Estimating the lives saved by safety belts and air bags. 2003. National highway transportation safety administration paper no. 500. http://www-nrd.nhtsa.dot.gov/pdf/nrd-01/esv/esv18/CD/Files/18ESV-000500.pdf
47. Habyarimana J, Jack W. Heckle and chide: results of a randomized road safety intervention in Kenya. Center for Global Development. 2009. Working paper no 169. http://www.cgdev.org/files/1421541_file_Habyarimana_Jack_Heckle_FINAL.pdf
48. Haddon W. On the escape of tigers: an ecologic note. Am J Public Health. 1970;60: 2229–34.
49. Haynes AB, et al. A surgical safety checklist to reduce morbidity and mortality in a global population. N Engl J Med. 2009;360:491–9.
50. Hazen A, Ehiri J. Road traffic injuries: hidden epidemic in less developed countries. J Natl Med Assoc. 2006;98:73–82.
51. Heng KW, et al. Helmet use and bicycle-related trauma in patients presenting to an acute hospital in Singapore. Singapore Med J. 2006;47:367–72.
52. Herbert HK, et al. Global health: injuries and violence. Infect Dis Clin North Am. 2011;25:653–8.
53. Herbert HK, et al. Patterns of pediatric injury in South Africa: an analysis of hospital data between 1997 and 2006. J Trauma Acute Care Surg. 2012;73:168–74.
54. Hijar MC, et al. Analysis of fatal pedestrian injuries in Mexico City, 1994-1997. Injury. 2001;32:279–84.
55. Hijar M, Trostle J, Bronfman M. Pedestrian injuries in Mexico: a multi-method approach. Soc Sci Med. 2003;57:2149–59.
56. Hijar M, et al. Quantifying the underestimated burden of road traffic mortality in Mexico: a comparison of three approaches. Traffic Inj Prev. 2012;13:5–10.

57. Houston DJ, Richardson LE. Motorcycle safety and the repeal of universal helmet laws. Am J Public Health. 2007;97:2063–9.
58. Howitt P, et al. Technologies for global health. Lancet. 2012;380:507–35.
59. Hung DV, Stevenson MR, Ivers RQ. Prevalence of helmet use among motorcycle riders in Vietnam. Inj Prev. 2006;12:409–13.
60. Hyder A, et al. Falls among children in the developing world: a gap in child health burden estimations? Acta Paediatr. 2007;96:1394–8.
61. Hyder AA, Muzaffar SSF, Bachani AM. Road traffic injuries in urban Africa and Asia: a policy gap in child and adolescent health. Public Health. 2008;122:1104–10.
62. Hyder AA, et al. Global childhood unintentional injury surveillance in four cities in developing countries: a pilot study. Bull World Health Organ. 2009;87:345–52.
63. Ian R, et al. School based driver education for the prevention of traffic crashes. Cochrane Database Syst Rev 2001;(3):CD003201
64. Iribhogbe PE, Odai ED. Driver-related risk factors in commercial motorcycle (Okada) crashes in Benin City, Nigeria. Prehosp Disaster Med. 2009;24:356–9.
65. Jagnoor J, et al. Unintentional injury mortality in India, 2005: Nationally Representative Mortality Survey of 1.1 million homes. BMC Public Health. 2012;12:487.
66. Jayaraman S, et al. First things first: effectiveness and scalability of a basic prehospital trauma care program for lay first-responders in Kampala, Uganda. PLoS One. 2009;4:e6955.
67. JEVIC. Kenya roadworthiness inspection criteria for vehicles exported from Japan to Kenya. 2012. http://jevic.co.jp/en/activities/regulatory-inspections/kenya/KENYA%20RWI%20 Inspection%20Criteria%20Mar2012.pdf
68. Joubert JB. A comprehensive analysis of the effectiveness of speed camera enforcement in decreasing the accident rate in the Johannesburg Metropolitan Area. In: Proceedings of the 30th southern African transport conference. 2011. p. 285–293. http://www.kr8.co.il/ BRPortalStorage/a/46/59/08-lagpxdQV0D.pdf
69. Juillard C, et al. Patterns of injury and violence in Yaounde Cameroon: an analysis of hospital data. World J Surg. 2011;35:1–8.
70. Kahane CJ. Fatality reduction by air bags: analyses of accident data through early 1996. NHTSA technical report. 1996. http://www-nrd.nhtsa.dot.gov/Pubs/808470.pdf
71. Kalayi GD, Muhammad I. Clothing burns in Zaria. Burns. 1994;20:356–69.
72. Karkhaneh M, et al. Effectiveness of bicycle helmet legislation to increase helmet use: a systematic review. Inj Prev. 2006;12:76–82.
73. Kendrick D, et al. Home safety education and provision of safety equipment for injury prevention. Cochrane Database Syst Rev 2007;CD005014.
74. Kendrick D, et al. Parenting interventions for the prevention of unintentional injuries in childhood. Cochrane Database Syst Rev 2007;CD006020.
75. Kenya Bureau of Standards. A guide to making your premises safe from fire 2012. Kenya Standard KS 2390. 2012. http://www.kebs.org/standards/review/KS2390-2012.pdf
76. Kenya Law Reports. The factories and other places of work (fire risk reduction) rules. 2007. Legal notice no. 59. http://www.kenyalaw.org/klr/index.php?id=570
77. Kenya Law Reports. The occupational safety and health act, 2007(b), No. 15. http://www. kenyalaw.org/klr/fileadmin/pdfdownloads/Acts/OccupationalSafetyandHealth(No.1 5of2007).pdf
78. Kenya Police. Role of motor vehicle inspection unit in enforcement of road safety regulations. 2012. http://www.kenyapolice.go.ke/Role_Mvihecle%20Inspection.asp
79. Ker K, et al. Post-license driver education for the prevention of road traffic crashes: a systematic review of randomised controlled trials. Accid Anal Prev. 2005;37:305–13.
80. Khan I, et al. Factors associated with helmet use among motorcycle users in Karachi, Pakistan. Acad Emerg Med. 2008;15:384–7.
81. Kobusingye O, Guwatudde D, Lett R. Injury patterns in rural and urban Uganda. Inj Prev. 2001;7:46–50.
82. Kobusingye OC, et al. Emergency medical systems in low- and middle-income countries: recommendations for action. Bull World Health Organ. 2005;83:626–31.

83. Kraemer JD, et al. Public health measures to control tuberculosis in low-income countries: ethics and human rights considerations. Int J Tuberc Lung Dis. 2011;15:S19–24.

84. Kraemer JD, Honermann BJ, Roffenbender JS. Cyclists' helmet usage and characteristics in central and southern Malawi: a cross-sectional study. Int J Inj Contr Saf Promot. 2012; 19(4):372–7.

85. Kulanthayan S, et al. Prevalence and determinants of non-standard motorcycle safety helmets amongst food delivery workers in Selangor and Kuala Lumpur. Injury. 2012;43:653–9.

86. Lari AR, et al. Epidemiology of childhood burn injuries in Fars Province, Iran. J Burn Care Rehabil. 2002;23:39–45.

87. Ledesma RD, Peltzer RI. Helmet use among motorcyclists: observational study in the City of Mar del Plata, Argentina. Rev Saude Publica. 2008;42:143–5.

88. Lewis IM, et al. Promoting public health messages: should we move beyond fear-evoking appeals in road safety. Qual Health Res. 2007;17:61–74.

89. Li G, Baker SP. Injuries to bicyclists in Wuhan, People's Republic of China. Am J Public Health. 1997;87:1049–52.

90. Liberian Ministry of Health and Social Welfare (MOHSW, National Malaria Control Program, Liberia Institute of Statistics and Geo-Information Services (LISGIS, ICF International. Liberia malaria indicator survey 2011. Monrovia: NMCP; 2012.

91. Liu BC, Ivers R, Norton R, Boufous S, Blows S, Lo SK. Helmets for preventing injury in motorcycle riders. Cochrane Database Syst Rev 2008;(1):Art. No.: CD004333. doi:10.1002/14651858.CD004333.pub3

92. Liu Q, et al. The gap in injury mortality rates between urban and rural residents of Hubei Province, China. BMC Public Health. 2012;12:180.

93. Liu Y, et al. Characteristics of paediatric burns in Sichuan Province: epidemiology and prevention. Burns. 2012;38:26–31.

94. MacPherson A, Spinks A. Bicycle helmet legislation for the uptake of helmet use and prevention of head injuries. Cochrane Database Syst Rev 2007;CD005401.

95. Malawi National Statistical Office (NSO), ICF Macro. Malawi demographic and health survey 2010. Zomba: NSO; 2011.

96. Malta DC, et al. The characteristics and factors of emergency service visits for falls. Rev Saude Publica. 2012;46:1–9.

97. Marucci-Wellman H, et al. A survey of work-related injury in a rapidly industrializing commune in Vietnam. Int J Occup Environ Health. 2009;15:1–8.

98. Mashreky SR, et al. Epidemiology of childhood burn: yield of largest community based injury survey in Bangladesh. Burns. 2008;34:856–62.

99. Maziak W, Ward KD, Rastam S. Injuries in Aleppo, Syria: first population-based estimates and characterization of predominant types. BMC Public Health. 2006;6:63.

100. Michael YL, et al. Primary care-relevant interventions to prevent falling in older adults: a systematic evidence review for the U.S. Preventive Services Task Force. Ann Intern Med. 2010;153:815–25.

101. Mock CN, et al. Incidence and outcome of injury in Ghana: a community-based survey. Bull World Health Organ. 1999;77:955–64.

102. Mock CN, Forjuoh SN, Rivara FP. Epidemiology of transport-related injuries in Ghana. Accid Anal Prev. 1999;31(4):359–70.

103. Mock C, et al. Childhood injury prevention practices by parents in Mexico. Inj Prev. 2002;8:303–5.

104. Mock CN, et al. Improvements in prehospital trauma care in an African country with no formal emergency medical services. J Trauma. 2002;53:90–7.

105. Mock C, et al. Injury prevention counselling to improve safety practices by parents in Mexico. Bull World Health Organ. 2003;81:591–8.

106. Mohamed N, et al. Analysis of factors associated with seatbelt wearing among rear passengers in Malaysia. Int J Inj Contr Saf Promot. 2011;18:3–10.

107. Mohan D, et al. Impact modelling studies for a three-wheeled scooter taxi. Accid Anal Prev. 1997;29:161–70.

108. Moshiro C, et al. Injury morbidity in an urban and a rural area in Tanzania: an epidemiological survey. BMC Public Health. 2005;5:11.
109. Mutto M, et al. The effect of an overpass on pedestrian injuries on a major highway in Kampala—Uganda. Afr Health Sci. 2002;2:89–93.
110. Naci H, et al. Distribution of road traffic deaths by road user group: a global comparison. Inj Prev. 2009;15:55–9.
111. Nagel CL, et al. The relation between neighborhood built environment and walking activity among older adults. Am J Epidemiol. 2008;168:461–8.
112. Ng CP, et al. Factors related to seatbelt-wearing among rear-seat passengers in Malaysia. Accid Anal Prev. 2013;50:351–60. doi:10.1016/j.aap.2012.05.004.
113. Nielsen K, et al. Assessment of the status of prehospital care in 13 low- and middle-income countries. Prehosp Emerg Care. 2012;16:381–9.
114. Noe R. Occupational injuries identified by an emergency department injury surveillance system in Nicaragua. Inj Prev. 2004;10:227–32.
115. Nzegwu MA, et al. Patterns of morbidity and mortality amongst motorcycle riders and their passengers in Benin-City, Nigeria: one-year review. Ann Afr Med. 2008;7:82–5.
116. Odebode TO, Abubakar AM. Childhood head injury: causes, outcome, and outcome predictors. Pediatr Surg Int. 2004;5:348–52.
117. Parbhoo A, Louw QA, Grimmer-Somers K. Burn prevention programs for children in developing countries require urgent attention: a targeted literature review. Burns. 2010;36:164–75.
118. Passmore J, et al. Impact of mandatory motorcycle helmet wearing legislation on head injuries in Viet Nam: results of a preliminary analysis. Traffic Inj Prev. 2010;11:202–6.
119. Paulozzi LJ, et al. Economic development's effect on road transport-related mortality among different types of road users: a cross-sectional international study. Accid Anal Prev. 2007;39(3):606–17.
120. Peck MD. Epidemiology of burns throughout the world. Part I: distribution and risk factors. Burns. 2011;37:1087–100.
121. Peek-Asa C, et al. The prevalence of non-standard helmet use and head injuries among motorcycle riders. Accid Anal Prev. 1999;31:229–33.
122. Perel P, et al. Noncommunicable diseases and injuries in Latin America and the Caribbean: time for action. PLoS Med. 2006;3:e344.
123. Perry MJ, et al. Emergency department surveillance of occupational injuries in Shanghai's Putuo District, People's Republic of China. Ann Epidemiol. 2005;5:351–7.
124. Pevin A, et al. Viet Nam's mandatory motorcycle helmet law and its impact on children. Bull World Health Organ. 2009;87:369–73.
125. Puvanachandra P, et al. Burden of road traffic injuries in Turkey. Traffic Inj Prev. 2012;12:64–75.
126. Ramani KV, et al. Study of blood-transfusion services in Maharashtra and Gujarat States, India. J Health Popul Nutr. 2009;27:259–70.
127. Republic of Zambia Road Transport and Safety Agency. Getting a driver's license is easy. http://www.rtsa.org.zm/index.php?option=com_content&view=article&id=6:rtsa-adopts-miss-zambia-&catid=1:announcements&Itemid=67. Accessed 10 July 2012
128. Retting RA, et al. Crash and injury reduction following installation of roundabouts in the United States. Am J Public Health. 2001;91:628–31.
129. Richburg KB. For China's driving test, be ready for almost anything. Washington Post. 2012.
130. Rivara FP, Tompson DC, Cummings P. Effectiveness of primary and secondary enforced seat belt laws. Am J Prev Med. 1999;16:30–9.
131. Roberts H, et al. Putting public health evidence into practice: increasing the prevalence of working smoke alarms in disadvantaged inner city housing. J Epidemiol Community Health. 2004;58:280–5.
132. Rosen E, Sander U. Pedestrian fatality risk as a function of car impact speed. Accid Anal Prev. 2009;41:536–42.

133. Rowland D, et al. Prevalence of working smoke alarms in local authority inner city housing: randomised controlled trial. BMJ. 2002;35:998–1001.
134. Runyan CW. Using the Haddon matrix: introducing the third dimension. Inj Prev. 1998; 4:302–7.
135. Russell KF, et al. graduated driver licensing for reducing motor vehicle crashes among young drivers. Cochrane Database Syst Rev 2011;(10):CD003300.
136. Shehu D, Iheh AT, Kuna MJ. Mobilizing transport for obstetric emergencies in northwestern Nigeria. Int J Gynaecol Obstet. 1997;59:173–80.
137. Smitha MW, et al. Effect of state workplace safety laws on occupational injury rates. J Occup Environ Med. 2001;43:1001–10.
138. Solagberu B, et al. motorcycle injuries in a developing country and the vulnerability of riders, passengers, and pedestrians. Inj Prev. 2006;12:266–8.
139. Spector JM, et al. Improving quality of care for maternal and newborn health: prospective pilot study of the WHO Safe Childbirth Checklist Program. PLoS One. 2012;7:e35151.
140. Spiegel R, et al. Motivating motorists to voluntarily slow down. J Prev Interv Community. 2010;38:332–40.
141. Thompson DC, Rivara FP, Thompson R. Helmets for preventing head and facial injuries in bicyclists. Cochrane Database Syst Rev 2000;CD001855.
142. Tiska MA, et al. A model of prehospital trauma training for lay persons devised in Africa. Emerg Med J. 2004;21L:237–9.
143. Tsai MC, Hemenway D. Effect of the mandatory helmet law in Taiwan. Inj Prev. 1999;5: 290–1.
144. Useh U, Moyo AM, Munyonga E. Wheelchair accessibility of public buildings in the Central Business District of Harare, Zimbabwe. Disabil Rehabil. 2001;23:490–6.
145. van Schoor O, van Niekerk JL, Grobbelaar B. Mechanical failures as a contributing cause to motor vehicle accidents—South Africa. Accid Anal Prev. 2001;33:713–21.
146. Vernick JS, et al. Effects of high school driver education on motor vehicle crashes, violations, and licensure. Am J Prev Med. 1999;16:40–6.
147. Vilasco B, Bondurand A. Burns in Abidjan, Cote D'Ivoire. Burns. 1995;21:291–6.
148. Vlahov D, et al. Perspectives on urban conditions and population health. Cad Saude Publica. 2005;21:949–57.
149. Vos R, et al. Albatros: an innovative low-cost wheelchair. Disabil Rehabil. 1993;15:44–6.
150. Wakefield MA, Loken B, Hornik RC. Use of mass media campaigns to change health behaviour. Lancet. 2010;376:1261–71.
151. Waters HR, Hyder AA, Phillips TL. Economic evaluation of interventions to reduce road traffic injuries—a review of the literature with applications to low and middle-income countries. Asia Pac J Public Health. 2004;16:23–31.
152. WHO. World report on road traffic injury prevention. 2004.
153. WHO. Helmets: a road safety manual for decision-makers and practitioners. 2006.
154. WHO. Drinking and driving: a road safety manual for decision-makers and practitioners. 2007.
155. WHO. WHO global report on falls prevention in older age. 2007. http://www.who.int/ageing/publications/Falls_prevention7March.pdf
156. WHO. Speed management: a road safety manual for decision-makers and practitioners. 2008.
157. WHO. A WHO plan for burn prevention and care. 2008. http://whqlibdoc.who.int/publications/2008/9789241596299_eng.pdf
158. WHO. Global status report on road safety. 2009.
159. WHO. Falls. 2010. http://www.who.int/mediacentre/factsheets/fs344/en/index.html
160. WHO. Compendium of new and emerging health technologies. 2011.
161. WHO. Burn prevention: success stories, lessons learned. 2011. http://whqlibdoc.who.int/publications/2011/9789241501187_eng.pdf
162. WHO. World health statistics. 2012.

163. WHO. Cost-effectiveness thresholds, CHOosing Interventions that are Cost Effective (WHO-CHOICE). http://www.who.int/choice/costs/CER_thresholds/en/index.html. Accessed 25 July 2012.

164. Williams AF, Ferguson SA. Driver education renaissance? Inj Prev. 2004;10:4–7.

165. Wilson C, et al. Speed cameras for the prevention of road traffic injuries and deaths. Cochrane Database Syst Rev 2010;(10):CD004607.

166. Winchester. A crack in the edge of the world. 2005.

167. Xuegun Y, et al. Prevalence rates of helmet use among motorcycle riders in a developed region in China. Accid Anal Prev. 2011;43:214–9.

168. Xia Z, et al. Fatal occupational injuries in a new development area in the People's Republic of China. J Occup Environ Med. 2000;42:917–22.

169. Yeung JHH, et al. Bicycle related injuries presenting to a trauma center in Hong Kong. Injury. 2009;40:555–9.

170. Yoshida S. A global report on falls prevention: epidemiology of falls. WHO ageing and life course. 2007. http://www.who.int/ageing/projects/1.Epidemiology%20of%20falls%20in%20older%20age.pdf

171. Zhuang X, Wu C. Pedestrians' crossing behaviors and safety at unmarked roadway in China. Accid Anal Prev. 2011;43:1927–36.

172. Hyder AA, et al. Estimating the burden of road traffic injuries among children and adolescents in urban south Asia. Health Policy. 2006;77(2):129–39.

Part III
Frameworks, Cases and Tools
to Address Urbanization and Health
Through Innovation

Chapter 11
The Millennium Cities Initiative: An Experiment in Integrated Urban Development

Susan M. Blaustein

Background

This chapter describes an innovation in urban development in Africa, how it emerged, and the importance of taking an integrated, multidisciplinary approach in order to effect durable advances in the public health and related sectors.

With urbanization rates skyrocketing even in the world's least industrialized countries, it is clear that smart, targeted approaches to urban development are urgently needed if the Millennium Development Goals (MDGs) are ever to be realized. Without linking farms to domestic, regional, and international markets, creating a continuum of care that will allow an expectant mother in a complicated labor to reach the tertiary care center in time to deliver her newborn safely, and providing a continuum also in education that will enable village girls and boys to continue their schooling through junior and senior high and beyond, these goals, however pragmatic and well crafted, cannot be achieved. For this reason, the Millennium Cities Initiative (MCI) was founded by Columbia University Earth Institute Director Jeffrey D. Sachs in 2006, as a counterpart to the Earth Institute's Millennium Villages Project. That innovative, integrated rural development project was designed as a proof-of-concept that with smart, cross-fertilizing inputs in agriculture, health, education, and essential infrastructure, even impoverished smallholder farmers

---

Electronic supplementary material: The online version of this chapter (doi: 10.1007/978-1-4899-7597-3_11) contains supplementary material, which is available to authorized users.

S.M. Blaustein, Ph.D. (✉)
The Earth Institute, Columbia University, 405 Low Library,
535 West 116th Street, New York, NY 10025, USA
e-mail: sblaustein@ei.columbia.edu

© Springer New York 2015
R. Ahn et al. (eds.), *Innovating for Healthy Urbanization*,
DOI 10.1007/978-1-4899-7597-3_11

across sub-Saharan Africa—often deemed "the poorest of the poor"—could attain the MDGs by the universally-embraced target date of 2015.[1]

Despite the grand and optimistic bet embodied in the Millennium Villages Project, it was clear even in 2005 that attaining the MDGs in isolated clusters of remote, previously hungry villages simply would not eradicate extreme poverty. By mid-2009, more of the world's population lived in cities than not. And while in 2010 the sub-Saharan population remained primarily rural, with 296 million people (39 %) living in urban areas, by 2050 that number is expected to rise to 1.1 billion, bringing the *global* percentage represented by sub-Saharan urban residents up dramatically, from 8 to 17 %.[2] Neither African cities, the continent, nor the global community is ready for the strain on social services, natural resources, and international security prefigured by such numbers.

The first presupposition, then, of the MCI was that a distinct and innovative set of diagnostics, interventions, and investments—akin to those enlisted in rural settings and at the national level, but custom-tailored to the exigencies of city life—would be essential if the MDGs are to be achieved in urban areas worldwide.

Second, *sustainable* development is not achievable by addressing deficits with regard only to education, health service provision, or infrastructure. All prescribed interventions, individually and/or in combination, need to address multiple sectors simultaneously, to realize those synergies and cross-fertilizing effects that are the key to transformational change.

Given these principles, as MCI's founders went about designing its strategy, program, and methodology, the question remained how to best achieve this vision of integrated urban development, given the many laudable but failed efforts at urban renewal, slum upgrading, and other antipoverty works; the burgeoning challenge of stemming abject privation in rapidly growing metropolitan areas; the diminishing and increasingly cautious allocation of resources on the part of donor governments and multilateral agencies; and some key differences among the cities themselves. The test case for this endeavor—sub-Saharan cities, chosen because of their spiraling growth and because they, like their nearby village counterparts, are perceived to be the furthest off-track from attaining the MDG—would also serve to demonstrate that if this integrated, evidence-based approach could work in these complex, severely underserved settings, it can work anywhere.

---

[1] This target was conceivable because of commitments made in 2005 by the Group of Eight, or G8, a regularly convening body of governments including what used to be the world's largest economies: France, Germany, Italy, Japan, the United Kingdom, the United States, Canada, and Russia. At its annual summit that year in Gleneagles, Scotland, the G8 promised $25 billion more per year to help the sub-Saharan region, deemed the furthest off-track, attain the MDGs on time. Due to a sluggish uptake of these promises, however, followed several years later by the global economic crisis, that much-needed assistance by and large has not come through. The G8 has since been supplanted by the Group of 20 (G20), as a more inclusive body more accurately representing emerging economic powerhouses and the global economy.

[2] World Urbanization Prospects: The 2009 Revision. New York: UN Population Division, 2010.

Strategy and Methodology

Research: Assessing the Gaps in and Costs of MDG Attainment

The first task in any challenging undertaking is to know the scope of the challenge(s) to be undertaken. How far off-track *are* these African cities, exactly, from realizing the MDGs in maternal and child health; reducing the infection rates of HIV/AIDS, TB, and malaria; attaining universal primary education and gender parity; providing reliable access to potable water and sanitation services; and protecting the environment? Moreover, what assets and attractions exist in each venue that might be enlisted in support of this effort and also attract income-generating investment, domestic and foreign? And what infrastructure deficits currently inhibit such investment and/or the attainment of the aforementioned goals?

Clearly, a set of diagnostics was required in all MDG-related areas, as well as in the business and investment arenas. For the social sector, MCI adopted the needs assessments and costing instruments developed for use at the *national* level by specialized task forces as part of the United Nations Millennium Project (UNMP), in the areas of public health, gender, education, and water/sanitation.[3] Given that the G8's 2005 commitment of $25 billion more per year for sub-Saharan Africa was conditioned on the beneficiary governments' transparent and accountable budgeting, MCI believed the detailed costing tools would also be useful for local governments to know the relative extent of the need in each sector, so they may budget, plan, and prepare proposals accordingly.

MCI's application of the needs assessment instruments to the Millennium Cities was these tools' first use at the subnational level, yielding a fairly rounded, high-level depiction of the social sector needs in each city. Roads, energy, and other civil infrastructures are obviously missing. Because these sectors' respective mandates, planning, and budget processes are essentially national in nature, they tend to take place within the relevant line ministries and consequently would seem to yield far less useful information at the municipal level. Some of this information has been captured (by our own industrial infrastructure survey), developed, and carried out by MCI in three Millennium Cities to help local authorities understand better the precise needs of small- and larger-scale manufacturers, other entrepreneurs, and

---

[3] The UN Millennium Project, led by Prof. Jeffrey D. Sachs, Earth Institute Director and UN Special Advisor on the MDGs to then-Secretary-General Kofi Annan, assembled some 260 scientists worldwide into 13 Task Forces to determine how each of the MDGs, and the targets within each overall goal, could best be achieved. UN Millennium Project officials, and more recently, UN Development Programme (UNDP) officials, then applied this knowledge to national-level planning in ten sub-Saharan countries and elsewhere. A number of these Millennium Project Task Forces devised these extremely useful need assessments, costing instruments, and sets of recommendations, enabling participating Millennium Project countries to understand precisely how far they need to go to attain each goal and the relative cost of doing so.

potential investors, with an eye toward improving mobility and energy access for all.[4]

MCI has also found the absence of neonatal and maternal mortality baselines to be a critical gap in the Millennium Cities' health records. We have undertaken, upon request from the local health authorities, to assist in producing such baselines in a number of sites, albeit with difficulty. Some of our constant challenges include: continued irregularity of institutional delivery and the lack of clear numbers on those mothers delivering outside of health facilities[5]; the lack of proper and homogenized data collection systems at public and private facilities; and the common overreporting of stillbirths, sometimes due to staff sensitivity in instances when a clinical error might have resulted in a newborn fatality that could have been prevented by a timely intervention. Yet it is impossible to measure progress toward the attainment of MDGs 4 and 5—child and maternal survival and health—without this information.

The most effective way MCI has found to institutionalize collection of these data is to work simultaneously at the ministerial, tertiary, and local facility levels. Our priorities are first, to modify labor/delivery reporting forms so that they capture this information more precisely; second, to educate midwives, nurses, other birth attendants, and community health workers, both at tertiary and primary care facilities and in more remote communities, as to the vital importance of accurate reporting; and third, to reach out to pregnant women in peri-urban and other remote neighborhoods to encourage antenatal care, institutional delivery, breast-feeding, proper nutrition, hygiene, inoculations, and regular postnatal care, so that the relevant information can be properly recorded and fed into health policy planning at the local, regional, and national levels.

Because the UNMP assessments and costing instruments are essentially top-down, supply-side tools, MCI has also developed its own comprehensive, poverty-related household survey intended to depict, in telling granularity, precisely what it is in each city that is keeping its residents trapped in extreme urban poverty. Is it, for instance, the lack of reliable public transport that compels an adolescent girl to walk to school, forcing her to eventually drop out when her father fears for her safety? Is it the lack of safe, close-in water points that keeps a mother out of the workforce because she is consigned to gathering water for her family twice a day, at an hour's walk, despite living deep within the city? Is it the lack of a competently equipped and staffed neighborhood clinic and/or an effective emergency referral and triage system at the municipal level that results in a maternal or newborn death when that mother in a compromised labor was not seen in time? And does the cruel paradox pertain here that the lack of available local job opportunities forces devoted fathers far from their families in order to provide for them?

---

[4] MCI has produced industrial infrastructure surveys for the Millennium Cities of Blantyre, Malawi; Kisumu, Kenya; and Kumasi, Ghana. All of these are available on the MCI website, at www.mci.ei.columbia.edu.

[5] In some cases, as in Malawi, this lack of clarity can be attributed in part to the prosecution and penalization of home deliveries, an unanticipated outcome of an aspirational law unmatched at the time it entered into effect.

These are the questions that MCI's truly integrated MDG-based household survey seeks to answer with the development and use of this detailed instrument, which has now been successfully piloted in Kisumu, Kenya, and in Blantyre, Malawi.[6]

Further bottom-up research has been carried out in support of our community-based development work. In a number of neighborhoods in the Ghanaian capital of Accra, MCI has undertaken local urban planning and economic development efforts,[7] and in Ghana's second largest city, Kumasi, MCI has overseen the preliminary design as well as the community and institutional work essential to building a comprehensive Women's and Girls' Center (see below for more on this initiative). In each case, MCI carried out focus groups, generally with structured questionnaires, to ascertain people's own assessments, grievances, plans, and aspirations regarding the issue(s) in question. These have ranged from the possible uses and adaptations for overgrown and currently abandoned railroad tracks to sanitation and waste disposal needs and practices; priorities for upgrading open-air food markets; and how to revive a nearly moribund, small-scale fishing industry in an era of dramatic environmental and industrial changes.

In the investment arena, MCI went far beyond the industrial infrastructure survey and commissioned reviews of the business climate and regulatory environment, both at the national and the regional or municipal levels, which were carried out pro bono in and for the Millennium Cities by partner law firms.[8] The intention here was to delve deeper into analysis of the situation at the *local* level than the excellent country-level information available in such volumes as the World Bank's *Doing Business* series.

In an effort to further understand the potential of local businesses, at MCI's request, the United Nations Industrial Development Organization (UNIDO) profiled small- and medium-sized enterprises in five Millennium Cities and posted profiles of promising firms seeking technical or financial partners[9] on the UNIDO website. To better evaluate the viability of seemingly promising investment opportunities and sectors, MCI has trained the investment promotion specialists in a number of Millennium Cities to conduct SWOT analyses that can then be shared with the national investment authorities, potential investors, and those local partners

---

[6] The Kisumu household survey for Kisumu, Kenya, is available at http://mci.ei.columbia.edu/files/2014/05/Kisumu_HH_Survey_Report_F2014.pdf. The survey instrument itself is available upon request.

[7] Including helping to select a site for a World Bank-funded bus rapid transit station project and comprehensive community upgrading in the neighborhoods of Nima, Ga Mashie, and Korle Gonno. Focus groups in these cases included residents, members of street vendors' and market associations, youth and mothers' associations, and the transport industry, as well as local, regional, and national ministry-level officials.

[8] The international law firms that carried out these regulatory reviews pro bono were Carter Ledyard & Milburn, Cravath, Swaine & Moore LLP, and DLA Piper.

[9] The five Millennium Cities where small- to medium-sized enterprises were profiled by UNIDO are Akure, Nigeria; Blantyre, Malawi; Kisumu, Kenya; Kumasi, Ghana; and Mekelle, Ethiopia.

seeking direct investment.[10] Finally, with the benefit of information obtained through a series of focus groups, interviews, literature reviews, and informal discussions, MCI and the global accounting firm KPMG separately identified and examined promising opportunities and sectors worth exploring further for potential domestic or foreign investment. The results of each of these studies, for a number of the Millennium Cities, have been published in a series of what MCI believes to be the first stand-alone City Investment Guides.[11]

Yet another investment-related instrument, a matrix to assess the relative sustainability of a given prospective investment, was developed under our Regional Partnership to Promote Trade and Investment in sub-Saharan Africa.[12] This project, funded by the Government of Finland, together with the Millennium Cities of Kumasi, Ghana; Mekelle, Ethiopia; and Tabora, Tanzania, aims to strengthen capacity in the area of investment promotion and bring job-generating investments to these three cities. This sustainability matrix, which was recently "test-driven" in several cities, including the Millennium City of Kisumu, is intended to assist local investment promotion specialists and policymakers in evaluating and comparing investment proposals and developing their own priority projects requiring outside investment.

For these innovative instruments and research findings to be useful and effective, one cannot overestimate the vital importance of capacity building: for experts working in the social sector to perform accurate data collection, diagnostics, and/or costing exercises, and for business and investment promotion specialists to strengthen their abilities to profile investments and target investors. The needs assessment and survey instruments utilized by MCI, however comprehensive, can provide only snapshots if they are not repeated at regular intervals so that progress can be monitored and trends detected. Without the ability to carry out a SWOT analysis or feasibility study, facilitate public-private sector dialogue on business-related issues affecting business and investment, or avail prospective and committed investors of the services they need, there can be no sustainable investment capable of creating good jobs and ultimately transforming whole communities. MCI's Regional Partnership to Promote Trade and Investment in sub-Saharan Africa was conceived and developed to achieve precisely these ends.

---

[10] A SWOT analysis, or SWOT matrix, is a methodology attributed to American management consultant Albert Humphrey, undertaken to appraise the relative Strengths, Weaknesses/Limitations, Opportunities, and Threats (ergo, "SWOT") pertaining to any business venture or potential investment project. After defining the project's aims, this structured technique then proceeds to identify and evaluate as positive or negative an array of pertinent internal and external factors that might affect the attainment of the stated aims.

[11] MCI's five investment guides are for the Millennium Cities of Blantyre, Malawi; Kisumu, Kenya; Kumasi, Ghana; Mekelle, Ethiopia; and Tabora, Tanzania; KPMG produced six investment guides, for Blantyre, Kumasi and Kisumu, Mekelle, and Tabora, with the sixth going beyond Akure to cover the whole of Ondo State, Nigeria.

[12] http://mci.ei.columbia.edu/mci/files/2012/12/Sustainable-FDI-Guidance-Paper-Kline.pdf, by John Kline, Georgetown University, commissioned by MCI.

Selected municipal staff in all sectors require thoughtful and thorough training, both in the uses of the assessment and targeting tools and in the processes of carrying them out. This labor-intensive process will prove its value as those charged with data gathering, policy formation, and attracting investors assume more responsibility for the outcomes in their respective departments and bring measurable successes or failures to the attention of their superiors, both within the city government and within those ministries and agencies providing resources and policy direction at the national level.

As is readily apparent from the examples given here, MCI does not operate in a vacuum and is completely reliant on a broad network of partners; from local, regional, and national government entities to universities in the Millennium Cities and the region, and to international agencies and multilateral organizations. The independent credibility of the UN Millennium Project, Development Programme and Industrial Development Organization, MCI's three international partner law firms, and KPMG adds a luster and a "Good Housekeeping Seal of approval" to its analytic findings that can serve to reinforce MCI's own claims in the minds of prospective public and private investors.

MCI Interventions: Meeting Need with Opportunity

In the course of MCI's initial diagnostic phase, certain urgent needs and programming gaps became apparent in such MDG-related areas as neonatal and maternal survival, access to potable water, sanitation services, and quality education. MCI has taken it upon itself to intervene where we have been invited by local authorities to help fill such gaps; where we have identified serious holes in coverage of especially vulnerable populations or underfunded government mandates in areas where MCI or a partner has competency; or where a timely opportunity has presented itself, often through a willing and capable partner. These interventions have generally been smaller-scale projects designed to solve the problems at hand which, if successful, can then be considered for replication and scaling both within the city, nationally, and well beyond. The following are examples of interventions triggered in each of the abovementioned ways.

Filling known gaps: MCI was asked by the head of the teaching hospital in Kumasi, Ghana, to bring in medical professionals to train in the areas of emergency medicine, neonatal emergency, infectious diseases, HIV/AIDS and nutrition, and lifestyle and heart disease. MCI turned to the Government of Israel's Agency for International Cooperation (MASHAV), in the Ministry of Foreign Affairs, which arranged for Israeli experts at Ben-Gurion University and Hadassah Hospitals to come to Kumasi to carry out the requested trainings. Israeli doctors have also trained medical students and practitioners in Kisumu, Kenya, and Mekelle, Ethiopia, in emergency medicine and infectious diseases, at the invitation of the local health authorities. American surgeons have trained in both cities on conducting complex urological surgical procedures.

In all cases, concrete interventions came with the training. In Kisumu, the Israeli agency MASHAV designed, built, and trained staff for the city's first-ever emergency ward. In Mekelle, the Israeli team dewormed all of the city's primary schoolchildren, learning in the process that the anticipated soil-transmitted helminths (e.g., *Ascaris*, hookworm, *Trichuris*, and tapeworm) turned out to be far less common among the children than had been assumed. (*Schistosoma mansoni* was actually much more common, and is generally treated with praziquantel.)[13] By alerting the city health authorities to the urgent need for praziquantel, this finding enabled the city to develop a timely public health response that addressed the actual challenge at hand, rather than the imagined one. In another example, the multiple missions of US-based surgeons to Kisumu, Kenya, and Mekelle, Ethiopia, organized by the Chicago-based Knock Foundation, have provided container-sized donations of state-of-the-art surgical equipment, complete with training in its use, as well as ordinary surgical and medical supplies and consumables that are often in short supply in these two cities.

In the arena of urban planning and design, MCI's main work in Accra is another example of responding to an urgent invitation to fill known gaps. Ghana's sprawling, rapidly growing capital has long since exceeded any residual mid-twentieth-century infrastructure planning. Brimming with approximately four million people, Accra is also home to a severely degraded environment, dangerously and increasingly overcrowded slums, sclerotic key arteries, and unhealthful and severely inadequate supplies of clean air, water, waste management capacity, and energy. Although MCI's mandate has directed us to strengthen the resilience, service delivery, and planning capacity in *secondary* cities (generally regional rather than national capitals), when the mayor of Accra came to us to ask for help in addressing some of these issues, MCI was able to identify a limited source of initial financing and promptly went to work. After over 2 years of working in Accra, MCI produced a substantial reservoir of research and, at the request of the mayor and the Accra Metropolitan Assembly (AMA) over which he presides, helped map (using geographic information systems or GIS), rationalize, plan, and propose detailed revitalizations of several of the city's longest neglected neighborhoods, always in cooperation with the communities themselves and in full cognizance of residents' most pressing issues and dreams.[14] Projects undertaken have included measuring and redesigning slum dwellings and open-air markets, analyzing the quality of locally sourced water in a cholera-riddled neighborhood and the composition of solid waste in another, conducting local economic development studies with an eye toward improving training and employment opportunities for youth and women, and organizing focus groups among local vendors regarding the proposed siting of a bus rapid transit depot.

---

[13] This work, carried out by Dr. Zvi Bentwich and his team from Ben-Gurion University, with support from the Government of Israel's Office of International Cooperation (MASHAV) and the NALA Foundation, is documented in more detail at: http://www.nalafoundation.org/.

[14] At the AMA's request, MCI focused its work in particular on the neighborhoods of Nima, Ga Mashie/Jamestown (Old Accra), and Korle Gonno.

A number of comprehensive publications linking economic opportunity and safe, healthful living to the physical space in specific neighborhoods have resulted from these studies, all of which are available on the MCI website. The work continues, both with regard to neighborhood-specific development in Accra and in Kumasi and expanding to examine regional mapping and planning issues.

Fulfilling unfunded government priorities: Two of MCI's most successful education projects have arisen in response to unfunded mandates put forth by the Government of Ghana: (1) there should be a functioning kindergarten or preschool attached to every primary school; and (2) computer technology and educational uses of the Internet should be taught in junior high school.[15] To address the first gap, MCI reached out once more to the Government of Israel's MASHAV and to the world-renowned specialists in early childhood education (ECE) training and curricula at the Mount Carmel Training Center (MCTC) in Haifa to help design a program. This highly successful project, organized and run by MCTC and MCI in tandem with the Kumasi Metropolitan Assembly, Metropolitan Education Directorate, and the local St. Louis Teaching College, is now in its fourth year, with 85 educators trained and 26 model preschools ("kindergartens") built. It serves an average of 3,500 preschoolers each day. With the continuing sponsorship by the Government of Israel, the trainings are being replicated for early childhood educators in Accra, with 45 teachers trained and 19 new preschools established. The carefully-tailored, comprehensive ECE curricular design is under consideration for full adoption by the certificate-granting national universities.

To fill the second unmet government commitment—to offer training in computer technology and to measure performance at all junior high schools—MCI designed its own program to fit the specific needs and circumstances pertaining to this level of schooling in Ghana. It has been amply demonstrated, both in the industrialized and developing nations, that simply providing computers to schools and assuming that students will become computer literate is an inadequate, wasteful, and counterproductive intervention. In impoverished settings with severe energy and Internet connectivity issues, where teachers receive very limited in-service professional development, the challenges are even more pronounced. Together with the Kumasi Metropolitan Assembly and Education Directorate, Ericsson, Airtel Ghana, and Teachers College, MCI designed a unique computer and connectivity training program—our School2School Connectivity Project—that (a) focuses on training the teachers before concentrating on the students; (b) helps teachers zero in on online educational resources that can feed directly into the specific science and math curricula they are expected to teach; (c) interjects and repeats, as necessary, training in proper maintenance of the computers and related equipment; (d) links teachers and students in Kumasi with their counterparts in New York to pursue joint projects and create new lesson plans; and (e) assists these new teams of partners in developing applications of these lessons that deepen understanding of the MDG.

---

[15] At the Form II level in junior high school, equivalent to the eighth grade in an American middle school.

Following up on serious holes in coverage of at-risk populations: Soon after starting to work in the Millennium Cities, it became distressingly clear to MCI that in nearly all Millennium City sites, there is little common practice of maintaining a safe and reliable blood supply at local health facilities. These health centers may have trained technicians, but they generally lack cold storage, electricity, and, indeed, running water. With postpartum hemorrhage as the region's primary killer of pregnant women, there is no doubt about the need for safe blood or its role in maternal survival. Vehicular accidents are Africa's biggest killer, and nearly all treatments for these, too, rely on access to safe blood. Though safe blood became an issue in the 1980s as the AIDS pandemic seized the world's attention, the lack of access to this resource remains insufficiently linked in the public mind to the inability to reduce maternal deaths or traffic accident-related deaths.

Together with MCI partner Physicians for Peace, a Norfolk, Virginia-based non-profit that sends medical practitioners worldwide to treat patients and to train in a wide range of skills; *l'Hôpital Nianankoro Fomba* in Segou, Mali; the National Blood Banking Authority of the Ministry of Health in Bamako, Mali's capital; the American Red Cross; the Centers for Disease Control; the nonprofit Safe Blood for Africa; and other organizations with complementary competencies, MCI has set out to demonstrate that a hub-and-spoke model for the safe collection and typing, separation and centrifugation, storage, dissemination, and administration of safe blood can work smoothly, save countless lives, and be sustainable and replicable, both across the project and across the continent.

This is not an easy project; to instill the culture of voluntary blood donation, testing, meticulous labeling, temperature-controlled storage, safe transfusions, facility maintenance, training, and repeat training in all these areas is complex and fraught with risk. For these and other mundane, bureaucratic reasons, the project has taken years to move from inception to implementation. But despite these delays, followed by the 2012 military coup and more recent strife in Mali, the facility has now been successfully outfitted, the Africa-based NGO Safe Blood for Africa oversaw the equipment's installation and conducted an extensive series of trainings of hospital practitioners—and Mali's first regional blood bank is fully operative.

Need and opportunity combined in another instance, when MCI addressed the stubbornly high neonatal mortality rates in Kumasi and across the central Ashanti region of Ghana. Because of the overcrowding of the neonatal intensive care unit (ICU) at the national teaching hospital in Kumasi, the Israeli neonatologists who had been invited to train hospital staff in neonatal emergency care were moved to design a low-cost, low-tech neonatal triage unit able to resuscitate newborns and treat such less urgent conditions as jaundice, low-grade infections, and difficulty in nursing. A Kangaroo Mother Care component was specifically added to work with mothers and premature infants.[16] The Government of Israel's MASHAV, with support from MCI and the Kumasi Metropolitan Health Directorate, funded and

---

[16] Kangaroo Mother Care, developed by Dr. Nils Bergman of the University of Cape Town, is a set of protocols embraced by the World Health Organization that has proven highly successful in supporting mothers and saving the lives of newborns and premature infants through the combination

built two such centers, locally known as Mother-Baby Units, or MBUs, in two underserved Kumasi sub-metros. Two more MBUs, also courtesy of the Government of Israel, are currently planned for other sub-metros at the request of city health authorities, who very much appreciate the effectiveness of these units in resuscitating and treating newborns on-site and for significantly decongesting the neonatal ICU, which can now dedicate more space, staff, and time to its gravely ill patients.

The recent development and promulgation by the American Academy of Pediatrics (AAP) of its Helping Babies Breathe™ (HBB) training protocol, a distillation of the AAP's proven, comprehensive set of protocols embodied in its Neonatal Resuscitation Program, gave MCI a further opportunity to strengthen capacity in newborn emergency care beyond the cohort previously trained by the Israeli practitioners. MCI developed a program to train health staff in HBB at every sub-metro health facility in *both* Millennium Cities in Ghana, Kumasi, and Accra[17] and to follow up with the mothers and babies over a 6-month period. With funding from Johnson & Johnson, in-kind support from the US-based nonprofit AmeriCares, and the cooperation of the Ghana Ministry of Health, Ghana Health Service, and the Accra and Kumasi Metropolitan Health Directorates, MCI trained 120 practitioners and resuscitated 68 newborns out of 2004 live births (3.4 % of our total). In Ghana's national insurance scheme, under which it is free for mothers to come in for monthly postnatal checkups and inoculations, MCI and our local partners were also able to follow up on 1,650 registered mother/baby pairs,[18] providing tips on infant and under-five health, hygiene, and nutrition to the mothers—thereby improving the likely health outcomes for the families as a whole.

I have described this sequence of interventions in some detail, because it is an excellent example of a dire need identified through research and consultation—in this case, the high neonatal mortality rate and unacceptably cramped ICU—that was met by a cascade of opportunities. The brilliance and ingenuity of the Israeli doctors and the generosity of their government, the timely development and effective dissemination of the AAP's HBB training protocols, the interest of Johnson & Johnson and AmeriCares in improving newborn survival, and Ghana's national insurance plan ensuring the ongoing, regular participation of the mother/baby pairs through the immediate postnatal period, combined to create a response that could not have been foreseen or planned. It was rather a function of the careful research illuminating this serious gap, coupled with the strong working relationships with relevant actors and institutions on the ground; the network of national and international partners able to contribute according to their abilities and means; and MCI's keen interest, tenacity, and flexibility in being able to maneuver between these quite different

---

of skin-to-skin contact, exclusive breast-feeding, early release from the hospital, and the intimate bonding that inevitably results.

[17] To help address the urgent need to reduce neonatal mortality in the Ashanti countryside, Millennium Villages Project health staff were also trained, as part of both the Israeli-led instruction in Kumasi and the training in HBB.

[18] The number of pairs attending the MCI workshops, however, decreased significantly over time, from the first monthly checkup/inoculation appointment to the fourth.

actors in the public and private arena to put together a replicable, scalable program that has already saved many new lives. Indeed, with renewed support from Johnson & Johnson, the project has been adapted this year for replication in northern Ethiopia, both in the Millennium Villages there and in the Millennium City of Mekelle.[19]

A further example relates to girls' education and empowerment, both of which significantly lag behind the MDG targets in all our sites. Together with MCI partner LitWorld and in close coordination with the local public school districts, MCI has created Girls' Clubs, or "LitClubs," in two of the Millennium Cities (Kisumu and Kumasi) and has trained female teachers in each city to serve as LitClub facilitators and role models for these adolescent and/or prepubescent girls. Activities focus on literacy strengthening; helping each child find her individual voice; connecting and sharing stories and poems, artwork, thoughts, and ideas with girls in other Girls' Clubs worldwide; and forging a sense of compassion, sisterhood, and mutual responsibility, both among LitClub members and with the larger community.

Eight Kisumu and 30 Kumasi teachers have been trained and have been running four Girls' LitClubs in Kisumu and 15 in Kumasi. Numerous girls have already been identified as at-risk, as the girls and their facilitators have opened up to each other in this; some girls were actually being "kept" by much older men, who may have paid a portion of their school costs, and others had endured domestic violence or abuse at home.

Both local school districts immediately embraced and understood the utility of the program, which deepens the existing health- and hygiene-related offerings for their female students, thereby addressing (at least in part) concerns about female student retention. The school districts are eager to scale this intervention citywide. Moreover, in the summer of 2012, the lead Kisumu teachers, backed by the Municipal Education Office and perceiving the need and opportunity to attend to the shockingly similar pressures and concerning issues affecting adolescent boys, worked with MCI staff and several Harvard Summer School students to train six more teachers and establish MCI's first three Boys' LitClubs, a number we hope to grow significantly in the coming years. LitWorld and MCI also perceived a tremendous appetite in Kisumu for a Mothers' Club and organized a hugely successful trial

---

[19] Other examples of MCI's taking advantage of opportunities to address identified needs include our sanitary pad-making project in Mekelle, conceived and implemented by Columbia University School of Nursing Clinical Instructor Mary Moran and her nonprofit organization, Girls2Women. The project, which has been adopted wholeheartedly by the Mekelle public schools, trains early adolescent girls to sew recyclable cotton sanitary pads, making it possible and affordable for them to remain in school during their menses. The other two examples are: (a) MCI partner CyberSmart Africa's work with interactive digital pens and smart boards in public middle schools in Louga, Senegal, and the nearby Millennium Villages, to hone learning skills and to help keep girls in school; and (b) MCI's extensive partnership with the Himalayan Cataract Project, furthest evolved in Mekelle, Ethiopia, and Kumasi, Ghana, where top ophthalmologists have by now carried out thousands of cataract repair and other eye surgeries, have trained local ophthalmologists to do the same, and are now opening a Regional Center for Eye Care Excellence in both sites, to be led by these now-seasoned local practitioners.

workshop, including many of the Girls' LitClub girls and their mothers, during which the palpable hunger for learning and the joy shared in this unusual, creative, intergenerational communication confirmed the transformational potential for this exciting intervention.[20]

In Kumasi, the ready availability of quality bamboo, combined with a resilient and attractive bike design created by Earth Institute colleagues, a feasibility study by KPMG, and an intrigued domestic investor who first heard of this possibility at a Kumasi Investment Day hosted by MCI at Columbia University in New York, has resulted in the construction of a state-of-the-art bicycle factory that has employed dozens of Kumasi residents. So far, hundreds of sturdy bikes ideally suited to the needs of local students, community health workers (CHWs), and farmers in rural areas have been produced. The Millennium Villages Project has considered purchasing dozens of bikes for its CHWs in a new MVP project in the north of Ghana, and MCI and MVP are considering planting some of this fast-growing bamboo in wetland areas near the MVP that have been severely degraded by large-scale corporate mining.

Again, these opportunities could not have been foreseen in MCI's project design. A renewable natural resource, constructive ingenuity, a certain dose of serendipity, and the zeal and commitment of a Ghanaian businessman to invest in his hometown were the recipe for the development of an exciting investment prospect brought to fruition.[21]

Bringing It All Together: Convening and Convergences

Stakeholder Consultations

Once the MDG-based needs assessments, investment-related research, and household surveys have been completed, MCI and city authorities work together to convene a diverse array of stakeholders to consider the findings and the estimated costs of implementing MCI's recommendations, weigh their foremost concerns and considerations, and determine together their top development priorities that can serve as the basis of a City Development Strategy (CDS) designed to achieve them. These priorities, thoughtfully mulled and debated by the assembled business leaders, youth, women, civil servants, academics, and NGO representatives, are then fleshed out into a full-fledged road map charting the city's forward growth and development.

This consultative process has been completed in five venues—Mekelle, Kumasi, Segou, Bamako, and Louga. While the proportion of representation from the private

---

[20] See below for more about MCI's and LitWorld's plans and pending financing, to grow the LitClubs program, for girls, boys, and their mothers.

[21] For more on MCI's bamboo bike project and the company, Bamboo Bikes Ltd., see http://mci.ei.columbia.edu/?id=bamboo_bikes, and http://bamboobikeslimited.com.

sector, NGO community, slum dwellers' associations, and regional government has varied from one set of consultations to another, the level of discussion has been uniformly high, with important insights voiced and heard by all present—from each city's mayor and chiefs to the modest street vendor. These open, cross-sectoral, cross-class discussions are already a rare and noteworthy event in most of the Millennium Cities[22]; what MCI tries to do, especially in the venues less accustomed to hearing the voices of the underserved, is to elicit, record, and underscore the comments from this constituency, with particular attention to the degree to which they reverberate with MCI's own evidence-based observations and findings. These consultations are at the heart of MCI's approach, constituting a vital reality check. As external technical advisors, professors, and students, it is critical for us to remember that we are, first and last, outsiders, with infinitely more to learn than we could possibly share. We have far less at stake than our local partners, in whose lives and whose children's lives, livelihood, and living conditions we are all engaged in action-oriented thought.

As at most times in this work, the risk of trampling on tradition, on cultural mores, and even, quite literally, on ancestors—as occurred last year with our architects in Accra's old Ga Mashie neighborhood—is severe. In the case of Ga Mashie, we learned early on that we could simply forget about our plan for a straightforward vertical densification of the residential compound, because the ancestors buried in each compound's central courtyard required direct, unimpeded access to the sky and the stars.

Nowhere are cultural practices more firmly held than in the intimate arena of reproductive health. One can, for instance, make a compelling case to a pregnant woman that she delivers institutionally during a private consultation at the clinic. However, if the woman's husband is not on board, she is a lot less likely to show up—unless her labor has already been compromised, at which point, by the time she arrives at the clinic, it may be too late. Of course, there are also more controversial health issues regarding family planning and genital cutting, where it has been demonstrated that engaging the relevant family and community actors early on—the elders, imams, mothers-in-law, aunties, and, of course, the midwives—results in the best chance of success in amending behavior in healthful ways.

After initial presentations of MCI's findings by city administrators together with MCI and a series of breakout discussion groups, MCI's stakeholder workshops conclude with plenary sessions in which all participants vote in a structured way for their preferred MDG-based priorities—the sectors, and the desired improvements within these sectors, that they believe will unlock the city's growth and release its potential. They may be thinking of the much-needed improvements to the water system, which are so critical to public health, industry, and tourism, or of new and better classrooms, labs, and libraries that everyone deems essential to the city's children and their common future. If the level of maternal mortality is especially high, they may wish to concentrate hoped-for donor resources on improving the

---

[22] With the possible exception of Kisumu and with its vibrant and highly conscienticized civil society sector.

continuum of care for pregnant women, including the maintenance of the requisite supply of drugs, safe blood and trained personnel to treat postpartum hemorrhage at the point of entry, and the health provider knowledge of when to refer to a tertiary facility if the mother's condition can no longer be handled on-site.

Challenges in facilitating these stakeholder consultations include reconciling competing sectoral interests and priorities; managing conflicts with other projects and priorities championed by the city's leadership[23]; and dealing with the possibility that subtle and less subtle pressures will be felt by the less well-suited, more marginalized groups to remain silent regarding their own needs and priorities, thereby allowing an agenda promoted by the ruling interests to prevail.

In MCI's experience, when all parties have reviewed together the priority areas to confirm their consensus on the most important issues facing the city, there has been a remarkable sense of unity, direction, and hope—uncommon sentiments for people otherwise divided by class, gender, and often ethnicity, united only by their geographic coordinates.

Preparing the City Development Strategy

Once this process has been concluded, MCI is prepared to furnish a template and initial list of stakeholder-selected priorities and recommendations as a sort of blank slate on which local authorities can take the lead in this important exercise in local autonomy and MDG-based city planning. In cases where other strategic plans may be under way, recently ended, or contemplated by the parties, MCI is prepared to review, elucidate, and align the various documents with the MDG-related agenda. A technical team of city officials will be best positioned to take up the assignment of fleshing out a full draft of the CDS and reckoning the approximate cost estimates issuing from MCI's initial needs assessments with updated, on-the-ground costs for the implementation of any of the recommended interventions.

When the provisional CDS has been drafted, reviewed by MCI, and revised by the technical team, it can then be submitted to a representative group of city stakeholders for discussion and validation. Upon completion of the final version, the CDS should be shared with regional and national government and with individual donors and multilateral agencies, as appropriate, in order to mobilize the resources necessary to filling the deficits singled out as blocking the strategy's timely realization.

MCI has helped with this process, as well as with setting up a donor round table for the city (in some cases in association with a Millennium City Investors' Day) to showcase and promote promising public and private sector investment opportunities. Official donors, multilateral agencies and development banks, corporations with an

---

[23] For example, a commercial development or infrastructure project brought in by an elected official may not be known to all stakeholders or may not fit with the more organic, participatory view of community upgrading and economic development envisaged by MCI and other on-the-ground partners.

interest in the country or region, and foundations are targets for these events, as are individual investors and philanthropists. Regional and national government—leadership as well as the relevant agencies—should play a key role as champions of their city's vibrancy and potential and, in many cases, as reliable counterparties for any prospective investment.

Innovations

As described above, in many areas, MCI has determined that a new approach, developed and tested by MCI and its partners, can fill the gap. The Early Childhood Education program, School2School Connectivity Project, Neonatal Survival Training program for health staff and new mothers, our approach to integrated urban planning and design, and our Girls' and Boys' LitClubs, are key examples.[24]

MCI has plans for further innovations, some of which constitute relatively modest expansions of our ongoing work, while others require additional resources.

The first major program undertaken by MCI—and now ready for expansion—is our pilot of an Urban Community Health Worker (CHW) training in Kisumu. Although training community health workers is commonly viewed as a cost-effective solution for the countryside, where few medical resources are generally available, it is MCI's contention that CHWs can be at least as effective, and a good deal more cost-effective, in urban areas, given the smaller distances and their ability to facilitate successful referrals and cover many more households in a given day. In urban settings, existing CHWs often focus on specific diseases or conditions, as they are generally trained by and accountable to individual, under-coordinated nongovernmental organizations with more limited mandates than what MCI has in mind. We intend for urban CHWs to be the frontline practitioners, just as in rural areas, but we wish for them to operate within a more tightly defined hub-and-spoke framework, with a more closely networked healthcare system and at least several reasonably well-equipped facilities serving as home base and backup.

A second initiative in regional GIS mapping and planning, coupled with capacity- and community-building and local governance strengthening, requires an infusion of resources to purchase the GIS equipment that will enable community and local government representatives to train in its uses and applications. Such an exercise will enable the community, urban policy planners, and environmental and emergency preparedness specialists to recognize the location and extent of pressing infrastructure gaps, schedule and budget essential repairs and upgrades, and learn

---

[24] Respectively, these projects were undertaken by the Mount Carmel Training Center, supported by the Government of Israel's Agency for International Cooperation (MASHAV), in Kumasi and now Accra; MCI, in partnership with Columbia University Teachers College, Ericsson, Airtel Ghana, and the Kumasi Metropolitan Education Directorate; MCI, in partnership with Johnson & Johnson, AmeriCares, the Ghana Health Service, and the Accra and Kumasi Metropolitan Health Directorates; MCI, together with the Earth Institute's Urban Design Lab and Center for Sustainable Urban Development, Accra Metropolitan Assembly, Kumasi Metropolitan Assembly, and Kwame Nkrumah University of Science and Technology; and MCI and LitWorld, together with the Kisumu Municipal Education Office and the Kumasi Metropolitan Education Directorate.

from local adaptations to chronic flooding and other impacts of climate change. Once equipped and trained in the uses of smartphones and/or other devices to carry out interactive GIS, ordinary residents will be able to report a flooded street or sewage line break to the City Hall, know that the information will appear immediately on the screens of the relevant officials, and expect a timely, effective government response. Based on the information gleaned, neighborhood consultations with local government officials to discuss the most pressing problems and plan viable remedies will not only improve communication and trust but can also enlist the community itself in the work of repairing or replacing inadequate civic infrastructure.

To deepen this involvement, MCI plans to engage the communities and residents themselves in the actual upgrading as part of their path to social and economic empowerment. The Urban Design Lab and MCI hope to mobilize—indeed, not only to mobilize but also to monetize as a tradable asset—the nearly boundless social capital inherent in each community. As an example, a mother interested in converting the front of her home into a retail storefront might trade an agreed amount of cooking or day care for an agreed amount of carpentry, plumbing, or electrical work to be carried out by a neighbor. We imagine a sort of exchange, to be guaranteed and perhaps run by a financial institution, wherein precise units of work, each with an attached monetary value, might be appraised and converted into currency or "credits" representing earned units of social capital that can be "spent" or reinvested in the new project.[25]

As mentioned, MCI and the Kisumu and Kumasi school districts hope to expand the Girls' and Boys' LitClubs program to cover many more girls and boys by establishing a number of Mothers' Clubs as a way to delivering to so many actual heads of families a range of services, including: livelihood, literacy, financial literacy, and ICT training that can lead to higher-income job opportunities; health care, screenings, and counseling; and advice on nutrition, family health, and hygiene.

MCI envisages taking the expansion of Girls' to Mothers' Clubs many steps further—to the creation of dedicated Centers for Women and Girls in several Millennium Cities, where Girls' and Mothers' Clubs and a comprehensive package of services and activities can be offered. In both Kisumu and Kumasi, services and activities addressing the declared needs of local women and girls are already well under way. In Kumasi, together with the women of the vibrant downtown Bantama neighborhood, Columbia's Urban Design Lab, Kumasi's Kwame Nkrumah University of Science and Technology, LitWorld, the Regional Ministry Department of Women, Global Fund for Women, African Women's Development Fund, Ghana's Association of Small-Scale Industries, and many other partners, we have also helped to plan, structure, and design such a Center, for which the city is now seeking financial and technical partners.

---

[25] Conceived by UDL faculty and MCI Advisory Committee member Geeta Mehta, a social capital credit system goes hand in glove with community upgrading while realizing other MDG-related objectives as well. As another example, youth in a poor community might support that community by paving or building a gutter in an alleyway that floods regularly, thereby earning SoCCs they can then use to start their own mobile phone repair shop or to enroll in a mobile phone repair or other technical training courses.

Strategically located near the open-air market at the heart of this thriving developing world city, the Kumasi Women's and Girls' Center will be run by indigenous women's organizations and vertically integrated with competent and committed national and international organizations able to provide meaningful, timely backstopping on a wide range of women's issues. The offerings currently envisaged, all of which have been recommended in the course of extensive consultations with local women, girls, and local authorities, include a sexual and reproductive health clinic, complete with rape counseling, emergency contraception, and family planning; a classroom to host training in literacy, financial literacy, computer literacy, mobile banking, savings, a myriad of job skills, and conservation-related activities; a day care and business center; and a large attractive space for meetings, speaker series, films, exhibitions, and concerts that can be rented out for weddings and other private and corporate events.

The purpose of these and similar such centers in Kumasi, Kisumu, and other partner venues is to empower women and girls and, through them, their communities, improving their lives and their options in irreversible, singularly transformative ways. Of course, the offerings, governance structures, and fund-raising modalities will vary widely from site to site. The research hypothesis here is that women and girls working together in a safe, dedicated space to address multiple priorities of vital interest to themselves, their families, and communities can effect lasting change through a synergistic assault on some of the symptoms and deep structures of the searing poverty they face every day—the poverty that so constrains their choices and their children's future. It is the hope of both the MCI and the Earth Institute and other international and local partners that establishing, piloting, and evaluating such Centers can lead to the confirmation and further championing of women as the primary delivery system for tangible progress toward achieving the MDGs.

Monitoring and Evaluation (M&E)

Due to its scope, levels of complexity, open-ended timetable, and pattern of city-specific evolution in response to identified need, MCI has not instituted a one-size-fits-all monitoring and evaluation component. We have put many tools in place, however, that give us feedback at multiple levels on the impact and effectiveness of our engagement with the individual cities and their residents.

First, MCI trains city employees in the relevant sector to work with the need assessment and costing instruments so that they can update the city's statistics on an annual basis, at least until the 2015 target date for MDG attainment. Obviously, MCI's published needs assessments cover education, gender, health, and water/sanitation, providing only a snapshot linked to a given moment of the city's capacity for service delivery in these sectors. These initial assessments have established certain baselines against which annual progress toward attaining the Goals in each area can be measured. The regional investment initiative, too, has established clear metrics against which progress is noted (most significantly, the ability to engage in investment profiling and promotion and the number of substantial, job-generating investments) in each of the participating Millennium Cities. Finally, many of the individual projects developed in response to specific gaps have their own M&E components, whether in our School2School Connectivity Project or the HBB training work described above. MCI is working to strengthen the reporting by the ultrasound trainees in Kumasi[26] and the health staff at Kumasi's two neonatal triage clinics (Mother-Baby Units, or MBUs). Although we are seeking data on symptoms, diagnosis, treatment, and follow-up, at this point the numbers of screenings, clinic visits, and the resulting decongestion of the neonatal ICU are the only data MCI and its partners have been able to obtain from our local colleagues on a regular basis.

Our MDG-based household survey is subjected to several layers of evaluation, few of them conventional. First is the validation of MCI's survey findings by the participating communities themselves, in what is apparently a rare instance of researchers returning to share their findings with those under scrutiny.[27] In our first pilot of this new instrument in Kisumu, Kenya, the 40+ community members with whom we held a workshop to review and give feedback on our findings—all were residents of one of three informal settlements where the study was carried out— were wonderfully responsive, exigent, and ultimately affirming of our conclusions, defining these, in many cases, with even greater precision than our own analysts had done.

These findings are now being translated into recommendations to policymakers at the level of the Kisumu City Council, city managers, and the new county government. As an example, while everyone is aware that transport is a major inhibitor for slum dwellers in the neighborhoods of Nyalenda A, Nyalenda B, and Obunga, it may be helpful to know that fixing the existing roads is a higher priority for residents than adding a walkway, bike path, or more buses. In Obunga, adding more bus routes is considered even more important than fixing the roads. In negotiations with private and public sector utilities and when preparing their annual budgets, it might also be useful for local officials to know that lack of access to clean water in these three neighborhoods is considered far less of a community-wide crisis than the dearth of sanitation and solid waste disposal facilities, which has resulted in the depositing of fecal matter and other wastes along footpaths and in drains, exacerbating the poor hygienic conditions and heightened rates among children of infection with waterborne diseases.

Having identified and confirmed the most severe deficits and priorities, MCI will assist community members in advocating for these upgrades in their community infrastructure and will follow up with the relevant municipal authorities. Two final

---

[26] The series of trainings has been conducted by the London-based International Society for Ultrasound in Obstetrics and Gynecology, with ultrasound equipment donated by Siemens.

[27] MCI was told by members of the community that although many researchers had come to Kisumu to investigate one aspect or another of their poverty, we were the first to return and share our findings with the study population.

measures of the usefulness of the survey findings will come in the form of: (1) a list of those recommendations that are actually budgeted and built/improved; and (2) an account of the impact on the community of each improvement.

MCI is now putting in place a robust M&E of the effectiveness of our Girls' LitClubs that will take into account not only any change in the girls' academic performance, but also their levels of confidence, sense of compassion and altruism, and the impact on their families. We will also examine effects of the program on the Girls' Clubs facilitators themselves, including changes in their effectiveness as teachers, sense of confidence and altruism, and the effect of their training and mentoring on their schools and communities. We are also developing a multilayered iteration of the planned Women's and Girls' Centers, including the selection of baseline indicators to be measured and an impact evaluation on the participating women and girls,[28] their families, and the surrounding community.

Dissemination, Replication, and Scaling Up

MCI publishes its research findings on the MCI website and in professional journals.[29] For our Regional Partnership to Promote Trade and Investment in sub-Saharan Africa, each participating city has created its own investment-related website, and each investment specialist has created his own log of activities, prospects, events, leads worth pursuing, and lessons learned, to be shared with city authorities and across the Regional Partnership. Additionally, MCI is developing an online toolkit to help cities attract investment. This virtual manual will spell out the steps for preparing materials, promoting investment opportunities and promising sectors, targeting and courting prospective investors, and providing effective aftercare services to ensure investors' ease of maneuvering and their satisfaction with their decision to invest in this venue.

Project-wide, MCI is also creating a new online "MCI Field Guide" that can serve as a "how to" for municipalities, agencies, NGOs, and individuals worldwide in everything from becoming a full-fledged Millennium City start-to-finish to replicating a MCI-designed project, such as our School2School Connectivity, Neonatal Resuscitation Training program, or Regional Partnership to Promote Trade and Investment in a new venue.[30]

Municipal officials worldwide, in poor countries and wealthy ones, can also search our field guide for the needs assessment and survey instruments MCI has used or generated, complete with manuals or relevant information for carrying them out in areas deemed to require urgent attention. Once these cities have measured how far

---

[28] In the Kumasi case, this would involve measuring also the impact of the designed physical space itself on the outcomes of the interventions among the women and girls.

[29] The MCI website, mci.ei.columbia.edu, is part of the Earth Institute website, at Columbia University.

[30] For projects carried out as part of a Millennium City program designed by a MCI partner, MCI directs interested parties to the appropriate organization or individual.

off-track the city is from attaining the MDGs in a particular area, they can design a package of targeted interventions expected to have a synergistic impact. Data, social sector, and investment analysts in local governments around the globe can read the MCI field guide to learn about valuable case studies in their particular fields of interest, including descriptions of best practices and lessons learned. This field guide is part of MCI's firm commitment to capacity building, which is the sine qua non of all field-based development work. Whole projects are clearly described and detailed so that they can readily be replicated and/or scaled, and pending resources and government commitment, a government's response to specific issues (e.g., neonatal survival) or to entire sectors (e.g., public health) can be reconfigured and rendered significantly more effective, based on the MDG-based prescriptions and recommendations enumerated in the needs assessments and household surveys.[31]

Conclusion

Overcrowded, underserved informal settlements have been part of the landscape since time immemorial. What has changed is that they have increasingly come to define the planet's present and are slated, should the current ratio of population growth to levels of investment persist, to be the face of its future. But as efforts continue, both to increase awareness of the scope of the challenges cities face and to gin up development assistance and private sector investment accordingly to meet these challenges, it is the *thinking* about urban poverty that urgently needs to be jolted into the twenty-first century. The essential integration of infrastructure with public health; the relevance of maternal survival not only to family nutrition but also to educational attainment, reductions in street crime, and improved economic outlook of entire communities; the centrality of clean water and adequate sanitation facilities to everything from child survival to student retention to the hopes of attracting tourists and foreign investors, all pose evidence of the utility of the fundamentally integrated, MDG-based conceptual framework that is at the heart of our work.

We live at a lucky moment, when the understanding, science, and technologies are readily available to devise transformative solutions to many of the seemingly chronic urban problems referenced in this chapter. There is no doubt that innovative action research, carried out by practiced groups and individuals from across the globe, will develop a repertoire of smart, effective interventions that can dramatically accelerate progress toward MDG attainment and the end of urban poverty, leapfrogging over many of the well-intentioned but inevitably inadequate single-sector fixes of the past. We require only the resolve, the tenacity, the treasury of willing and capable partners, and, first and last, the compassion, so that we might keep going, despite the many daunting obstacles, to see the cities where we are working through such transformations to a more humane, just, and healthier world.

---

[31] The remaining constraints on rapid progress generally align with those interventions and/or policy changes that cannot take place solely at the municipal level.

Chapter 12
Diagnostic Innovations in Developing Urban Settings

Patrick Beattie, Matthew Stewart, and Charles Mace

Health in Developing Urban Settings

There is a significant body of literature highlighting the importance of point-of-care diagnostics in improving health in developing countries [1]. Access to effective healthcare options can be severely limited in the developing world by the (typically) large distance between villages and appropriately stocked clinics and poor accessibility to skilled clinicians and physicians. This problem is often exacerbated by inadequate access to clean water, sanitation services, and a reliable source of electricity. The development of diagnostic tests, designed specifically for use in low-resource settings, would thus meet a substantial need. Urban and rural settings in the developing world are often beset by a lack of resources. The unique characteristics and different diagnostic needs of each setting, however, must be considered. Much attention is given to novel diagnostics designed for primary care settings in rural areas where patients are geographically far from the formal healthcare system, while urban areas are largely ignored. To understand the importance—and future—of diagnostics in developing urban settings, it is necessary to first understand the distinct ecosystem present there.

While the world is becoming more urbanized, there are significant differences behind the reasons for urbanization and the effects of urbanization on a city's residents in developed- and developing countries. Developed country urban areas and developing country urban areas have very different standards of public health, environmental health, and city planning. Between developing urban areas, there is important variability. For example, while urbanization appears to correlate with economic opportunities in many Latin and South American countries, this trend does not hold in Africa, where urbanization is more often driven by high fertility rates and people

P. Beattie, B.S.E. (✉) • M. Stewart, Ph.D. • C. Mace, Ph.D.
Diagnostics for All, 840 Memorial Drive, Cambridge, MA 02139, USA
e-mail: pdbeattie@gmail.com

© Springer New York 2015
R. Ahn et al. (eds.), *Innovating for Healthy Urbanization*,
DOI 10.1007/978-1-4899-7597-3_12

269

fleeing rural poverty. More importantly, developing urban areas have not benefited from the health improvements afforded by better housing and sanitation—as has occurred in developed urban areas. Instead, developing urban areas contend with an increasing burden of noncommunicable diseases in addition to persistent infectious disease. According to a 2000 World Health Organization article, the environmental change precipitated by urbanization has created novel environments for the spread of pathogens not typically found in those areas, adding to the burden of existing infectious disease. Unregulated slums in large cities, in particular, are susceptible to these effects [2].

An additional problem in developing urban areas is the large disparity between high-income and low-income populations. Income disparity without an engaged middle class can undermine public health services, leaving low-income patients with few affordable health options. High-income communities are typically more engaged in government and public decision-making than those in low-income groups, and they also are able to insulate themselves from the dangerous risk factors common in cities (e.g., pollution, poor health services, poor nutritional content of food). There is thus little incentive to improve public health systems that would benefit all levels of society. Without a middle class that is politically engaged but unable to afford the insulating solutions of the wealthy class, the unengaged poor are left with suboptimal public health systems and the burden of paying for health services through the private sector [2]. Therefore, affordable healthcare options are just as important in developing urban areas, as patients rely more on private providers of health care. Likewise, assumptions that point-of-care diagnostics are unnecessary in urban areas (where the distance to healthcare facilities is not as great as in rural areas) do not hold, though for different reasons that are outlined below. Other characteristics of an ideal diagnostic for rural settings, while still favorable, might be deprioritized depending on how health care is provided. To identify which characteristics are important in urban areas, we must first look at the types of diseases needing to be diagnosed.

Disease Classification and Diagnostic Needs

Diseases can be classified as either *communicable* or *noncommunicable*. Communicable diseases are those caused by pathogenic microorganisms (i.e., viruses, bacteria, and protozoa) and can be transmitted between people or animals, whereas noncommunicable diseases are those that cannot be transmitted to others. Both types of diseases can present as an acute sickness or a chronic, persisting affliction. Communicable and noncommunicable diseases present the healthcare system with very different challenges in terms of diagnosis and treatment. Communicable diseases primarily require diagnostic tools to identify a causative agent in order to inform proper treatment, while noncommunicable diseases, especially those of a chronic nature, require diagnostic tools for ongoing patient monitoring as well as initial diagnosis. Though the diagnostic requirements for each disease type differ, management of each disease type in developing urban settings would greatly benefit from innovation.

Communicable Diseases

Communicable diseases can spread through a population by a number of different mechanisms that result in the transmission of pathogens to humans: (1) direct transmission between people via contact with contaminated bodily fluids (e.g., rhinovirus or *M. tuberculosis*); (2) indirect transmission through environmental contamination, often with an origin in the feces of humans or animals (e.g., Giardia parasites or *E. coli* bacteria); (3) by a vector through a relatively unaffected host organism (e.g., malaria parasites carried by mosquitoes); or (4) by infected animals (e.g., rabies virus). Zoonotic pathogens—those agents transmitted to humans from nonhuman origins—account for greater than 60 % of infectious diseases that affect humans [3, 4]. In the case of zoonotics, the value of diagnostic tests rises beyond monitoring populations of animals (e.g., livestock and companion animals) to protecting human health, food sources, and the livelihood of farmers.

The focus of a diagnostic for a communicable disease is on the identification of a causative agent to inform clinicians and guide the selection of a treatment. Once an appropriate treatment has been determined, the need for further diagnosis is minimal; notable exceptions include chronic communicable diseases (e.g., hepatitis C), which might require ongoing monitoring [5]. In rural settings, a rapid diagnosis is important, because patients must travel long distances to centralized health facilities, and patient follow-up is difficult [6]. If they do not receive a diagnosis with their initial visit, it is unlikely that they will receive their results. These limitations, especially physical distance, do not necessarily apply in developing urban settings, but the need for rapid identification of communicable disease is just as important. In one study, less than 10 % of the patients testing positive for syphilis using a non-rapid diagnostic in Nairobi received treatment [7]. Additionally, poor public health and high population densities mean that hospitals are typically overburdened, and the time to treatment and quality of care can suffer [8]. One way to alleviate some of this burden is to push screening for communicable diseases to primary care facilities or the home through the use of point-of-care diagnostics. This strategy would allow for efficient triage outside of the hospital, separating those who need hospital follow-up from those who can self-treat. This potential improvement in care provision is dependent on innovations to bring the high quality of testing found at centralized hospitals to point-of-care platforms available outside of the hospital.

Below, we describe the potential for low-cost diagnostic tests to improve health care in developing urban settings using two model communicable diseases: enteric disorders and HIV/AIDS.

Enteric Disorders

Diarrhea, caused by infections from enteric pathogens, is a leading cause of mortality and morbidity worldwide [9] and affects young children disproportionately [10, 11]. The reduced availability of clean water and unsanitary living conditions in many developing urban environments (e.g., slums) exacerbates the spread of enteric diseases. The physiological symptoms of enteric disorders are easy to diagnose (e.g., abdominal pain and/or diarrhea [12]), but infection by a number of pathogens [13]—bacteria (e.g., enterotoxigenic *E. coli*), viruses (e.g., rotavirus), and protozoa (e.g., cryptosporidium)—are known to cause this very common condition. Proper treatment requires identifying the cause of the symptoms. Antibiotics, for example, will not cure viral diseases and, when administered prophylactically, can lead to drug resistance [14] or advantageous colonization by dangerous flora [15]. Therefore, it is important for clinicians to use diagnostic tests to identify the specific pathogen before selecting a method of treatment. Two common test methods include molecular diagnostics and standard microbial culture techniques. These methods, however, are difficult to implement in low-resource settings, because they are either too expensive (e.g., PCR amplification of a gene sequence) or require well-equipped, centralized laboratories with highly trained personnel (e.g., culture). In many cases, easy-to-use point-of-care tests to classify the pathogenic microorganisms would be sufficient to influence healthcare decisions and select a course of treatment.

HIV and AIDS

Infection with HIV ultimately leads to AIDS, an incurable disease. While AIDS is no longer considered to be acutely fatal, it remains a global epidemic and affects developing urban environments disproportionately. The causes for this disparity are related to living conditions in comparison to those in rural or established urban settings: inhabitants of developing urban centers become sexually active at a younger age, have more sexual partners, and are less likely to adopt preventative strategies [16]. AIDS can be managed with a carefully administered therapeutic program to slow the progression of the disease and treat opportunistic disorders. Over six million people in the developing world are treated with highly active antiretroviral therapy (HAART) [17], antiretroviral drugs that inhibit a number of the important pathways in the replicative life cycle of the HIV virus. The result of effective treatment is a decrease in the number of HIV particles in the blood and an increase in the number of CD4+ cells that can be found in the blood; diagnostic tests for these markers can be used as a prognosis of the efficacy of HAART (vide infra). Another use of diagnostics in the treatment of HIV is to monitor the side effects of HAART. Antiretroviral drugs may cause hepatotoxicity [18]; therefore, rapid point-of-care diagnostic assays for liver function would help healthcare workers determine the safety and efficacy of treatment regimens.

Noncommunicable Diseases

Noncommunicable diseases are the predominant cause of death worldwide. According to a 2012 WHO World Health Statistics report, mortality rates from noncommunicable diseases are rising and account for approximately 60 % of deaths per year in low- and middle-income countries [19]. Therefore, these diseases are a major threat to global health and economic development. While noncommunicable chronic diseases, such as cardiovascular disease, cancer, and diabetes may have once been thought of as developed-world problems, the reality is that the developing world accounts for the majority of this burden. In a 2007 paper in *The Lancet*, Abegunde et al. state that in 2005 over 80 % of global deaths from chronic diseases occurred in low- and middle-income countries and that the overall burden of chronic diseases was quickly increasing, driven by rapid population growth in developing urban areas [20]. According to the same paper, the cost of doing nothing to address the issues of heart disease, stroke, and diabetes—in terms of reduced economic output—will be $84 billion over a 10-year period, with millions of people unnecessarily dying during that time period. Requiring patients to utilize healthcare facilities for ongoing management of their disease is inefficient and unsustainable.

Unlike communicable diseases, whose causative agents are identifiable, the causes of noncommunicable diseases are more difficult to diagnose. Sources of noncommunicable diseases may be environmental, genetic, or due to lifestyle choices. Diseases caused by environmental factors—or those that cannot be directly controlled by an individual—include acute toxicity from the ingestion of heavy metals (e.g., tainted water supply) and the effects of malnutrition. Genetic diseases include autoimmune disorders (e.g., lupus or celiac disease), hemophilia, and sickle cell anemia. Diseases that arise from the lifestyle choices of an individual include cirrhosis (liver damage linked to alcoholism) and emphysema (lung damage linked to smoking tobacco). While it may be instructive to classify the causes of noncommunicable diseases in this way, a great number of them are caused by a combination of factors. Examples of such noncommunicable diseases include diabetes mellitus type 2 (lifestyle choices and genetics) [21], allergies (environmental and genetics) [22], and cancer (environmental, lifestyle, genetics) [23].

According to a 2005 analysis of the disability-adjusted life years (DALY) burden—a measure of the costs of mortality and morbidity—in developing countries, the most burdensome noncommunicable diseases are: cardiovascular diseases, diabetes, cancer, and chronic respiratory diseases [24]. Notably, an important factor in the large DALY burden for each of these diseases is their chronic nature, requiring ongoing monitoring and care. A prime example of this is diabetes, where a single test might identify a patient as diabetic, but one or more blood glucose tests per day are needed to maintain an individualized plan to manage a patient's health. The need for continual monitoring in parallel with an extended period of treatment creates a vastly different model of healthcare provision than that encountered during the management of communicable diseases. If patient monitoring is limited to health facilities, the patient burden on the health facility will continue to increase, overwhelming the facility and reducing quality of care for all patients. Despite the physical proximity to healthcare facilities in developing urban areas, at-home diagnosis and monitoring solutions must become an integral part of the healthcare system.

For certain noncommunicable diseases (e.g., cardiovascular disease, many cancers), initial diagnosis requires highly skilled personnel and centralized facilities with specialized instrumentation. Access to these resources is restricted in most developing urban areas, due to heavily constrained healthcare budgets. The emerging field of biomarker discovery, however, is reforming this paradigm by enabling the development of rapid, point-of-care diagnostic tests for noncommunicable diseases. A prominent example is the quantitative measurement of cardiac troponins as a means to diagnose cardiac health [25]. Immunoassays for troponin have been developed successfully for a number of laboratory [26] and point-of-care platforms [27]. These point-of-care technologies, however, rely on portable electronic instruments and individual test cartridges. The high costs associated with these components have limited their penetration in developing world markets.

Diabetes

For many reasons, diabetes can be considered the archetypal noncommunicable disease. There are methods to diagnose, monitor, and manage diabetes, and diagnostic tests are available and in use globally. Before the first blood glucose reader was introduced in 1970, monitoring of glucose levels by patients was limited to urine dipsticks. This was suboptimal, as urinalysis could only detect blood glucose levels elevated above the renal threshold and with an inherent delay in the results. Despite these limitations in at-home monitoring, it was not until the mid-1970s that at-home use of blood glucose readers was considered, and even then, there were significant concerns as to their accuracy, ease of use, and affordability [28]. The concerns have been addressed through technological advances, and at-home blood glucose monitoring is now an integral part of managing diabetes in developed countries. Similar diagnostic strategies exist in the developing world, but significant challenges still remain due to the economic strain of frequent testing and treatment. The costs associated with diabetes—due to the aggregate prices of consultation, syringes, insulin, and testing—can be massive in comparison to an individual's yearly income. For example, the cost of treating diabetes can account for up to 75 % of yearly wages for those living in developing urban settings [29]. Further complications arise for individuals with tuberculosis infections, as there is a strong link between diabetes and an increase in the risk of developing active and difficult-to-treat tuberculosis [30]. Proper diagnostic tests for each disease would generate valuable, actionable information toward providing individualized health care, and affordable at-home monitoring solutions would improve service provision at overburdened hospitals.

Cancer

One of the most difficult diseases to diagnose in a point-of-care or low-resource environment is cancer. Environmental (e.g., melanoma caused by sunlight), lifestyle (e.g., lung carcinoma caused by smoking), and genetic factors (e.g., lymphomas) can cause cancer, which is a leading cause of death worldwide [31]. Tumors commonly are located within the body, and, as a result, cancers are diagnosed using sophisticated imaging technology—X-ray, computed tomography (CT), and positron emission tomography (PET) are three such techniques—that is not typically available in the developing world. A combination of tumor biopsy and microscopy is a more accessible approach but requires significant expertise and infrastructure to employ. The majority of cancer cases in the developing world are detected at an advanced and untreatable stage—due to inadequate screening and early diagnosis services [32]. Biomarkers may be useful diagnostically for some cancers, such as prostate cancer (prostate-specific antigen) and ovarian cancer (CA-125). While the accuracy and specificity for these biomarkers are still in question [33, 34], a bladder cancer biomarker (NMP-22) [35] has been validated clinically and is used in FDA-approved point-of-care diagnostic assays (NMP22 BladderChek, Alere). It is apparent that true point-of-care diagnostic tests—using a combination of new methods to obtain biospecimens, biomarker discovery and validation, and technology development—would find immediate use in diagnosing and combating cancer.

Solutions to Better Diagnosis in Developing Urban Areas

There are several possible ways to improve the health of patients suffering from chronic or noncommunicable diseases in developing urban areas. For example, improving the existing healthcare system, reducing income disparity or improving the voice of low-income urban dwellers, and reducing environmental and behavioral risk factors, could improve patient health [2, 36]. Another method to improve patient care would be to empower patients and improve treatment efficiency through at-home diagnosis and monitoring tools. As the incidence of noncommunicable diseases continues to rise in developing urban areas, the development of novel, affordable, at-home diagnostics will become immensely important to prevent over-burdening of hospitals and the associated impacts on patient care.

Characteristics of an Ideal Test

The World Health Organization Sexually Transmitted Diseases Diagnostics Initiative (WHO/SDI) developed the ASSURED criteria to determine if diagnostics are suitable for deployment in limited-resource settings [37]. ASSURED stands for Affordable, Sensitive (i.e., low probability of false negatives), Specific (i.e., low probability of false positives), User-friendly (i.e., easy to use, requiring minimal training), Rapid and Robust (i.e., short time to a result, stable and reliable at ambient conditions), Equipment-free, and Deliverable to end users. These settings, however, place more demanding design challenges on diagnostics that are not as critical in developed urban areas with reliable sources of power, refrigeration, supply chains, and trained personnel. Although these criteria were created to evaluate diagnostics for resource-limited rural settings, many of these criteria are also relevant for diagnostics designed for use in developing urban areas.

The *affordability* of a diagnostic is particularly important to consider when designing Point of Care (POC) tests for developing urban areas. As stated in the introduction, while urban areas have relatively more wealth than rural areas, there is a great disparity in wealth that causes urban dwellers to rely more on private providers of health care, which means affordability is still important. Ideally, the final cost of the diagnostic should be pennies and include the cost of materials, manufacturing, packaging, shipment, and storage. Manufacturing tests in a developing urban area for local distribution and use reduces a number of these costs and has the added benefit of bolstering the local economy. The cost of materials can be minimized by using relatively inexpensive components, such as plastics and paper-based materials.

Clinical *sensitivity and specificity* are two important performance characteristics of diagnostic devices. These characteristics are evaluated by comparing the results of the test to the results of a reference standard test (i.e., a "gold standard") for the same panel of samples. The clinical sensitivity is defined as the probability that a sample shown to be positive by the gold standard test will also test positive using the test under evaluation. The clinical specificity is defined as the probability that a sample shown to be negative by the gold standard test will also test negative with the test under evaluation. Designing POC diagnostics with both high sensitivity and specificity is desirable. Diagnostic tests should also provide reproducible results. The reproducibility or precision of a test is often reported as the coefficient of variation (CV), which is the standard deviation of a measurement normalized by the mean. This value is typically reported as a percentage; an ideal diagnostic has a %CV of zero. Although this goal cannot be achieved realistically, diagnostic manufacturers strive to minimize this value and generally achieve CVs less than 10 %. For example, Roche's handheld Accutrend® Plus meter measures blood glucose and cholesterol levels with a %CV of ~3 % [38], and Abbott's i-STAT measures cardiac troponin I in blood with a %CV of ~8 % [39].

User-friendliness is another characteristic that is important, regardless of the setting, and is especially critical for tests designed for home use by patients to reduce the burden on hospitals. A user should be able to administer a test successfully with little to no technical training. Ideally, the test should require as few steps as possible, little to no sample preparation, and be minimally-invasive and self-contained. The results should be available within minutes of applying the sample, and the readout should be clear and have a low likelihood of misinterpretation. A rapid time to result enables users to take immediate action to manage a chronic condition or illness or prevent spread of infectious diseases. Diabetics self-monitoring blood glucose is a classic example where rapid time to result is important for the effective management of a disease.

An ideal POC diagnostic should also be *robust* and dependable. Diagnostics often contain biological reagents that can lose activity when exposed to harsh environmental conditions. In developed urban areas, tests are transported and stored in controlled environments (i.e., the cold chain) that prolongs a product's lifetime. In developing urban areas, however, reliable refrigeration and controlled environments may be lacking (e.g., brownouts), and tests may be exposed to harsh conditions ranging from freezing to tropical temperatures that degrade device performance. Therefore, reagent stability is an important consideration when designing tests for developing urban areas. One method of improving the activity of reagents is to dry and store them on fibrous membranes with additional stabilizers, such as proteins and sugars.

POC diagnostics for use in limited-resource settings should require *no external equipment* and little to no power to operate. These characteristics are less important in developing urban areas where adequate infrastructure exists and there is often access to relatively consistent power. However, requiring equipment often increases cost significantly, which could limit availability of the diagnostic or restrict it to well-funded hospitals instead of primary care or at-home testing. One of the aims of innovation in diagnostics for developing urban areas is to push diagnosis and monitoring into primary care and at-home testing in order to reduce burden on hospitals. Therefore, the cost of required external equipment can be very important, even in urban areas.

Ultimately, a diagnostic must be adopted by its target population in order to generate a benefit. Barriers to adoption can include an unintuitive user interface, operational complexity, or something as fundamental as failing to avoid cultural taboos. An example of a product failing after market introduction due to this simple, yet vital, consideration is the mosquito bed net [40]. In this case, users in certain sub-Saharan regions of Africa were expected to sleep under white bed nets, a color culturally associated with those who had recently died. In this case, simply changing the color of the nets addressed this taboo. By involving potential end users through user-centered design, diagnostic developers can minimize the risk that their product will not be used for cosmetic or other nontechnical reasons.

This section has shown that while an *ideal* test follows the ASSURED guidelines, not every characteristic must be met in order for a diagnostic device to be useful in developing urban areas. In addition to considering these criteria, innovative groups must also work closely with end users to identify the most important characteristics of a test and ensure that the user interface is intuitive and that the test is culturally acceptable and perceived as useful. If these additional criteria are not considered, a diagnostic test may not achieve widespread adoption.

Technologies

As previously discussed, there exists a real need for innovative diagnostic technologies that will allow for diagnosis and monitoring to be moved from overburdened hospitals to primary care facilities and at-home testing. Because of the unique challenges of providing health care in developing urban areas, innovation at the technology level is critically needed. The sections below describe POC tests that are commercially available or in development at the time of publication of this chapter. The advantages and disadvantages of each test or diagnostic platform will be discussed in context of its utility in developing urban areas.

Commercial POC Tests

Several technologies already on the market could have a positive impact in developing urban areas if their current limitations are addressed.

Electrochemical Readers

Glucometers

Untreated diabetes and its associated complications are burdens on budgets, families, and healthcare systems worldwide. Although diabetes mellitus type 2 is often considered a disease of the developed world, it is a growing global problem [41]. The burden of diabetes in developing urban areas can be reduced through the use of glucometers. The glucometer is a POC diagnostic device that enables diabetic patients to regularly monitor and control blood glucose levels—through insulin therapy and/or diet—to prevent acute and late-stage complications of the disease. It is one of the most ubiquitous and commercially successful POC tests on the market in developed countries.

Early POC blood glucose test technologies were developed in the mid-1960s by the Ames Division of Miles Laboratories (now part of Bayer) [42]. Its test strips, marketed as Dextrostix®, contained dried enzymes and chromagens that produced a visible, colored product in the presence of glucose. The user applied a drop of blood to the reagent-impregnated zone of the test strip, waited 1 minute, rinsed the blood from the strip, and matched the color of the test zone to a calibrated, color-coded read guide. Two examples of tests on the market that use visual color matching to estimate blood glucose levels include the BETACHEK® Visual by National Diagnostic Products and the Chemcard™ Glucose Test by Chematics, Inc.

These tests are affordable, use robust reagents, do not require external equipment or power, are portable, and provide rapid test results (~3 minutes). The tests are convenient to use in any location, deliverable to end users, and reported to be accurate and reproducible. According to company product literature, an independent study showed that the BETACHEK® has a high level of accuracy compared to a reference method ($R^2=0.977$) and a low percent coefficient of variation (<5 %). Although these tests have many advantages, they require multiple user steps to obtain results, and the visual readout by color matching is subject to user interpretation.

Most glucometers on the market today consist of battery-operated, hand-held electronic readers and single-use, disposable test strips. To measure blood glucose levels, the user inserts a test strip into the meter and applies a finger-stick drop of blood to the end or side of the strip. The digital display provides visual numeric readout of blood glucose levels. These glucometers are cost-effective, accurate, and easy to use. User interaction is minimized, and blood glucose measurements are obtained visually or audibly within seconds.

Glucometers use electrochemical measurements to determine blood glucose levels, and the electrodes and reagents necessary for these measurements are printed directly on a disposable test strip. A finger-stick drop of blood is delivered to the reagents and electrodes on the strip via passive wicking through a microfluidic capillary. Today's meters require less than 1 μL of blood and provide results in 5 seconds [43]. The prevalence of diabetes and the need for frequent blood glucose measurements create a high demand for glucose test strips. The strips are produced at a scale of approximately 10^{10} test strips per year, with single manufacturing lines producing roughly 10^6 test strips per hour [44]. These large manufacturing scales are achieved using well-established, high-precision printing and lamination technologies that drive the manufacturing cost down to pennies per test strip.

Digital glucometers have several advantages for disease management in developing urban areas, because they satisfy most of the ASSURED criteria. Although the electronic readers require batteries, they generally have low power consumption and long battery lifetimes. The main disadvantage of this technology is the pain associated with finger sticks to obtain blood samples for analysis.

Given the frequency of testing, maximizing user comfort has been (and will continue to be) a key focus in the development of glucometers. Requirements of blood sample volumes, and thus lancing depths, have been reduced to minimize the discomfort associated with finger sticks. Many glucometers function with blood drawn from alternative sites, such as the arm or thigh [45]. Another approach to reducing the discomfort associated with lancing devices and blood sampling is developing minimally invasive or noninvasive measurement techniques, such as sampling interstitial fluids or transcutaneous spectroscopy [43]. These devices have the potential to make continuous blood glucose measurements and enable closed-loop insulin dosing. Scientists are also developing ways to reappropriate electronic glucometers to measure analytes other than glucose in whole blood, such as cholesterol and lactate [46]. This approach involves making test strips with appropriate chemistries for a specific metabolite and determining the correlation between glucometer response and metabolite levels using standards.

Cholesterol/Triglycerides

Cardiovascular disease is emerging as a social and economic burden on the people and healthcare systems in developing countries [47]. Devices similar to glucometers are available for measuring triglyceride and cholesterol levels in blood, which are important markers for cardiovascular disease risk assessment. Two commercially available systems include Roche's Accutrend Plus and Polymer Technology Systems, Inc.'s CardioChek Plus. Both devices consist of handheld electronic meters and separate, disposable test strips that can measure a number of different analytes. The test strips contain enzymes and reactive dyes that produce changes in the reflectance of the test strip in the presence of analyte. The meters convert reflectance to a clinically relevant value, and the user reads the test result from the digital display. Both the CardioChek Plus and Accutrend Plus are FDA-approved and

CLIA-waived. These devices have similar advantages and disadvantages as glucometers; however, cholesterol and triglyceride levels do not need to be measured as frequently as blood glucose levels.

Lateral Flow

The lateral flow or immunochromatographic strip test is a well-established diagnostic platform developed to enable low-cost, rapid POC testing. The tests are designed for single use and enable qualitative or semiquantitative visual detection of a variety of analytes including proteins, small molecules, antibodies, nucleic acids, and viruses [48]. One of the earliest and quintessential lateral flow tests is the home pregnancy test. Most lateral flow tests do not require the addition of external reagents, making them straightforward to perform and user-friendly. The user simply adds sample, waits several minutes, and looks for the appearance of colored lines (i.e., sample and control lines) in the test window. Figure 12.1 shows a schematic of a traditional lateral flow test.

The main benefits of lateral flow tests are their simplicity of use and of readout. The user is typically required just to apply the sample (and perhaps a chase fluid), and the natural wicking potential of the material begins the test. Specifically, a liquid sample is applied to the sample pad, and the fluid wicks into the device by capillary action. The sample picks up a visual labeling agent or detection conjugate (e.g., antibody-gold nanoparticle or antibody-latex particle conjugates) stored in dry form in the conjugate pad. In a sandwich assay, binding between the conjugate and target analyte in the sample occurs as the fluid moves through the membrane. As the sample wicks along the membrane, the analyte-conjugate complexes are bound by antibodies or other capture agents immobilized at the test line on the membrane. At sufficient densities, the captured conjugates form a visible colored line on the membrane that is read by eye. Gold nanoparticle conjugates appear pink or red, and polystyrene or latex particle conjugates are typically dyed red or blue. The absorbent pad wicks excess sample and conjugate from the membrane. Lateral flow tests include a control line that should also be visible after running a sample. A lack of color at the control line indicates an invalid test. The user needs only to determine whether there is color present or not in the test area, meaning that even untrained users can perform these tests with relatively high accuracy.

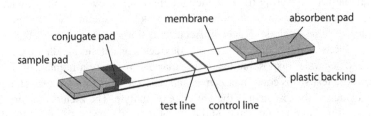

Fig. 12.1 Schematic illustration of the components of a lateral flow test

Lateral flow tests meet many of the ASSURED criteria, making them well suited for POC testing in developing urban areas. The tests are affordable (they are composed of relatively inexpensive plastic materials and porous membranes), and they are easily manufactured at high volumes and low cost using established printing, cutting, and lamination technologies. In many cases, the most expensive components of lateral flow tests are the biomolecular reagents; however, this cost can be minimized through high-volume production. Since the tests use capillary action to drive fluid flow and results are visually read, no expensive external equipment or power is needed. This makes lateral flow tests compact, portable, deliverable to end users, and easy to operate. The tests are also generally robust, can be shipped without refrigeration, and be stored for more than a year when appropriately sealed in pouches with desiccant [49]. A variety of biological samples are compatible with lateral flow tests including blood, plasma, urine, stool, and saliva. Samples with higher viscosity, such as stool or saliva, however, must be either mixed with a diluent or buffer before testing or chased with additional liquid to help it travel along the membrane.

Although lateral flow platforms have many attractive features, these diagnostic tools have several notable constraints. For example, detecting multiple analytes (i.e., multiplexing) on one test strip can be challenging, because different reagent sets can potentially interfere with one another, and the optimal test conditions (e.g., pH, blocking agents, and surfactants) for one reagent set may not be suitable for a different reagent set. It is also challenging to test limited sample volumes on lateral flow tests without the addition of a diluent or buffer. Lateral flow tests also have limited quantitative analysis capabilities.

Traditional colloidal gold lateral flow tests are typically limited to low nanomolar visual detection limits [50]. Greater analytical sensitivity (100–1,000-fold more) can be achieved using external readers, alternative conjugate labels (e.g., fluorophores), or additional signal enhancement techniques such as silver amplification of gold nanoparticle conjugates [6, 47]. These approaches, however, can increase assay cost and/or complexity.

In addition to pregnancy, other examples of commercially available lateral flow tests include assays for infectious diseases (e.g., influenza, HIV, dengue fever, hepatitis, gonorrhea, syphilis, chlamydia, and malaria), cardiac markers, and illicit drugs.

Emerging Technologies

Although glucometers and lateral flow tests are powerful diagnostic platforms, there is a need for more advanced POC devices that can perform complex, multistep laboratory-based analyses (e.g., immunoassays, cell counts). Ideally these systems should be portable, highly automated, and require little to no user interaction to obtain results. Devices that perform several laboratory procedures (e.g., sequential reagent addition, mixing, washing, and detection) are often referred to as "lab-on-a-chip" or "micro-total analysis systems." Microfabrication and microfluidics have emerged as promising technologies to achieve this goal. The sections below describe lab-on-a-chip technologies developed or in development that have potential for improving health in developing urban areas. The interested reader can find a comprehensive survey of companies using microfluidic and lab-on-a-chip technologies in a recent review article by Chin and colleagues [51].

Microfluidic Technologies

Microfluidic-based diagnostics are lab-on-a-chip devices that test for single or multiple analytes in less than a milliliter of sample. This is typically achieved by creating tiny (<1-mm-wide) channels in glass or plastic and using specially designed analyzers to move the sample and other fluids in a predefined manner to perform analyses. The origin of microfluidic device development dates back to the 1970s; however, it was not until the 1980s that academic interest in microfluidics began to intensify [52]. The main benefits of microfluidic technologies are their ability to manipulate small volumes of fluid, perform several analyses from one sample (i.e., multiplexing), perform complex operations (e.g., mixing and splitting), and achieve a higher assay sensitivity than lateral flow devices. Unfortunately, this typically comes at increased cost; most microfluidic diagnostics require an analyzer and fine-tolerance manufacturing. This section will outline some of the plastic- or glass-based microfluidic technologies currently in development that could have a large positive impact in developing urban areas.

Small Molecule Analyzers

Abbott's i-STAT blood analyzer is an example of a successful, commercially available POC diagnostic that uses active microfluidic technology. The i-STAT is used in over 1,800 hospitals worldwide and gives clinicians access to laboratory-quality data within minutes at the POC, which allows them to make critical treatment decisions in real time. The system consists of a handheld, battery-operated analyzer and single-use, disposable test cartridges to perform several different clinical chemistry tests and/or immunoassays. The cartridges have microfluidic channels for sample handling and microfabricated thin-film electrodes for making electrochemical measurements. Each cartridge contains stored calibrant and is designed to perform one or more (i.e., a panel) quantitative diagnostic tests on <100 μL of blood, including measurements of blood gases, electrolytes, lactate, glucose, creatinine, hemoglobin, hematocrit, coagulation parameters, and cardiac markers. The i-STAT has several features that make it easy to use and effective in emergency and critical care applications: no sample pretreatment steps, automated calibration, bar code scanning for automatic loading of user or patient information, a docking unit for downloading test results for electronic record keeping, and wireless transmission and sharing of test results. This device meets many of the ASSURED criteria; however, the high price of the analyzer limits the settings where it would be economical. Reduction in overall cost and cartridges designed specifically for the needs of primary care facilities in developing urban areas would make this technology much more useful by allowing for the transfer of care from hospitals to primary care facilities. In its current form, however, this powerful technology is not a practical solution for at-home testing or for use in many urban and rural areas of the developing world (due to its cost).

Quantitative, Rapid Immunoassays

Immunoassays are a category of tests that detect the presence or amount of an analyte through the use of immune system antibodies selected to bind to the target analyte. Several technologies on the market are based on immunoassay principles. For instance, the previously mentioned lateral flow tests use immunoassay detection. Immunoassays can be performed in formats that are qualitative (e.g., lateral flow tests) or quantitative (e.g., enzyme-linked immunosorbent assays, ELISAs). ELISAs can be performed using a variety of biological samples and are often highly sensitive, but they are not well-suited for POC testing applications in developing urban areas. ELISAs require costly reagents, well-equipped labs, and trained personnel, and it can take hours or longer to obtain results. Claros Diagnostics recognized the limitations of traditional immunoassays for developing world applications and was founded in 2004 to create a low-cost, easy-to-use POC diagnostic platform that can perform complex, multistep immunoassays in minutes with high sensitivity and specificity. The platform consists of a photometric analyzer and inexpensive disposable plastic assay cassettes that contain networks of microfluidic channels and reagents to perform quantitative immunoassays. The analyzer uses pneumatic actuation to combine sample (whole blood or urine) and reagents in a controlled manner to perform multistep immunoassays with silver enhancement chemistries to achieve high analytical sensitivities. The analyzer comes in both a benchtop and battery-operated handheld unit.

In 2010, Claros obtained CE marking for a prostate cancer immunoassay test and is currently pursuing FDA approval with CLIA waiver for the US market. The platform has also been used to successfully diagnose HIV and syphilis in field trials in sub-Saharan Africa [53]. Although the technology was initially designed to offer a relatively low-cost method of acquiring lab-quality immunoassay test results at the POC in developing countries, the technology has also proven attractive for use in developed countries. Claros was acquired by Opko Health in 2011 and will expand its testing capabilities to include panels for infectious diseases, cardiology, neurodegenerative diseases, companion diagnostics, and women's health. The Claros platform strives to provide improved sensitivity and quantitative results when compared to lateral flow but with increased cost. Similar to the i-STAT, the higher cost and need to purchase an analyzer means that this technology will have limited utility in an at-home testing setting. Instead, with the development of test cartridges specifically aimed toward the needs of developing countries and depending on final cost, it has the potential to positively impact health care delivery at primary healthcare facilities in urban (and rural) settings.

Cell Analyzers

In addition to small molecule and immunoassay detection, microfluidic devices are being developed to perform cell-type analyses. One company developing POC diagnostics for cell-type analysis using a microfluidic platform is Daktari Diagnostics, Inc. Daktari is developing a robust, portable CD4+ cell-counting system (Daktari CD4) that allows physicians in remote settings to monitor the immune status of patients. Measuring CD4+ cell count is particularly important for monitoring the progression of HIV and AIDS and the effects of therapeutic treatments (e.g., highly active antiretroviral therapy). Flow cytometry is traditionally used to measure CD4+ cell counts in centralized laboratories. However, this testing is limited to only the best supported urban hospitals, because flow cytometers are expensive to purchase and maintain and require highly skilled personnel to prepare and test samples. A CD4+ cell diagnostic suitable for primary healthcare facilities would enable monitoring of HIV+ patients to be moved away from overburdened hospitals. This would result in more efficient screening for those patients in need of further care and streamline care provided at the hospitals.

The Daktari CD4 consists of a portable analyzer and disposable plastic microfluidic cartridges with on-board reagents stored in blister packs. The system uses a combination of microfluidic cell chromatography, cell lysis, and impedance spectroscopy to provide CD4+ cell counts from a finger-stick drop of blood. Sample preparation and reagent delivery are automated, thereby minimizing the need for user interaction. In comparison to flow cytometry, the Daktari CD4 system is more suitable for use in developing urban areas—it is more user-friendly, less expensive, and provides faster results. The Daktari CD4 is in development and undergoing performance evaluations.

An alternative approach to rapid CD4+ cell counting is being developed by Zyomyx. The Zyomyx platform uses separation by sedimentation and cell stacking in a disposable high-precision capillary to estimate cell counts. A measurement is performed by mixing a finger-stick drop of blood with antibody-particle conjugates (1-μm particles) and injecting the mixture into a closed-end glass capillary filled with a high-density medium. Results are interpreted visually within tens of minutes. This system has several advantages over competing technologies, including low cost, rapid time to results, no need for external equipment or power and it is simple to use. Given these advantages, this system has the potential to greatly improve the treatment and health of patients in developing urban areas.

Paper Microfluidic Devices

Within the last 5 years, paper-based microfluidics have emerged to provide an attractive platform for the development of easy-to-use, low-cost, portable, and disposable diagnostics for POC testing in resource-limited settings. Paper microfluidic devices were originally developed by Andres Martinez and Professor George Whitesides at Harvard University to address several limitations of traditional glass- or plastic-based microfluidics. Paper-based microfluidics leverage the natural wicking properties of paper to drive fluid flow. Wicking eliminates the need for power or external pumps to actuate fluids and run samples, which reduces the cost of the tests and makes them compact, portable, easy to operate, and useful for at-home monitoring. Paper is also readily available, inexpensive, and relatively easy to manufacture and process. Despite all of these benefits, one significant limitation of paper is that a sample wicking through the paper will travel radially unless somehow constrained. This makes it difficult to control fluid flow and therefore perform anything other than simple assays, such as those performed on unidirectional lateral flow test strips. Martinez and Whitesides were able to overcome this limitation by patterning hydrophobic barriers in paper to direct fluid flow along desired paths [54].

Several methods to pattern paper have been developed in recent years. The original method described by Martinez et al. involved UV curing of a photosensitive polymer, SU8 [54]. Methods using other photosensitive polymers were subsequently developed by Whitesides [55]. Fenton et al. [56] and Fu et al. [57] describe cutting methods as a means of patterning paper (in these cases the edges of the substrate act as barriers). Li et al. [58] describe a method of patterning hydrophilic channels in a hydrophobic paper using plasma treatment. A very simple method called wax printing, described by Lu et al., uses a commercially-available printer and an oven to create hydrophobic barriers [59]. A version of this process developed by Carrilho et al. [60] and Diagnostics For All is described in more detail below.

The wax printing method of patterning paper leverages existing commercial printers with solid-ink technology, such as the Xerox ColorQube. This method of fabrication is scalable and can provide the volumes of devices needed to reach global markets. Figure 12.2 shows the process for making wax-patterned paper-based microfluidics using a solid-ink printer.

Devices are designed on a computer using standard graphics software, and the hydrophobic wax walls of the microfluidic channels are printed onto the surface of a sheet of paper. The printed paper is then heated to above the melting point of the wax so that it permeates through the thickness of the paper to create hydrophobic barriers. Channels patterned in this way wick microliter volumes of fluids by capillary action and distribute the fluids into test zones where independent assays take place, similar to the SU-8 patterned device shown in Fig. 12.3. Many different types of paper or porous materials can be patterned using this technique—including materials composed of cellulose, nitrocellulose, and nylon—such that the properties of the membrane can be selected for specific applications (e.g., filtering, wicking fluids, and storing reagents) and sample types (e.g., urine, feces, blood, or saliva).

More complex microfluidic networks are made by stacking layers of patterned paper and affixing them to one another with layers of patterned adhesive (Fig. 12.4) [61]. These multilayer microfluidic devices enable control of wicking fluids in three dimensions and provide access to a variety of fluidic operations, including splitting, incubation, and mixing. Figure 12.4 shows an example of a multilayer device with four sample inlets that divide each sample into an array of 16 individual detection zones on the bottom face of the device (256 detection zones total). The length of each fluidic channel connecting the sample inlet and the detection zones is equal

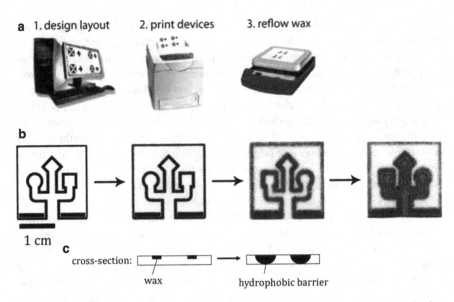

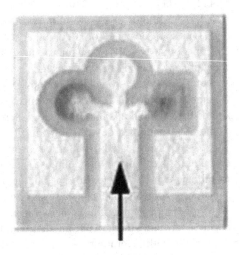

Fig. 12.2 Patterning hydrophobic barriers using wax printing. (**a**) Devices are prepared using inexpensive equipment: device layouts are designed using computer software (*1*), a commercially available printer prints solid wax ink onto paper (*2*), and a hot plate or other heat source reflows the wax to create hydrophobic channels throughout the thickness of the paper (*3*). (**b**) Demonstration of a three-channel device advanced from concept to working prototype. (**c**) Cross-sectional schematic illustration of a device before and after heating to reflow printed wax. Adapted with permission from Carrilho et al. [60]. Copyright 2009 American Chemical Society

Fig. 12.3 Single-layer patterned paper diagnostic test for glucose (*left*) and protein (*right*) in urine. The *arrow* indicates the direction of sample flow when dipped in urine. Reprinted with permission from Martinez et al. [54]. Copyright 2007 Wiley-VCH Verlag GmbH & Co. KGaA, Weinheim

and ensures equal distribution of sample into each of the detection zones. The parallel nature of the fluidic conduits in this platform makes it particularly well-suited for multiplexed assays. Each detection zone, for example, could contain unique, independently optimized sets of reagents to perform a number of different assays on a single input specimen. Further complexity has been integrated into the paper

Fig. 12.4 Three-dimensional multilayer patterned-paper microfluidic device that splits single input samples into 16 equal volume detection zones on the bottom of the device. This design enables multiplexed detection of multiple analytes in parallel. Reproduced with permission from Martinez, A.W. et al. *Proc. Natl. Acad. Sci.* 105, 19606 (2008). Copyright 2008 National Academy of Sciences, USA

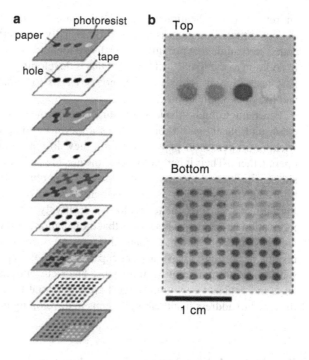

platform with the development of timing gates [62], valves [55, 61], and batteries [63]. Quantitative results can also be obtained by imaging test results using a scanner, digital camera, or mobile camera phone and analyzing the results with image analysis software. The latter method allows for integration with the powerful and promising field of telemedicine [64].

In addition to the colorimetric readouts demonstrated above, much work has been done proving the compatibility of paper microfluidics with electrochemical analyses. By screen printing conductive inks, such as silver/silver chloride or carbon black, electrodes can be patterned on the paper microfluidic devices [65]. These electrodes can be used for a variety of purposes, including electrochemical analysis of glucose [66], analysis of other analytes (e.g., cholesterol) using modified commercial glucometers [46], or to provide heat to specific areas of the paper microfluidic device [65].

Paper-based microfluidics is a highly-flexible diagnostic platform that is compatible with a number of different assay formats and readouts, and it is now moving from academia toward the market. Diagnostics For All (DFA), a nonprofit based in Cambridge, Massachusetts, is building off of the developments of the Whitesides Group at Harvard University; DFA aims to develop specific diagnostic tools for developing countries [67]. Traditional clinical chemistry assays and immunoassays have been successfully demonstrated on the patterned paper platform using electrochemical and colorimetric readouts. DFA's lead rapid diagnostic test is a colorimetric clinical chemistry assay for measuring liver transaminase levels from a finger-stick drop of whole blood [68, 69]. This low-cost, disposable test is targeted to help detect potentially fatal medication-induced liver damage in patients taking antiretroviral medications (e.g., HIV patients) in resource-limited settings. Semiquantitative readout is achieved by visually comparing test results to a color-coded read guide that provides clinically actionable information at the point of care. In addition to the liver function test, DFA is developing several other clinical chemistry tests as well as several immunoassay tests for human health and agriculture and livestock applications.

Paper microfluidic devices are attractive, because they offer the capabilities of glass- and plastic-based microfluidics to perform complex assays but rely on the wicking properties of paper; therefore, they do not require external equipment to operate them. Their inherent low cost means that if they can demonstrate the requisite sensitivity and specificity, they have the potential to be of great utility in decentralized testing situations, such as primary healthcare facilities and at-home testing. Furthermore, because the technology is relatively new, there is still a great deal of innovation happening. This means that the capabilities of paper microfluidic devices are constantly expanding in many different ways, including providing quantitative results, performing assays not yet capable in simple rapid formats, and improving sensitivity through amplification steps. Their current characteristics, inherent low cost, and constant evolution suggest great potential for paper microfluidic devices designed to address healthcare problems in developing urban settings.

The Potential for Innovative Technologies

Developing urban areas face a sometimes daunting combination of disease burden and financial limitations on care. When viewed from a traditional, centralized healthcare delivery model, the potential for high-quality care of all residents can seem bleak. However, the same constraints making centralized healthcare models infeasible push for new models of healthcare delivery and drive the development of new, innovative technologies. As presented in this chapter, new microfluidic technologies that address the constraints of developing urban areas are in development and have the potential to greatly improve patient care and hospital efficiency. Furthermore, because several of these technologies are being developed specifically for developing countries—with involvement from potential end users—adoption could be higher than technologies developed for centralized healthcare models. In this respect, developing urban areas act as incubators for new technological innovation that could eventually move to developed countries if patient demand for at-home testing rises.

References

1. Hay Burgess DC, Wasserman J, Dahl CA. Global health diagnostics. Nature. 2006;444:1–2.
2. McMichael AJ. The urban environment and health in a world of increasing globalization: issues for developing countries. Bull World Health Organ. 2000;78:1117.

3. Taylor LH, Latham SM, Woolhouse ME. Risk factors for human disease emergence. Philos Trans R Soc Lond B Biol Sci. 2001;356:983–9.
4. Jones KE, Patel NG, Levy MA, Storeygard A, Balk D, Gittleman JL, Daszak P. Global trends in emerging infectious diseases. Nature. 2008;451:990–4.
5. Wada M, Kang KB, Nishigami T, Shimoyama T. Importance of pretreatment viral load and monitoring of serum hepatitis C virus RNA in predicting responses to interferon-alpha2a treatment of chronic hepatitis C. Hanshin Chronic Hepatitis C Study Group. J Interferon Cytokine Res. 1997;17:707–12.
6. Mabey D, Peeling RW, Ustianowski A, Perkins MD. Tropical infectious diseases: diagnostics for the developing world. Nat Rev Microbiol. 2004;2:231–40.
7. Temmerman M, Mohamedalf F, Fransen L. Syphilis prevention in pregnancy: an opportunity to improve reproductive and child health in Kenya. Health Policy Plan. 1993;8:122–7.
8. Van Lerberghe W, De Béthune X, De Brouwere V. Hospitals in sub-Saharan Africa: why we need more of what does not work as it should. Trop Med Int Health. 1997;2:799–808.
9. World Health Organization. Cause-specific mortality: regional estimates for 2008 [Online]. 2011. http://www.who.int/healthinfo/global_burden_disease/estimates_regional/en/index.html. Accessed 24 Aug 2012.
10. Bryce J, Boschi-Pinto C, Shibuya K, Black RE, The WHO Child Health Epidemiology Reference Group. WHO estimates of the causes of death in children. Lancet. 2005;365: 1147–52.
11. Fischer Walker CL, Black RE. Diarrhoea morbidity and mortality in older children, adolescents, and adults. Epidemiol Infect. 2010;138:1215–26.
12. Lewis SJ, Heaton KW. Stool form scale as a useful guide to intestinal transit time. Scand J Gastroenterol. 1997;32:920–4.
13. Trier JS. Acute diarrheal disorders. In: Greenberger NJ, Blumberg RS, Burakoff R, editors. Current diagnosis & treatment: gastroenterology, hepatology, & endoscopy. 2nd ed. New York: McGraw-Hill; 2012. p. 45–63.
14. Austin DJ, Kristinsson KG, Anderson RM. The relationship between the volume of antimicrobial consumption in human communities and the frequency of resistance. Proc Natl Acad Sci U S A. 1999;96:1152–6.
15. Blondeau JM. What have we learned about antimicrobial use and the risks for *Clostridium difficile*-associated diarrhoea? J Antimicrob Chemother. 2009;63:238–42.
16. Van Donk M. "Positive" urban futures in sub-Saharan Africa: HIV/AIDS and the need for ABC (A Broader Conceptualization). Environ Urban. 2006;18:155–75.
17. World Health Organization. Progress report 2011: global HIV/AIDS response [Online]. 2011. http://www.who.int/hiv/pub/progress_report2011/en/index.html. Accessed 24 Aug 2012.
18. Kontorinis N, Dieterich D. Hepatotoxicity of antiretroviral therapy. AIDS Res. 2003;5: 36–43.
19. World Health Organization. Cause-specific mortality: regional estimates for 2008 [Online]. 2011. http://www.who.int/healthinfo/global_burden_disease/estimates_regional/en/index.html. Accessed 24 Aug 2012.
20. Abegunde DO, Mathers CD, Adam T, Ortegon M, Strong K. The burden and costs of chronic diseases in low-income and middle-income countries. Lancet. 2007;370:1929–38.
21. Marx J. Unraveling the causes of diabetes. Science. 2002;296:686–9.
22. Björkstén B. Genetic and environmental risk factors for the development of food allergy. Curr Opin Allergy Clin Immunol. 2005;5:249–53.
23. Kolonel LN, Altshuler D, Henderson BE. The multiethnic cohort study: exploring genes, lifestyle and cancer risk. Nat Rev Cancer. 2004;4:519–27.
24. Boutayeb A, Boutayeb S. The burden of noncommunicable diseases in developing countries. Int J Equity Health. 2005;4:2.
25. Wu AHB, Apple FS, Gibler WB, Jesse RL, Warshaw MM, Valdes R. National academy of clinical biochemistry standards of laboratory practice: recommendations for the use of cardiac markers in coronary artery diseases. Clin Chem. 1999;45:1104–21.
26. Melanson SEF, Tanasijevic MJ, Jarolim P. Cardiac troponin assays: a view from the clinical chemistry laboratory. Circulation. 2007;116:e501–4.

27. Bingisser R, Cairns C, Christ M, Hausfater P, Lindahl B, Mair J, Panteghini M, Price C, Venge P. Cardiac troponin: a critical review of the case for point-of-care testing in the ED. Am J Emerg Med. 2012;30(8):1639–49. doi:10.1016/j.ajem.2012.03.004.
28. Clarke SF, Foster JR. A history of blood glucose meters and their role in self-monitoring of diabetes mellitus. Br J Biomed Sci. 2012;69:83–93.
29. Beran D, Yudkin JS. Looking beyond the issue of access to insulin: what is needed for proper diabetes care in resource poor settings. Diabetes Res Clin Pract. 2010;88:217–21.
30. Jeon CY, Murray MB. Diabetes mellitus increases the risk of active tuberculosis: a systematic review of 13 observational studies. PLoS Med. 2008;5:e152.
31. World Health Organization. World health statistics 2012 [Online]. 2012. http://www.who.int/gho/publications/world_health_statistics/2012/en/index.html. Accessed 24 Aug 2012.
32. American Cancer Society. Global cancer facts & figures, 2nd ed. [Online]. 2011. http://www.cancer.org/acs/groups/content/@epidemiologysurveilance/documents/document/acspc-027766.pdf. Accessed 30 Aug 2012.
33. Ploussard G, de la Taille A. Urine biomarkers in prostate cancer. Nat Rev Urol. 2010;7:101–9.
34. Moore RG, MacLaughlan S, Bast Jr RC. Current state of biomarker development for clinical application in epithelial ovarian cancer. Gynecol Oncol. 2010;116:240–5.
35. Soloway MS, Briggman JV, Carpinito GA, Chodak GW, Church PA, Lamm DL, Lange P, Messing E, Pasciak RM, Reservitz GB, Rukstalis DB, Sarosdy MF, Stadler WM, Thiel RP, Hayden CL. Use of a new tumor marker, urinary NMP22, in the detection of occult or rapidly recurring transitional cell carcinoma of the urinary tract following surgical treatment. J Urol. 1996;156:363–7.
36. Stephens C. The urban environment, poverty and health in developing countries. Health Policy Plan. 1995;10:109–21.
37. Peeling RW, Holmes KK, Mabey D, Ronald A. Sex Transm Infect. 2006;82(Suppl V):v1–6.
38. Accutrend® Plus System Specifications; 2012. www.poc.roche.com
39. Cardiac Troponin I product information; 2012. www.abbottpointofcare.com
40. Urdea M, et al. Requirements for high impact diagnostics in the developing world. Nature. 2006;444:73–9.
41. Venkat Narayan KM, et al. Diabetes: the pandemic and potential solutions. In: Jaminson DT, et al., editors. Disease control priorities in developing countries. Washington, DC: World Bank; 2006. p. 591–603.
42. History of Bayer Healthcare Diabetes Care; 2012. www.bayerdiabetes.com
43. Hönes J, Müller P, Surridge N. Diabetes Technol Ther. 2008;10 Suppl 1:S10–26.
44. Gubala V, et al. Anal Chem. 2012;84:487–515.
45. Newman JD, Turner APF. Biosens Bioelectron. 2005;20:2435–53.
46. Nie Z, Deiss F, Liu X, Akbulut O, Whitesides GM. Integration of paper-based microfluidic devices with commercial electrochemical readers. Lab Chip. 2010;10:3163–9.
47. Gaziano TA. Cardiovascular disease in the developing world and its cost-effective management. Circulation. 2005;112:3547–53.
48. Posthuma-Trumpie GA, Korf J, van Amerongen A. Anal Bioanal Chem. 2009;393:569–82.
49. Yager P, Edwards T, Fu E, Helton K, Nelson K, Tam MR, Weigl BH. Microfluidic diagnostic technologies for global public health. Nature. 2006;442:412–8.
50. Gordon J, Michel G. Clin Chem. 2008;54:1250.
51. Chin CD, Linder V, Sia SK. Commercialization of microfluidic point-of-care diagnostic devices. Lab Chip. 2012;12:2118–34.
52. Gravesen P, Branebjerg J, Jensen OS. Microfluidics—a review. J Micromech Microeng. 1993;3:168–82.
53. Chin CD, et al. Nat Med. 2011;17(8):1015–20.
54. Martinez AW, Phillips ST, Butte MJ, Whitesides GM. Patterned paper as a platform for inexpensive, low-volume, portable bioassays. Angew Chem Int Ed. 2007;46:1318–20.
55. Carrilho E, Phillips ST, Vella SJ, Martinez AW, Whitesides GM. Paper microzone plates. Anal Chem. 2012;81:5990–8.

56. Fenton EM, Mascarenas MR, López GP, Sibbett SS. Multiplex lateral-flow test strips fabricated by two-dimensional shaping. ACS Appl Mater Interfaces. 2008;1:124–9.
57. Fu E, Lutz B, Kauffman P, Yager P. Controlled reagent transport in disposable 2D paper networks. Lab Chip. 2010;10:918.
58. Li X, Tian J, Nguyen T, Shen W. Paper-based microfluidic devices by plasma treatment. Anal Chem. 2012;80:9131–4.
59. Lu Y, Shi W, Jiang L, Qin J, Lin B. Rapid prototyping of paper-based microfluidics with wax for low-cost, portable bioassay. Electrophoresis. 2009;30:1497–500.
60. Carrilho E, Martinez AW, Whitesides GM. Understanding wax printing: a simple micropatterning process for paper-based microfluidics. Anal Chem. 2009;81:7091–5.
61. Martinez AW, et al. Programmable diagnostic devices made from paper and tape. Lab Chip. 2010;10:2499–504.
62. Noh H, Phillips ST. Metering the capillary-driven flow of fluids in paper-based microfluidic devices. Anal Chem. 2010;82:4181–7.
63. Thom NK, Yeung K, Pillion MB, Phillips ST. "Fluidic batteries" as low-cost sources of power in paper-based microfluidic devices. Lab Chip. 2012;12:1768–70.
64. Martinez AW, et al. Simple telemedicine for developing regions: camera phones and paper-based microfluidic devices for real-time, off-site diagnosis. Anal Chem. 2008;80:3699–707.
65. Siegel AC, Phillips ST, Wiley BJ, Whitesides GM. Thin, lightweight, foldable thermochromic displays on paper. Lab Chip. 2009;9:2775.
66. Nie Z, et al. Electrochemical sensing in paper-based microfluidic devices. Lab Chip. 2010;10:477–83.
67. www.dfa.org
68. Vella SJ, et al. Measuring markers of liver function using a micro-patterned paper device designed for blood from a finger stick. Anal Chem. 2012;84(6):2883–91. doi:10.1021/ac203434x.
69. Pollack NA, et al. Sci Transl Med. 2012;4:152ra129.

Chapter 13
Innovations in Global Health Professional Education: Implications for Urbanization

Leana S. Wen

Narrative History of Health Professional Education

Developed through literature review and through conversations with each field's prominent leaders and historians, this section presents a narrative history of medical, nursing, and public health education. We describe the major global innovations chronologically and then organize them based on their impact and implications for urbanization. Many of these "organization" and "teaching" innovations are described from the US perspective, because they originated there. The more recent innovations originate from other countries, including many developing countries. These will also be described, along with their impact for the future of urbanization worldwide.

Medical Education

That Abraham Flexner was the single most important factor in shaping the course of medical education in the twentieth century is incontrovertible. The state of medical education and medical practice in the late 1800s was appalling, devoid of science, standards, and regulation. As the President of Harvard University, Charles Eliot remarked in 1870: "The ignorance and general incompetence of the average graduate of American Medical Schools, at the time when he receives the degree which turns him loose upon the community, is something horrible to contemplate. The whole system of medical education in this country needs thorough reformation" [1].

Medical schools had existed in the United States since the late 1700s, with the University of Pennsylvania, Harvard University, and Johns Hopkins University

L.S. Wen, M.D., M.Sc., F.A.A.E.M. (✉)
Baltimore City Health Department, 1001 E. Fayette Street, Baltimore, MD 21202, USA
e-mail: health.commissioner@baltimorecity.gov

© Springer New York 2015
R. Ahn et al. (eds.), *Innovating for Healthy Urbanization*,
DOI 10.1007/978-1-4899-7597-3_13

among the first universities in the world to start affiliated medical schools. Medical education had become a lucrative business, as more and more students sought to gain entrance. Unfortunately, there were few standards for what constituted a "medical school," and by the late 1800s, for-profit enterprises masquerading as educational institutions had proliferated by the dozens. This is an account of what Flexner witnessed when he traveled by horse, train, and buggy, to audit these establishments [2]:

> These enterprises—for the most part, they can be called schools or institutions only by courtesy—were frequently set up regardless of opportunity or need, in small towns as readily as in large, and at times, almost in the heart of the wilderness. No field, however limited, was ever effectually preempted. Wherever and whenever the roster of untitled practitioners rose above half a dozen, a medical school was likely at any moment to be precipitated. Nothing was really essential but professors...
>
> The teaching was, except for a little anatomy, wholly didactic. The schools were essentially private ventures, money-making in spirit and object. Income was simply divided among the lecturers, who reaped a rich harvest besides, through the consultations which the loyalty of their former students threw into their hands... No applicant for instruction who could pay his fees or sign his note was turned down... Accordingly, the business throve.

Flexner also had some critical things to say about the few legitimate medical schools that he visited. About Harvard Medical School, he noted:

> The stethoscope had been in use for over thirty years before its first mention in the catalogue of the Harvard Medical School in 1868-69; the microscope is first mentioned the following year.

At the end of the report, Flexner made three major recommendations, all three of which form the basis of how US medical education functions today. First, he recommended that there be no more for-profit schools and that all existing schools be linked to universities and teaching hospitals. Second, the admitted students must meet certain qualifications, including a rigorous undergraduate science education. Third, Flexner believed that scientific research should form the basis of all medical school teaching and that medicine should be taught by those who are actively involved in original scientific investigation [2].

Flexner's report was damning. Because the report addressed the lay public, there was public outrage about sham schools and quacks profiteering at the expense of the health and well-being of the nation. Not surprisingly, the impact was swift and significant: from 1910 to 1935, 89 of the 155 institutions that Flexner surveyed closed their doors. As the number of medical schools decreased, admission became more competitive, and only students with qualified undergraduate degrees were granted entrance. The intertwining of medical training with universities and academic medical centers became complete. Medical students would receive training at university-affiliated teaching hospitals rather than at local clinics or home-based apprenticeship settings. Medical schools and their affiliated hospitals were to become engines of cutting-edge research, and medical training would be at the forefront of science.

In the first half of the twentieth century, this system of integrating teaching, clinical care, and scientific investigation worked well—so well that this was the model of medical education that spread around the world [3]. Clinical research was still predicated on direct interaction with patients, and those most gifted in clinical research tended to be the most talented clinicians and teachers. However, as scientific advances became more increasingly specialized and more technology-based, the cutting edge of science transitioned more and more from the wards to the laboratory. Those who were first-rate clinician-teachers found it difficult to also be first-rate researchers and vice versa. There was also increasing pressure for clinicians to increase their "clinical productivity" so as to generate increased revenue for their academic centers. Clinical teaching became divorced from the apprenticeship model, and medical students began to lose the benefit of learning from a master teacher. Students gradually lost hold of their ties to their community and strayed from their initial purpose of advocating for their patients and their communities.

Though initially and primarily a US phenomenon, the Flexner Report's effects were worldwide. The creation of the China Medical Board by the Rockefeller Foundation and the establishment of Peking University Medical College in the People's Republic of China represented the first application of the Flexnerian model in a developing country and marked the beginning of globalization of the Flexner Report [4]. There are several other examples of successful long-term collaborations between developed and developing countries. In 1948, the University of London helped establish the Medical School of Nigeria's University of Ibadan; graduates from Ibadan were able to receive the MBBS degree recognized by the General Medical Council of Great Britain, and Ibadan became the model for all of Nigeria's other medical schools [5, 6].

Much has evolved in US and international medical education since Flexner. The concept of Graduate Medical Education (GME) is arguably one of the other major developments in twentieth century medical education, requiring doctors to go through post-medical school apprenticeship training through residency programs. Initially pioneered by major US academic centers in the 1950s, GME has spread throughout the world. Although not technically part of "medical school" training, GME is now an integral part of medical training worldwide, mandating post-medical school clinical training and routes to specialization [7].

The 1970s saw explicit challenges to the Flexner model. Before Flexner, there was very little reliance on science; after Flexner, medicine became integrally intertwined with it, to the detriment of losing the "art" of medical practice. In the 1970s, medical schools began experimenting with models of medical education that would bring the art—and the patient—back into clinical teaching. An example is Canada's McMaster University developing the concept of problem-based learning, in which students learned in teams about cases instead of the traditional classroom lecture approach [8]. Since then, PBL has been adopted by prominent institutions, such as Harvard Medical School. As evidence accumulates for the superior professional competencies of those trained in PBL, more medical and health professional schools are beginning to rely on it for their core curriculum. This is a good example of global diffusion of a concept of medical education [9]. A related innovation is the use of standardized patients, not only to evaluate students on scientific know-how, but also to test their competency in communication and professionalism.

Another development away from the traditional Flexnerian approach has been the focus on community-oriented primary care (COPC). At the turn of the last century, it had been necessary to tie medical training to academic centers, as these were the only places with the rigor required to couple medicine with science. In the 1980s, an opposing phenomenon arose: educators realized the need not only to have innovative methods of medical education but to shift the location of education from the ivory tower to the community and to shift the focus away from increasingly sub-specialized science to primary care.

Developing countries have led the way in ensuring that training opportunities occur in rural and underserved areas. For example, Walter Sisulu Medical School in South Africa was an early adopter of the instructional design of COPC to improve primary healthcare delivery and teaching. Students are taught to incorporate COPC principles, such as prevention and promotion, into their daily routines. From the first year, students visit community resources like traditional healers and community health centers. They undertake a study of a community by visiting family homes, and most gain fluency in native dialects such as Khosa. There are now more than 500 graduates in primary care practice in the Eastern Cape, and a study of career destination of graduates shows that the majority are serving in rural and peri-urban areas [10].

Even the United States, traditionally a bastion of specialist academic training, has experimented with the branch campus movement and the establishment of osteopathic schools that are not associated with an academic center. A.T. Still School of Osteopathic Medicine in Arizona, for example, has a particularly innovative model of medical education. After the first year of medical school, students are assigned to one of 11 community health centers spread out across the country for their preclinical and then clinical education. Students are fully integrated into their community and are trained as apprentices by master educators at each site [11]. This and other efforts herald the return to a pre-Flexner education—though with a much improved approach. In Flexner's time, community-based training was not possible, as the training available outside academic centers was questionable; Walter Sisulu and A.T. Still are testament to adaptation and optimization of progress in the modern setting.

Not only has community-based teaching introduced students to the problems most relevant to what they will see in practice, it is helping to produce more physicians with less financial investment. This has been a particularly useful development as, since the 1990s, there has been increasing recognition that our society is facing a global health workforce shortage. Many reports have been written about the critical shortage of the most precious health resource: our healthcare workers. Several countries are using methods, including teaching outside academic centers as a way to address the impending shortage.

Loan repayment-for-service programs have also been a helpful addition to reduce the financial burden on students choosing medicine and to improve diversity in the workforce (an idea that was foreign during Flexner's time). The National Health Service Corps is a loan repayment program that has been in existence for over 30 years. In exchange for paying for medical students' tuition, it obligates trainees to practice primary care in an underserved urban or rural community for an equivalent number of years after residency. It is one of several programs that has been successful not only in addressing the shortage of primary care physicians in underserved communities but also in encouraging those who are truly committed to service to a career in the health professions.

Another innovation that has tremendous potential is the pipeline program, one of the most successful of which is the Sophie Davis School in New York City. Established in 1973 to address the growing deficit of underrepresented minority physicians in the United States, the Sophie Davis School is unique in its early recruitment, vigorous pipeline, and impressive retention of minority health professional students. It recruits almost exclusively from inner-city high schools in New York City and provides a combined undergraduate and medical education free of charge. More than 90 % of the students who attend Sophie Davis come from the lowest income tax bracket. Of the over 1,400 graduates, 25 % are African-American, 8 % are Latino, 28 % are Asian-American, and 39 % are white—a diversity of representation not seen in any other US medical school. The pipeline and aggressive early recruitment of Sophie Davis offers a model not just for the United States and developed countries but also for developing countries who wish to prioritize diversity and representation of their healthcare workforce [12]. Such programs may be particularly important in providing opportunities to students from urban slums and in encouraging them to seek a career in the health professions and to return to serve the needs of their communities.

Another dramatic example of human resource capacity building through free medical education is the *Escuela Latinoamericana de Medicina* (ELAM), or Latin American School of Medicine. Founded in the aftermath of Hurricane Mitch in 1998, ELAM, which is operated by the Cuban government, recruited 11,000 students from marginalized communities in 29 countries to study medicine, free of charge. It has become the largest and most diverse medical school in the world. In fact, its students are all international students from outside Cuba and are drawn primarily from Latin America, the Caribbean, and Africa. In addition, ELAM draws exclusively from marginalized communities, with an extensive selection process to ensure that selected students will return to serve their communities after the 6-year education. The free tuition, accommodation, board, and small stipend enable such students to attend medical school. ELAM's structure and mission provide an important model as we consider sustainable ways to ramp up the global healthcare workforce. As it is already producing doctors who are exported throughout the developing and developed world, ELAM is contributing directly to the global diffusion of health resources and information [13, 14].

A final concept that is gaining much traction is task shifting to allow for increasing scope of practice by lower-level practitioners. This development is calling upon physicians to be trained, such that they can be placed in a more educational and supervisory role than before. In resource-poor settings facing a deficit of physicians, nurses can be called upon to perform initial assessments, history taking, physical exams, and laboratory investigations and doctors only for the most difficult cases. Community health workers can perform many screenings and public health interventions. The emerging role of task shifting in global medical education cannot be overemphasized, especially as the global brain drain represents a major concern for many developing countries heading into the twenty-first century [15].

Medical education	
Organizational innovations	Teaching innovations
Collaborations to begin training programs with global input	Graduate medical education
Twinning between developing country and developed country	Problem-based learning
Increasing access to education through "free" medical education and recruitment of underrepresented minorities	Standardized patients
Task shifting	Teaching and testing of competency not only on science but on communication and professionalism
	Community-oriented primary care

Nursing Education

The theme of nursing education over the twentieth century can perhaps be character-ized as "from humanistic practice to university training." Perhaps the closest equiva-lent to Flexner for nursing education is Florence Nightingale, who in the mid-1800s (incidentally well before Flexner's time) began to exhort that good nursing care depended on having an educated group of nurses [16]. The first formal nursing edu-cation programs began in the 1850s in London as a 2-year hospital-based training program. Others quickly followed suit throughout the world. In the 1860s, organized nursing with hospital-based training began to become standard in Western countries, with the United States and UK leading the way followed by the Scandinavian countries and Germany. Due to the work of the Rockefeller Foundation and various missionary groups, the concept of organized nurses spread to the former colonies throughout Asia and Africa. In 1899, the International Council of Nurses was founded by nurse leaders of US, UK, and Scandinavian countries. It was modeled after the International Women's Organization, and its goal was to push for training and global standards, specifically to standardize curriculum [17].

Part of the advocacy work of the International Council of Nurses was to push for government licensing of nursing to further standardize practice and ensure safety. Interestingly, the first governments to license nurses were not the traditional power-houses in the developed world but South Africa and Puerto Rico (historically this has to do with the licensing of physicians, which was occurring at the same time in these two areas) [18]. The licenses also extended to visiting nurses, a model that began in the late 1800s by Lillian Wald. Nursing has traditionally had a strong com-munity pull, with home-based work still among the most popular positions.

In the 1920s, the Rockefeller Foundation attempted to duplicate the Flexner study by forming the Committee for the Study of Nursing Education. This so-called Goldmark Report found that existing nursing programs in the United States were inadequate. Interestingly, they discussed the role of the nurse with public health, with a proposal for work that combined clinical care of the sick with teaching of hygiene [19]. This part of the report was controversial, but other parts of the report calling for university-based nursing programs led to the foundation of the Yale School of Nursing as the first autonomous school of nursing that emphasized nursing as an academic discipline.

The next major breakthroughs in nursing education followed this trend, with nursing education relocating from the hospital to the university. By the 1950s, dozens of universities in the United States and Europe had schools of nursing. The University of Alexandria was the first of such universities in the Middle East. Since then, education at the Bachelor's level has become standard in most Western countries. The European Union countries now mandate standardized nursing educa-tion at the Bachelor's level; many Latin American countries, Cuba, and Botswana have followed suit [20].

Due to its proliferation of community college programs, the United States stands alone in developed countries as still having half of its nursing graduates with associ-ate rather than bachelor's degrees. At the same time, it is also in the United States that the highest proportion of nurses has advanced, master's or doctoral-level training. In the 1960s, as an outgrowth of Medicare and Medicaid, the nurse practitioner came into existence with nursing being available on the graduate level to expand scope of practice, including individual, unsupervised primary care practice in the community.

Nurse practitioners (and in developing countries, senior nurses and nurse trainers) play a central role in community-based and primary care. Discussions continue on the scope of practice of nurses. In Cuba, for example, nurses can see patients inde-pendently of doctors [21]. In Uganda, nurses are frequently trainers of community health workers such as birth attendants [22]. Such discussions of task shifting and integration of nursing care with public health will be instrumental in the next century of health professional innovation. This is particularly relevant to areas facing human resource shortages, including many urban areas.

Nursing education	
Organization innovations	Teaching innovations
Progression from hospital-based training to the university to Bachelor's level	Community college and post-baccalaureate programs for mature students
Nurses having scope of practice to see patients without doctors	Nurse practitioners
Attempts to increase scope of practice in developing world	Nursing training that is founded in population-based and primary care-based public health

Public Health Education

The roots of modern public health education lie in the nineteenth century, when the germ theory and sanitation movement provided impetus for microbiology and then population health to gain the same scientific credibility and societal recognition as medicine. In the early twentieth century, in 1913, the Harvard-MIT School for

Health Officers was founded as the first university-based school devoted to the teaching of public health. The Johns Hopkins University School of Public Health followed shortly behind. From 1916, the Rockefeller Foundation assisted with the development of several other US public health schools such as Columbia and Yale. They also helped establish some overseas ventures, including schools in Chile and Tokyo, with varying success.

While the US public health schools began developing, the London School of Hygiene and Tropical Medicine concurrently started in 1924 and flourished. Their focus was always, from the very beginning, on global health, with its mandate from the Royal Charter to send graduates to work in developing countries.

The success and failure of various public health education programs offer interesting lessons. For example, some of the most successful schools of public health have been ones that began independently of medical schools. While this allowed these independent public health schools (Harvard and Hopkins are both examples) to develop into strong entities in their own right rather than subject to funding pressures of academic medical centers, this may have led to the accidental dissociation between medicine and public health in the United States. How to integrate medicine and public health has been an ongoing debate. The Welch-Rose report of 1913 was the first to touch on the topic, and the New York Academy of Medicine and the Institute of Medicine, among others, have investigated this issue [23, 24].

Importantly, this issue of lack of interprofessional integration between medicine and public health is primarily a United States issue. In other countries, public health schools have not developed nearly to the extent US schools have, and since they are mainly departments under medical schools (i.e., department of community and preventive medicine) and many doctors work in public health, there is less separation. The flip side of this is that most other public health schools do not have the reach and impact of the separate schools of public health. Also, while the focus of other countries' public health schools has not been on leadership and research in the same way as US and UK schools, they have had perhaps as useful of a mission to develop public health professionals to work in their indigenous contexts.

There have been many specific seeds of innovation in public health education. For example, Mexico's Institute of Public Health was founded as a training ground for the Ministry of Health and then developed into a public health school with more academic rigor. In its retention of graduates after their doctoral training, the United States added to its strong academic and research mission [25].

Various programs are beginning to increase access to public health education. South Africa's National School of Public Health initiated a distance IT program. By using a primarily online teaching curriculum and limiting compulsory classroom time to four 2-week blocks, students of 16 African countries have been able to take the course. In just 5 years of the IT/distance course, the number of graduates from this public health school has exceeded the number of graduates from all six other public health schools combined [26]. Some issues relating to its dropout rate and lack of computer literacy must still be worked out; also it is not clear whether graduates have gone on to work on resolving public health issues in sub-Saharan Africa. Nevertheless, such a model taking advantage of technological resources to transcend national borders offers much potential, especially for those who lack the means to travel outside their home countries for public health education.

Another example of increasing public health education is through shorter-term courses. Brazil's story is colloquially referred to as how one public school turned into 40 because that, in fact, is its history. One public health school, the Sergio Arouca National School of Public Health (*Escola Nacional de Saude Publica Sergio Arouca*) in conjunction with the Oswaldo Cruz Foundation set up a short, 6-month public health course in each of Brazil's 27 states. These courses then each turned into public health schools [27]. Brazil now has one of the highest concentrations of public health training programs in the world. This model of short courses turning into core public health curricula is another good example of ramping up human resources for public health. It also illustrates how collaboration can be useful in public health education, with "private" representing both nonprofits and potentially for-profit enterprises.

Another area that has been called the greatest unfulfilled educational opportunity in public health is the lack of clinical curriculum for public health students. Bangladesh's James P. Grant School of Public Health at BRAC University is a non-governmental organization collaboration that has as part of its curriculum a required hands-on project in the community [28]. Lessons can be learned from BRAC and developing countries' programs to incorporate a practical, applied-learning experience that is the equivalent of clinical experience in medicine to public health training. Not only would this enhance public health education; it serves as a method to involve other health professions in interprofessional collaboration and can be extended to international contexts to improve global interconnectedness.

Another example of transcending national borders is direct collaboration between two schools or institutions in different parts of the world. A recent "twinning" project that focuses on interdisciplinary education is the Johns Hopkins University (USA) and Makerere University College of Health Sciences (Uganda) collaboration on the African Health Education Initiative. Funded by a $5-million grant from the Gates Foundation, the initiative is a 10-year-long process that involves the faculties of medicine, nursing, and public health at both schools to build upon the educational capacity of Makerere University, Uganda's largest university. The project is based on the principles of long-term sustainability and consistency with Uganda's national health priorities [29]. One critique of using this example is that it is a relatively new initiative, and results are still unknown; however, it is an example of a twinning collaboration that holds much promise as it takes advantage of a developed country's curriculum in the context of a developing country's health needs. This new model also standardizes public health education and makes it accessible to the many people who practice public health but have never received formal training in it.

Public health education	
Organizational innovations	Teaching innovations
Collaboration with academic institutions	Requirement of hands-on applied work
Collaboration with NGOs	Distance IT learning
Twinning initiatives	Certificate programs
Short-term courses in public health	

Ongoing Challenges and a Proposal for Reform

To commemorate the 100th anniversary of the Flexner Report, the Lancet published guidelines by a global independent Commission that aimed to establish the twenty-first century vision for the education of health professionals [30]. This Commission report emphasized the move beyond professional silos to new models of interprofessional collaboration and proposed many important innovations for moving health professional education into the twenty-first century.

A separate Lancet Commission of young health professional leaders from around the world[1] published an accompanying critique of the report that discussed its lack of emphasis to service and social accountability in health professional training [31]. The reforms of the nineteenth and twentieth centuries have been remarkable in improving the technical aspects of health care and health education, the report said, but many challenges remain—and these challenges require an entire reexamination of the mission of health professional education.

Perhaps the most important challenge is the neglect of the moral aspect of health professional education. The World Health Organization suggests that health professional training should feature social accountability, namely, "the obligation to direct their education, research and service of activities towards addressing the priority health concerns of the community, region and/or nation that they have a mandate to serve" [32]. Students entering the health professions have strong ideals that must be fostered during training and sustained within systems of practice. Such education must not only involve caring for the individual patient but must also instill the importance of community and the ethic of practicing in areas of greatest need.

Unfortunately, we are far from achieving this goal. Economic factors, such as the high cost of medical education and the commoditization of health care, have disincentivized young graduates everywhere from entering much-needed primary care fields [33]. In developed countries, there is a dearth of providers in underserved rural and urban areas; in developing countries, the "brain drain" has resulted in far worse shortages [15]. Moreover, one of the unintended effects of the Flexner Report is the disproportionate focus on basic science, leading to an unbalanced curriculum that has over 90 % of students reporting that they are not sufficiently trained in public health and problems facing their community [34]. Additional studies have shown that as students go through training, their idealism erodes away, with an accompanying decline in service orientation and empathy toward their patients [35, 36].

Heading into the twenty-first century, it is critical not only to make changes regarding the technical aspects of health professional education but also to transform and redirect the focus of health professional education toward social accountability. Only then can the emerging challenges in urbanization and global health be addressed. As the commission of young professionals proposed, here are five key steps for every

---

[1] The chapter author served as chair of this commission.

medical school and health professional training program to help align their training with emerging societal need:

1. *Establish an explicit social mission.* Studies have shown that having social accountability as the guiding principle will have transformative effects on every step of the subsequent training, from recruitment to curriculum design to choice of eventual career [37]. Regulatory bodies should measure social accountability and use it as a metric for excellence and accreditation and incentivize inclusion of social accountability into the mission statement [38]. Health professional schools located in urban areas should have an explicit mission statement to train students prepared to address challenges in urbanization. Graduates must be ready to serve the community in which they are trained.

2. *Integrate community learning and service into the curriculum.* Experiences with Cuba, South Africa, China, and the United States, among others, demonstrate that students who spend more time in community settings have a much higher rate of returning to the community to practice [38]. For doctors to truly serve as advocates for their communities, an irreplaceable part of training needs to occur in the community and directly deal with understanding and addressing community concerns. Those students training in urban areas—the majority of students worldwide—have a ready-made platform to commence and conduct their training of urban community and service learning.

3. *Emphasize the importance of primary care.* While few question the centrality of primary health care to the health system, too few young health professionals are entering primary care fields. Preferential recruitment of those committed to primary care principles is critical, as is fostering of the commitment through teaching COPC principles and incorporating apprenticeship models with primary care practitioners. Health systems also need to incentivize practice as primary care providers. This is just important as important in rural settings where there are few practitioners, as there are in urban settings, where the number of practitioners may be high but the proportion of those willing and able to serve the urban poor remains low.

4. *Provide a service option in exchange for free health professional education.* The concept of debt repayment in exchange for service has existed in virtually every country in the form of various loan repayment options [39]. The example of Cuba's ELAM that has recruited tens of thousands from marginalized communities, and compulsory service programs, provide important models for training a health workforce to serve communities most in need [40]. Schools in urban areas need to pay particular attention to recruiting those students who show potential and provide opportunities for them to seek higher education opportunities. Such students are far more likely to return to their urban communities to serve those most in need.

5. *Engage young health professionals in social accountability throughout the continuum of their training.* Altruism is not a concept that holds true only during training; it should last through the entirety of one's career [41]. Postgraduate programs should help young professionals identify mentors who can serve as role

models for social responsibility and help guide trainees to careers in public service. Reflective practice and continuing education can help to reinforce such concepts. Those practicing in urban communities should be encouraged to reach outside their ivory tower and specialty practices to recruit new trainees and practice their art and science in the most underserved areas. This key element of social accountability needs to be modeled from the first day of health professional training and throughout the continuum of education and practice.

The nineteenth and twentieth centuries saw remarkable growth and innovations in medical, nursing, and public health education. More interdisciplinary change is needed into the twenty-first century, but a far more fundamental reform is due that is rooted in the meaning and purpose of the health professions. Particularly as the world evolves and there are new and emerging challenges to urbanization and global health, the next generation of young health professionals needs to continue to uphold the concept that service is the highest calling of our profession. Reform to the healthcare workforce is the most fundamental change that must occur to meet societal needs. Every country's system of education and practice should endeavor to train the next generation of health professionals as socially responsible agents of change.

References

1. The American Experience. People and events. http://www.pbs.org/wgbh/amex/murder/peopleevents/e_medicine.html. Accessed 1 Sept 2012.
2. Flexner A. Report on medical education in the United States and Canada: a report to the Carnegie Foundation for the Advancement of Teaching, Bulletin No. 4. New York: The Carnegie Foundation; 1910.
3. Ludmerer KM. A time to heal. Oxford: Oxford University Press; 1999.
4. China Medical Board. China Medical Board and Peking Union Medical College: a shared history. http://www.cmbfound.org/index.php?option=com_content&view=article&id=49:cmb-and-peking-union-medical-college-a-shared-history&catid=11&Itemid=104. Accessed 1 Sept 2012.
5. Ibrahim M. Evaluation of the current role of Nigerian medical schools in the training of medical graduates. Niger Postgrad Med J. 2008;15 Suppl 1:22–30.
6. Ibrahim M. Medical education in Nigeria. Med Teach. 2007;29(9):901–5.
7. Wen LS, Geduld HI, Nagurney JT, Wallis LA. Africa's first emergency medicine training program at the University of Cape Town/Stellenbosch University: history, progress, and lessons learned. Acad Emerg Med. 2011;18(8):868–71.
8. Neville AJ. Problem-based learning and medical education forty years on. A review of its effects on knowledge and clinical performance. Med Princ Pract. 2009;18(1):1–9.
9. Schmidt HG, Vermeulen L, ver der Molen HT. Long-term effects of problem-based learning: a comparison of competencies acquired by graduates of a problem-based school and a conventional medical school. Med Educ. 2006;40(6):562–7.
10. Toward Unity for Health Network. Reassessment report for renewal membership; 2006. http://www.the-network.org/reassessment/files/95000b.doc. Last accessed 8 Jan 2010.
11. Medical Education Futures Study. AT still study sheet. http://www.medicaleducationfutures.org/ATStill. Accessed 1 Sept 2012.
12. Roman Jr SA. Addressing the urban pipeline challenge for the physician workforce: the Sophie Davis model. Acad Med. 2004;79(12):1175–83.

13. Huish R. Going where no doctor has gone before: the role of Cuba's Latin American School of Medicine in meeting the needs of some of the world's most vulnerable populations. Public Health. 2008;122(6):552–7.
14. Mullan F. Affirmative action, Cuban style. N Engl J Med. 2004;351(26):2680–2.
15. Mullan F. The metrics of the physician brain drain. N Engl J Med. 2005;353(17):1810–8.
16. Nightingale F. Notes on nursing. What it is, and what it is not. 1st American ed. New York: D. Appleton and Company; 1860.
17. Editorial. The International Council of Nurses. Old Nurses J. 1969;11(8):3–4.
18. Marks S. Gender and caring in South Africa. Some lessons from history. Adler Mus Bull. 2011;37(1):3–14.
19. Goldmark J. Nursing and nursing education in the United States: report of the committee on the study of nursing education. New York: Commissioned by the Rockefeller Foundation; 1923.
20. Bridgman M. Patterns of collegiate nursing education. Nurs Outlook. 1953;1(9):525–8.
21. Martinez N. Developing nursing capacity for health systems and services research in Cuba, 2008–2011. MEDICC Rev. 2012;14(3):12–8.
22. Nabudere H, Aslimwe D, Mijumbi R. Task shifting in maternal and child health care: an evidence brief from Uganda. Int J Technol Assess Health Care. 2011;27(2):173–9.
23. Welch WH, Rose W. Institute of hygiene: being a report to the General Education Board, Rockefeller Foundation. 1915. http://www.deltaomega.org/documents/WelchRose.pdf. Accessed 10 Apr 2015.
24. Institute of Medicine. The future of public health. http://www.nap.edu/openbook. php?isbn=0309038308. Accessed 1 Sept 2012.
25. Frenk J. The new public health. Annu Rev Public Health. 1993;14:469–90.
26. World Health Organization. Training of public health workforce at the National School of Public Health: meeting Africa's needs. Bull World Health Organ. 2007;85(12):949–54.
27. World Health Organization. How Brazil turned one public health school into 40. Bull World Health Organ. 2007;85(12):912–3.
28. School of Public Health. BRAC. http://sph.bracu.ac.bd/. Accessed 1 Sept 2012.
29. The Johns Hopkins University. Johns Hopkins and Uganda's Makerere University to Collaborate on African Health Education Initiative; 2008. http://www.hopkinsglobalhealth.org/about/news_center/headlines/2008/JHU-Makerere-12-1-08.html. Last accessed 8 Jan 2010.
30. Frenk J, Chen L, Bhutta ZA, et al. Health professionals for a new century: transforming education to strengthen health systems in an interdependent world. Lancet. 2010;376(9756):1923–58.
31. Division of Development of Human Resources for Health, World Health Organization. Defining and Measuring the Social Accountability of Medical Schools. Geneva: World Health Organization; 1995. http://whqlibdoc.who.int/hq/1995/WHO_HRH_95.7.pdf. Accessed 12 Dec 2010.
32. Wen LS, Greysen SR, Keszthelyi D, Bracero J, de Ross PDG. Social accountability in health professional education. Lancet. 2011;378(9807):e12–3.
33. Morrison G. Mortgaging our future—the cost of medical education. N Engl J Med. 2005;352(2):117–9.
34. Agrawal JR, Huebner J, Hedgecock J, et al. Medical students' knowledge of the US healthcare system and their preferences for curricular change: a national survey. Acad Med. 2005;80(5):484–8.
35. Hojat M, Mangione S, Nasca TJ, et al. An empirical study of decline in empathy in medical school. Med Educ. 2004;38(9):934–41.
36. Wen LS, Baca J, O'Malley P, Bhatia K, Peak D, Takayesu JT. Implementation of small group reflection rounds at an emergency medicine residency: a pilot study. CJEM. 2013;15(3):175–7.
37. Mullan F, Chen C, Petterson S, et al. The social mission of medical education: ranking the schools. Ann Intern Med. 2010;152(12):804–11.

38. Boelen C, Woollard B. Social accountability and accreditation: a new frontier for educational institutions. Med Educ. 2009;43(9):887–94.
39. Council on Graduate Medical Education. Eighteenth report: new paradigms for physician training for improving access to healthcare. http://www.COGME.org. Accessed 12 Dec 2010.
40. Frehywot S, Mullan F, Payne PW, Ross H. Compulsory service programmes for recruiting health workers in remote and rural areas: do they work? Bull World Health Organ. 2010; 88(5):364–70.
41. Wallenburg I, van Exel J, Stolk E, et al. Beyond trust and accountability: different perspectives on the modernization of postgraduate medical training in the Netherlands. Acad Med. 2010;85(6):1082–90.

Chapter 14
The Case for Comprehensive, Integrated, and Standardized Measures of Health in Cities

Patricia L. McCarney and Anita M. McGahan

After decades of unprecedented migration into urban areas, the iconic demographic development of the twenty-first century is indigenous growth of cities.[1] The world's urban population is projected to reach 4.2 billion by 2020, and the urban slum population is expected to increase to 1.4 billion by 2020. While 10 % of the world's population lived in cities in 1900, 53 % of the world's population now resides in an urban area, and by 2050 this number is expected to exceed 75 %. As a planet, we are about midway through this transition. The world is said to have crossed the so-called rural–urban divide in 2007.

---

[1] This demographic transition was noted very early in its history by Lewis Mumford (1956) in his seminal work "The Natural History of Urbanization," in *Man's Role in Changing the Face of the Earth* (Edited by William L. Thomas). Many documents from the international development agencies have tracked this transition with one of the more important ones being produced by the UN in 2001 and titled *Cities in a Globalizing World: Global Report on Human Settlements* (UNCHS 2001).

P.L. McCarney, Ph.D.
Department of Political Science, Global Cities Institute, John H. Daniels Faculty of Architecture, Landscaping, and Design, University of Toronto, 170 Bloor St. West, Suite 1100, Toronto, ON, Canada M5S1T9

A.M. McGahan, Ph.D. (✉)
Rotman School of Management, University of Toronto, 105 St. George Street, Toronto, ON, Canada M553E6
e-mail: anita.mcgahan@rotman.utoronto.ca

© Springer New York 2015
R. Ahn et al. (eds.), *Innovating for Healthy Urbanization*,
DOI 10.1007/978-1-4899-7597-3_14

Percentage of World Population

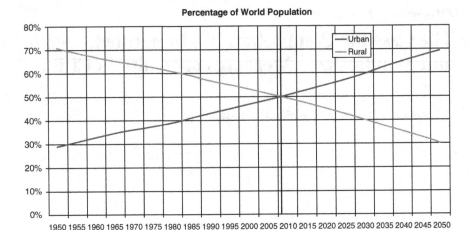

Source: UN Department of Economic and Social Affairs (2007): *World Urbanization Prospects: The 2007 Revision Population Database*

Most of this demographic shift is occurring in low- and middle-income countries (LMICs). Nations such as Canada are already through much of the transition. In the mid-1870s, Canada was 20 % urban and 80 % rural, whereas by 2005, this balance had reversed to 80 % urban and 20 % rural. Other relatively HICs have moved through similar transitions, including Brazil (now 86 % urban), the United States (82 %), Australia (89 %), United Kingdom (90 %), and Jordan (78 %). In global terms, it is the LMIC nations that are emerging as pivotal actors in this demographic transition. Virtually all of the world's future urban population growth is predicted to occur in less-developed countries. Cities of the developing world will absorb 95 % of population growth and will be home to 80 % of the world's urban population.

This global transition is also marked by a growing number of exceptionally large cities. In a UN ranking of city agglomeration by population, it was found that by 2005, the number of megacities (defined by the UN as greater than ten million) had increased to 20, and it is projected that there will be 22 megacities in 2015. With 35 million residents in 2005, the metropolitan area of Tokyo was by far the most populous urban agglomeration in the world. Tokyo was followed by Mexico City and New York-Newark, each with 19 million residents, and São Paulo, with 18 million people. In 2005, megacities accounted for about 9.3 % of the world's urban population [1]. By 2015, 17 of these 22 megacities will be in the LMICs [1].

Thus, one out of every three people living in cities in 2020 will live in impoverished, overcrowded, and insecure living conditions (UN-Habitat 2007). Global health risks, policy challenges in health services, and other health issues find particular expression in the world's cities as they grow. The relationships between health and other city conditions are increasingly complex and entangled—social cohesion, safety, security, and stability are being challenged by social exclusion, inequities, and shortfalls in basic services. Health is one manifestation of a city's complex conditions in each of these areas.

City leaders around the world have expressed intensified interest in the mechanisms available for supporting and promoting the health of both new and established residents.

This stems in part from the recognition that, in many ways, the path toward healthier cities is entwined with more effective governance and innovation in local urban policy. As the globe's population has congregated in major urban centers, the nature of health-care needs for urban populations has also changed. The health of a city's residents depends on critical infrastructure, the maintenance of water and sanitation systems, the availability of affordable housing, the protection of spaces for physical activity, the extent of pollution, and the strength of the economy, among many other conditions. Thus, the governance of a city has a profound impact on the health of its inhabitants. Understanding this link requires a broader scope of inquiry and a more nuanced understanding of what factors are worthy of attention in the urbanized and urbanizing setting. In other words, improving the health in any city must account for the complexity of layered conditions in the city, including its governance profile.

At the same time as cities are growing, healthcare industries are globalizing. A crisis of cost is occurring in many regions of the world [2]. Innovations carry the potential to sustain and improve quality of life and quality of health, but they must also be affordable both as investments and in operation. As a result, particular attention has focused on the opportunities for frugal or low-cost innovation in cities in which per capita income is lower than the global average. Healthcare innovation represents the convergence of both municipal and health policy. The challenge is in simultaneously innovating to improve the health of the poor while assuring that such innovation is locally relevant, given the complex fabric of issues unique to each city [3].

Meeting both the localized needs of a city's urban population and tapping the potential of global health innovations requires a comprehensive understanding of the complex condition of a city, as well as its prospects for improving health. In this paper, we argue that standardized city indicators, developed in partnership with city leaders to establish a common, accepted methodology for measuring health and other urban conditions, can unlock an understanding of each city's unique and shared health challenges and thus enable cross-city learning. This understanding is a prerequisite for effective action to improve the health of urban populations.

Nothing about the development or interpretation of standardized indicators is or should be simple. Such metrics must be developed collaboratively—through consultation with city leaders—to achieve legitimacy and relevance. The complexity of a city's conditions defies a ranking-based interpretation of such standards. Instead, comparisons must be accompanied by a detailed and qualitative interpretation of the relative circumstances of cities. The task of developing standard metrics must therefore be undertaken with sensitivity and commitment.

At the same time, the need for such measures is significant. The growth of major urban settings has many implications for the health of their inhabitants. Our ability to understand these effects has been hindered by a lack of comprehensive metrics for meaningfully measuring health in cities. While some data on health are available, we know little about the strategies and dynamics of improvements in health in settings where migration has been significant and/or where indigenous growth has occurred. We know even less about returns on major civic investments in health.

Thus, in spite of the obvious relevance of health metrics, the relationship between urbanization and health has remained under-discussed and under-studied.

With a view to addressing this gap, this paper will seek to make the case for integrated assessments of the relationship between health and urbanization. In making this case, we will briefly review the connections between various facets of city conditions and health. The core of our argument is that the evolution of cities has introduced new layers in our interpretation of urban health, new complexities in governing cities with respect to health services, and new research challenges to measure and monitor health in cities. How do we address this multiple layering and new complexity? How do we account for the unique health circumstances of each city while exporting best practices and fostering mutual learning across city boundaries? We argue that we can only obtain answers to these questions through a much broader and more comprehensive framework for assessing health than is available today, and we highlight a leading initiative based at the University of Toronto—namely, the Global City Indicators Facility (GCIF).

Facets of a Comparative Measurement Framework for Cities and Health

Historically, measures of the health of populations have fallen into two broad categories. The first category involves involves hard measures of medical capacity. This refers to quantitative assessments of factors such as the number of doctors per capita, the number of hospital beds, and gross expenditures on health services. The second category involves cross-sectional measures of population health with respect to specific outcomes such as infant mortality rates, life expectancy at birth, and maternal mortality. In this sense, all measures of health have been tied directly to traditional health sector indicators.

Recent emphasis on public policy and the social determinants of health has led to greater emphasis on project-specific assessments, in particular "evidence-based" analysis of the incremental impact of particular interventions on population health. Yet despite impressive efforts to improve understanding of the impact of particular programs, the applicability of these analyses has been limited primarily because the context for each intervention differs. In addition, the metrics relevant to a particular program reflect its idiosyncratic goals and thus differ by project, making comparability across studies difficult to achieve.

While these approaches are certainly not without merit, we recognize that there are a number of opportunities to develop comparative metrics that can inform the implementation of programs and policies. Without comparability, city leaders cannot assess the performance of their municipality's programs. However, developing "comparable" metrics must allow for the complexities associated with health factors, such as the levels of inequality and poverty within a city, the degree of participatory local governance, and the impacts of environmental, economic, and social conditions. As a result, we propose quantitative comparative analysis—both in cross section

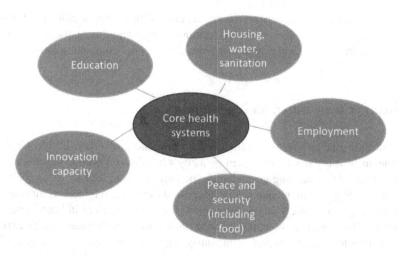

Exhibit 14.1 Facets of city life

and longitudinally—interpreted through integration with qualitative assessments of the complexities of each city's conditions with a view to exposing a more holistic picture of the status of health in cities (Exhibit 14.1).

This kind of comprehensive system of comparative, system-based assessments must include of the following facets of city life that have been documented as relevant to public health.

Education

Education is among the most important determinants of health in a city's landscape [4]. The correlation is sufficiently strong as to support the view that education—and especially the primary education of girls—is one of the most effective forms of preventative medicine [5]. Literacy, quantitative skills, and the ability to communicate effectively provide a city's youth with the capacity to envision alternatives related to personal health, such as avoidance of violence, the pursuit of nutrition, and a basic capability to self-diagnose illnesses such as malaria. Education is critical to one's ability to obtain meaningful employment and is essential for building a population with the ability to problem solve, think critically, and behave resourcefully.

As literacy and education are so closely tied to socioeconomic status, increased education reduces poverty and thus allows communities to overcome economic barriers to access to health [6]. By cultivating an understanding of the consequences of behavioral choices and of alternatives, education can dramatically reduce the spread of communicable diseases such as malaria and sexually transmitted diseases such as HIV/AIDS. It has the effect of improving maternal health, child health, and newborn survival. A comprehensive examination of the health of cities must therefore account for such factors as levels of primary-school enrollment, the rates of male and female attendance, and primary and secondary school completion rates.

Housing, Clean Water, and Sanitation

Safe and affordable housing is an integral component of urban health. Chronic homelessness is often a direct burden on a city's healthcare system.[2] The absence of safe and affordable housing engenders desperation and can lead to vulnerability to violence, poor nutrition, mental health issues, and exposure to infectious disease [7]. Poor housing is also frequently accompanied by practices such as in-home, open-pit cooking and inadequate separation of water and sanitation facilities, which expose city dwellers to carcinogens and perniciously drug-resistant waterborne diseases [8]. In short, access to housing is significant both to the physical and mental health of a population. Variability in the quality of available housing may exacerbate the health impacts of inadequate housing. For example, increases in the value of housing may be accompanied with reduced options for shelter. Poorly maintained, low-income housing may be only marginally healthy due to problematic air quality, pervasive mold, disease-amenable dampness, and inadequate emergency equipment.

Employment

The rate of employment is among the most significant determinants of health within a population. Of course, an immediate impact of employment is normally income, which confers direct benefits on workers who almost invariably use income to improve nutrition, personal security, and housing. Employment also confers other benefits on workers, such as social support, the prospects of long-term security, and mobility [9]. While sound and secure employment can have immediate and long-term benefits to a person's health, in environments where employment is less safe or secure, the adverse impact on one's health can be significant [10]. Unemployment or underemployment may harm one's health by prohibiting access to necessary care or by undermining nutrition or housing. Dangerous and stressful jobs and workplaces with minimal safety and security measures may also materially reduce a worker's prospect of health.

---

[2] Consider, for example, the Vancouver Coastal Health organization's adoption of a "housing first" strategy to address health issues in the city's notoriously impoverished downtown east side. The belief that housing is not only significant in providing immediate physical wellbeing but also dramatically reduces the prevalence of many health issues drove the innovative policy. The goal was to reduce the rates of homelessness in the area and simultaneously reduce the burden of preventable illnesses on the local healthcare facilities.

Peace and Security

Beyond the simple threats of physical danger and violence that are posed by the presence of conflict and civil unrest, the absence of peace and security impacts health in many other ways [11]. One of the most immediate is food insecurity [12]. When cities are engaged in or subjected to conflict, the regular importation of food-stuffs is almost always disrupted and may even be halted. Health conditions suffer accordingly and may become acute in regions already at risk due to malnutrition. Similarly, conflict may disrupt access to health facilities—for example, when civilians cannot leave their home for travel to hospitals or clinics due to the risk of injury en route. In contexts where movement is limited due to conflict, access to medicine, clean water, and heating fuel may also be limited. Lack of access to antibiotics or painkillers can trivialize the entire operational capacity of a medical team, as we have seen in many humanitarian crises (and recently in Homs, Syria) [13].

In cities where conflict or destabilization progresses, the likelihood of "medical flight" increases. Medical flight occurs when medical professionals or medical NGOs withdraw from a city, either voluntarily or on command, out of concern for safety. In 1995, humanitarian medical organizations left the city of Goma in the Democratic Republic of Congo (then Zaire), due in part to a belief that their medical contributions were having the effect of perpetuating conflict by enabling the health of the perpetrators of crimes [14]. The decision to depart was, however, adverse for thousands of Goma residents who no longer had access to any medical facilities [14].

Innovation Capacity

The presence of industry and the ability to develop a local economy or participate in regional or global markets are not only beneficial for employment but also increase a particular city's capacity to innovate and therefore achieve comparative advantage [15]. Over time, the ability of a city to flourish depends in a detailed way on the micro-dynamics of exchange among residents and the unique character of the city that emerges. Innovative cities and the ideas they spawn stimulate exchange that heightens a city's value added in the broader region and around the world, which ultimately makes the city economically sustainable.

Where there is capacity to innovate, there is greater achievement of context-specific solutions to health issues. The high-cost health solutions used in developed nations may not be sustainable or similarly effective in less-developed contexts [15, p. 17]. Low-cost innovations that have the ability to permeate health systems and practices in developing countries will have a far greater impact than externally imposed short-term, high-cost solutions [15, p. 25]. However, where there is no capacity or support for this type of innovation within a city, the potential benefits to population health are lost—which can have dire consequences in nations that already face health burdens from many of the aforementioned determinants of health. For example, this would certainly be true of Haiti, Somaliland, and South Sudan.

Designing a Comparative Measurement Framework for Cities and Health

Comparative health measures for cities and a broadened basis for a more informed contextual analysis for health in cities requires a platform of city data that is comparative and globally standardized across cities. The processes by which such a set of metrics is developed are crucial to their legitimacy and usefulness. Similarly, a careful interpretation of the metrics that integrates qualitative assessments and reflects the unique conditions of each city's context is central to carrying out an apolitical assessment.

The Global City Indicators Facility (GCIF) has been established to respond to the urgent need for a globally standardized set of city indicators. Headquartered at the University of Toronto, the GCIF hosts a network of some 250 cities worldwide and provides a globally standardized system for data collection that allows for comparative knowledge and learning across cities globally (see Exhibit 14.2).

The GCIF is currently developing a Global City Indicators Standard within the framework of the International Organization for Standardization (ISO) to ensure a

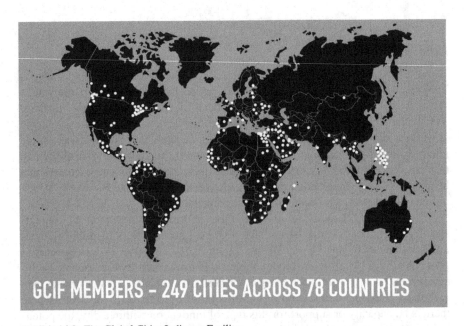

GCIF MEMBERS – 249 CITIES ACROSS 78 COUNTRIES

Exhibit 14.2 The Global Cities Indicator Facility

consistent and standardized methodology for city indicators. This work is being undertaken with the Technical Committee on Sustainable Development in Communities (TC268) to develop a new series of standards for a holistic and integrated approach to sustainable development.

The development of the indicators has only begun. No comprehensive assessments are yet publicly available, but the discourse surrounding the construction of the database has already yielded a number of important insights regarding the design of a comparative measurement framework. The prospective power of these indicators, in this age of urbanization, is in the hands of city managers, politicians, health planners, researchers, business leaders, designers, and other professionals who seek to promote livable, tolerant, healthy, sustainable, economically attractive, and prosperous cities globally.

One critical facet of the GCIF's work is the necessity of partnerships in the interpretation of the data generated through an assessment of any city's profile. The GCIF assists cities in drawing comparative lessons from other cities locally and globally. The GCIF online platform enables cities to compare and learn from other cities relative to their peer groups. Cities can sort themselves into relevant peer groups, for example, according to their *population size* or *region* in order to draw comparative lessons. Cities can also sort themselves into other comparative peer groups such as climate type, land area, GDP per capita, or gross operating budget. This comparative approach creates a knowledge network that connects cities and builds global partnerships.

As these collaborations develop, city leaders such as mayors and city managers increasingly ask for comparative analysis: How are we doing relative to our peers? How can we learn from our peers in order to better plan for the future?

The Challenge of Knowing Where to Draw the Line

The GCIF indicators are structured around 20 themes and measure a range of city services and quality of life factors which can support and provide a framework for health planning in cities. The current set of global city indicators was selected based on a pilot phase with nine cities and from significant input from the current member cities, ensuring that these indicators reflect city information needs, interests, and data availability. A subset of these indicators related to health is included as Exhibit 14.3 in the GCIF Profile titled *Health in the City*.

This profile includes a platform of health indicators for cities according to themes: Governance; Economy; Demographics; Demand for City Services; Environmental Stressors; Healthy Living Space; Potential Health Hazards; Access to Information, Education, and EMS; and Level of Healthcare Service.

A central challenge in the development of this list of indicators is in "drawing the line," i.e., identifying which facets of city conditions will *not* be considered an element of health. City leaders involved in the project naturally favored measures that reflected the unique conditions of their urban environments. Several GCIF

GCIF City Profile – Your Health in the City

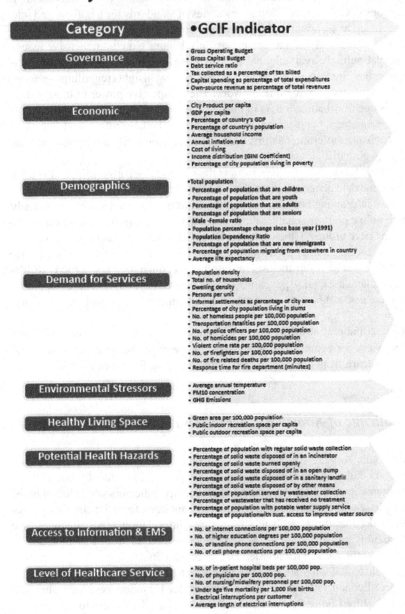

Category	•GCIF Indicator
Governance	• Gross Operating Budget • Gross Capital Budget • Debt service ratio • Tax collected as a percentage of tax billed • Capital spending as percentage of total expenditures • Own-source revenue as percentage of total revenues
Economic	• City Product per capita • GDP per capita • Percentage of country's GDP • Percentage of country's population • Average household income • Annual inflation rate • Cost of living • Income distribution [GINI Coefficient] • Percentage of city population living in poverty
Demographics	•Total population • Percentage of population that are children • Percentage of population that are youth • Percentage of population that are adults • Percentage of population that are seniors • Male -Female ratio • Population percentage change since base year (1991) • Population Dependency Ratio • Percentage of population that are new immigrants • Percentage of population migrating from elsewhere in country • Average life expectancy
Demand for Services	• Population density • Total no. of households • Dwelling density • Persons per unit • Informal settlements as percentage of city area • Percentage of city population living in slums • No. of homeless people per 100,000 population • Transportation fatalities per 100,000 population • No. of police officers per 100,000 population • No. of homicides per 100,000 population • Violent crime rate per 100,000 population • No. of firefighters per 100,000 population • No. of fire related deaths per 100,000 population • Response time for fire department [minutes]
Environmental Stressors	• Average annual temperature • PM10 concentration • GHG Emissions
Healthy Living Space	• Green area per 100,000 population • Public indoor recreation space per capita • Public outdoor recreation space per capita
Potential Health Hazards	• Percentage of population with regular solid waste collection • Percentage of solid waste disposed of in an incinerator • Percentage of solid waste burned openly • Percentage of solid waste disposed of in an open dump • Percentage of solid waste disposed of in a sanitary landfill • Percentage of solid waste disposed of by other means • Percentage of population served by wastewater collection • Percentage of wastewater that has received no treatment • Percentage of population with potable water supply service • Percentage of population with sust. access to improved water source
Access to Information & EMS	• No. of internet connections per 100,000 population • No. of higher education degrees per 100,000 population • No. of landline phone connections per 100,000 population • No. of cell phone connections per 100,000 population
Level of Healthcare Service	• No. of in-patient hospital beds per 100,000 pop. • No. of physicians per 100,000 pop. • No. of nursing/midwifery personnel per 100,000 pop. • Under age five mortality per 1,000 live births • Electrical interruptions per customer • Average length of electrical interruptions

GCIF Health Profile

Global City Indicators Facility
www.cityindicators.org

Exhibit 14.3 GCIF health profile

conferences were held to negotiate metrics among members of the facility to achieve a balance that allowed both comparability and captured systematically-relevant nuances of cities under varying circumstances. For example, after considerable discussion and reflection, conference participants elected to include measures of the stability of electricity as a critical component of the health system—primarily because frequent and long outages have a direct impact on health needs.

The Challenge of Accurately Measuring Change

Effective measurement requires not only cross-sectional validity but also inter-temporal series that support an understanding of how the circumstances of a city develop over time. The measurement of change in critical variables is central to the identification of a particular policy with a particular outcome.

Measuring health indicators accurately in these settings is complicated by many factors, including the absence of consistent systems of citizen registration, mortality, clinical outcomes, police action, school enrolments, and the quality of water, to name only a few. As the quality of measurement systems improves, accuracy depends not only on capturing contemporaneous metrics on each relevant dimension but also on tracking progress in the measurement itself. Such tracking is essential to the avoidance of attribution bias in improvements. In other words, an observed improvement in childhood education, may be partly due to actual improvement in school systems and partly due to better mechanisms of assessment. Understanding the difference is central to understanding the payoff to investments in health improvements. The challenge of effective implementation of systems for tracking improvement requires, in impoverished settings where the demand for resources is high, the diversion of crucial capabilities to tracking metric quality.

The Challenge of Comprehensiveness

The demographic transition occurring globally in cities is also marked by shifting age cohorts and, more generally, marked by aging populations in major geographic regions. Significant advancements in human development and public health have resulted in higher living standards and a global population that lives longer [16]. Statistics indicate that the global life expectancy rate has risen from 47 years in the 1950s to 65 years at the turn of the new millennium [17]. In Japan, a highly developed country, the average life expectancy is over 80 years, and by 2050, it is expected that those under the age of 20 will be outnumbered by those over the age of 80 [17]. Although these factors suggest major gains in human capabilities and knowledge, they also bring about a new set of challenges. Global population growth coupled with increased life expectancy rates indicate that aging is emerging as a pressing policy and development issue [18]. The number of senior citizens (aged 60 and over) will grow from 11 % in 2006 to 22 % by 2050 [1]. For the first time in human history, seniors will outnumber children aged 0–14 years [1].

This demographic shift brings with it a new set of policy challenges, particularly at the city level, and a new demand for metrics that account for these changes. This is especially true for LMICs, which must deal with the effects of an aging population in addition to the burdens of poverty. According to UN-Habitat, "in developing countries the share of older people in urban communities will multiply 16 times from about 56 million in 1998 to over 908 million in 2050. By that time, older people will comprise one fourth of the total urban population in less developed countries" [19]. In Africa, aging is not visible in most policy dialogue and so tends to be de-prioritized in terms of budgetary allocations, thereby increasing the vulnerability and marginalization of older Africans [20]. These predictions indicate that policy decisions at the city level are becoming increasingly vital to the state of the world's aging population. Evidence-based decision-making facilitated by indicators will prove invaluable in maneuvering through this demographic transition.

Early Insights

The issues raised in the implementation of a system of comprehensive, integrated, and standardized measures of health in cities reflect a larger and more fundamental question regarding urbanization. The rapid growth of cities and the transformation of nations to urban predominance raise a core set of challenges in the governance of cities. Governing frameworks and constitutions, created under historic circumstances of largely rural societies, are increasingly contested with the rise of cities. Key questions arise in cities worldwide and in almost all nations: What are the relative roles of national and local governments in managing cities? In particular, how should responsibilities and fiscal powers be distributed between different tiers of government, as an increasing proportion of a country's population is concentrated in cities? In terms of health, what multilevel governance model is preferred, and how does one determine answers to this governance arrangement locally?

The devolution of powers to the municipal level is often argued as a means by which to achieve good urban governance. Granting municipal governments control over revenues and expenditures, raised and spent locally for local benefit, aids in the improvement of a city's "livability" through improved performance and effective delivery of city services.

Empowering municipal governance is made more complex, however, by the growth of the urban population, its geographic spread across existing municipal boundaries, and its diversity. The actual economically functional areas of cities and their competitive geographic concentrations have rendered existing municipal boundaries and structures of governance outdated and ill equipped to confront the challenges of cities in the twenty-first century. In the UN-Habitat's *State of the World's Cities Report 2008/2009*, McCarney and Stren argue that governance across vast and multiple jurisdictional boundaries is plagued with fragmentation in policy, decision-making, management, and implementation. Poorly understood and poorly governed cities can neither deliver services nor support sustainability, poverty alleviation, and prosperity agendas. A growing challenge will be how to determine appropriate governance structures for managing urban areas and the inter-jurisdictional issues that megacities engender [21]. New systems of urban governance are required for inclusive and healthy cities that can deliver on the economic, social, and environmental promise of urbanization.

The effectiveness of governance is the determining factor in whether a population will be passive recipients of health interventions or active participants in a healthy city. Effective health governance in the face of rapid urbanization can only be achieved when decisions are supported by accurate, timely, and relevant information about both health conditions and the effectiveness of health interventions. The decentralization of the administration of effective health policy depends crucially on the development of a skilled workforce steeped in an understanding of the complexities of achieving desired health outcomes, plus a workforce equally skilled in the administration of health protocols. Effective health interventions should and must be targeted at elements of city conditions that are most relevant to the city's health profile: education, housing, water, sanitation, peace and security, and innovation systems. Targeting efforts at specific root causes while tailoring them to the constraints of a city's capacity is only manageable when information is readily available about a city's performance. Where the operations of governance have access to increased information, more informed decision-making becomes possible. This will require more extensive research and analysis of the indicators discussed above and the contextualization of this information within the governance of a given city.

Even as the GCIF develops, data limitations at the city level and the difficulties of translation of metrics into city management and informed policy point to critical challenges for the future. Already we envision the need for a deeper examination of the factors that shape health and the extent to which they can be measured comprehensively. There is reason to believe that education, empowerment, and innovation are mutually complementary and can best be understood not separately but in an integrated model of city dynamics. The GCIF contributes to the improved health of cities by sparking interactions among city leaders on the precise elements of such a model.

Acknowledgement   Thanks to Kerry Paterson for capable and thoughtful research assistance.

References

1. UN. Population ageing. New York: Department of Economic and Social Affairs, Population Division. United Nations; 2006.
2. Dillon K, Prokesch S. Global challenges in health care: is rationing in our future? HBR Blog Network. http://blogs.hbr.org/cs/2010/04/global_challenges_in_health_ca.html (April 5, 2010). Accessed 9 May 2013.

3. Widdus R, White K. Combating diseases associated with poverty: financing strategies for product development and the potential role of public-private partnerships. August 2004. http://www.globalforumhealth.org/filesupld/ippph/CombatingDiseases.pdf

4. Feinstein L. Quantitative estimates of the social benefits of learning, 2: Health (depression and obesity). London: Centre for Research on the Wider Benefits of Learning; 2002. http://www.learningbenefits.net/Publications/ResReps/ResRep6.pdf#search=%22quantitative%20estimates%20of%20the%20social%20benefits%20of%20learning%22

5. Benoit C, Shumka L. Gendering the health determinants framework: why girls' and women's health matters. Vancouver: Women's Health Research Network; 2009. p. 9–11.

6. Marmot M. Social determinants of health inequalities. Lancet. 2005;365(9464):1099–104.

7. Centre for Research on Inner City Health. Housing vulnerability and health: Canada's hidden emergency. Toronto: St. Michael's Hospital; 2010. p. 1–3.

8. WHO. Health Impact Assessment. Housing and health. 2010. http://www.who.int/hia/housing/en/. Accessed 9 May 2013.

9. Public Health Agency of Canada. What makes Canadians healthy or unhealthy?—population health approach. Government of Canada. 2013. http://www.phac-aspc.gc.ca/ph-sp/determinants/determinants-eng.php#employment Accessed 9 May 2013.

10. WHO. Health impact assessment. The determinants of health. http://www.who.int/hia/evidence/doh/en/index.html. Accessed 9 May 2013.

11. WHO. The Ottawa Charter for Health Promotion, Ottawa. 1986. http://www.who.int/healthpromotion/conferences/previous/ottawa/en/index.html. Accessed 9 May 2013.

12. WHO. Health Impact Assessment. The Determinants of Health; Food and Agriculture. http://www.who.int/hia/evidence/doh/en/index3.html. Accessed 9 May 2013.

13. Doctors Without Borders. How we work. http://www.doctorswithoutborders.org/aboutus/activities.cfm. Accessed 9 May 2013.

14. Orbinski J. An imperfect offering; humanitarian action in the twenty-first century. Toronto: Anchor Canada; 2008. p. 262–3.

15. Council on Health Research for Development. Beyond aid: research and innovation as key drivers for health, equity and development, Forum 2012, South Africa. 2012. p. 6–7.

16. Brasilia Declaration on Ageing. World Health Organization. 1997, No. 4:21.

17. Leithäuser G. A city for all generations—focusing on ageing population. World Urban Forum IV—Dialogue 6. Nanjing, China. 2008.

18. UN. United Nations Madrid international plan for action on ageing. New York: Department of Economic & Social Affairs, Division for Social Policy and Development. United Nations; 2002.

19. UN-Habitat. Living conditions of low-income older people in human settlements. A global survey connection with the International Year of Older People 1999. Nairobi: UN-Habitat; 1999.

20. Nadalamba A, Chikoko M. Aging population challenges in Africa. AFDB Chief Economist Complex. 2011;1(1). www.afdb.org/fileadmin/uploads/afdb/Documents/Publications/Aging%20Population%20Challenges%20in%20Africa-disribution.pdf

21. McCarney P, Stren R. Metropolitan governance: Governing in a city of cities in UN-HABITAT, state of the world's cities 2008/200. London: Earthscan; 2008.

Index

© Springer New York 2015
R. Ahn et al. (eds.), *Innovating for Healthy Urbanization*,
DOI 10.1007/978-1-4899-7597-3

Printed in the United States
By Bookmasters